Geriatrics

Editor

MARY GARDNER

AF834446

VETERINARY CLINICS OF NORTH AMERICA: SMALL ANIMAL PRACTICE

www.vetsmall.theclinics.com

March 2026 • Volume 56 • Number 2

ELSEVIER

1600 John F. Kennedy Boulevard • Suite 1800 • Philadelphia, Pennsylvania, 19103-2899
http://www.vetsmall.theclinics.com

VETERINARY CLINICS OF NORTH AMERICA: SMALL ANIMAL PRACTICE Volume 56, Number 2
March 2026 ISSN 0195-5616, ISBN-13: 978-0-443-43216-3

Editor: Stacy Eastman
Developmental Editor: Niharika Saxena

Publishing Office: *Veterinary Clinics of North America: Small Animal Practice* (ISSN 0195-5616) is published bimonthly by Elsevier Inc., 1818 Market Street, Philadelphia, PA 19103, United States. Periodicals postage paid at New York, NY and additional mailing offices. USA POSTMASTER: Send address changes to *Veterinary Clinics of North America:,* Elsevier Customer Service Department, 3251 Riverport Lane, Maryland Heights, MO 63043, USA. Months of issue are January, March, May, July, September, and November. Subscription prices are $419.00 per year (domestic individuals), $100.00 per year (domestic students/residents), $528.00 per year (Canadian individuals), $571.00 per year (international individuals), $100.00 per year (Canadian students/residents), and $220.00 per year (international students/residents). For institutional access pricing please contact Customer Service via the contact information below. To receive student/resident rate, orders must be accompained by name of affiliated institution, date of term, and the *signature* of program/residency coordinator on institution letterhead. Orders will be billed at individual rate until proof of status is received. Foreign air speed delivery is included in all *Clinics* subscription prices. All prices are subject to change without notice. Orders, claims, and journal inquiries: Please visit our Support Hub page https://service.elsevier.com for assistance.

Reprints. For copies of 100 or more of articles in this publication, please contact the Commercial Reprints Department, Elsevier Inc., 360 Park Avenue South, New York, NY 10010-1710. Tel.: 212-633-3874; Fax: 212-633-3820; E-mail: reprints@elsevier.com.
Veterinary Clinics of North America: Small Animal Practice is also published in Japanese by Inter Zoo Publishing Co., Ltd., Aoyama Crystal-Bldg 5F, 3-5-12 Kitaaoyama, Minato-ku, Tokyo 107-0061, Japan.

Veterinary Clinics of North America: Small Animal Practice is covered in *Current Contents/Agriculture, Biology and Environmental Sciences, Science Citation Index, ASCA, MEDLINE/PubMed (Index Medicus), Excerpta Medica, and BIOSIS.*

Contributors

EDITOR

MARY GARDNER, DVM, ACPEV
CEO and Co-Founder, Lap of Love Veterinary Hospice, North Palm Beach, Florida, USA

AUTHORS

LAUREN ADELMAN, DVM
Diplomate of the American College of Veterinary Internal Medicine (Small Animal Internal Medicine); Internal Medicine Specialist, Canada West Veterinary Specialists and Co-Founder, Senior Dog Veterinary Society, Vancouver, British Columbia, Canada

LEILANI X. ALVAREZ, DVM
Diplomate, American College of Veterinary Sports Medicine and Rehabilitation; Senior Veterinarian, Director, Department of Integrative and Rehabilitative Medicine, Schwarzman Animal Medical Center, New York, New York, USA

NIKKI E. BENNETT, PhD
Postdoctoral Scholar, Department of Psychological Sciences, Kent State University, Kent, Ohio, USA

MARK D. CARLSON, DVM
Associate Veterinarian, Chief of Surgery, Stow Kent Animal Hospital, Kent, Ohio, USA

TYLER CARMACK, DVM, CVA, CHPV, CVFT, CTPEP, CPEV, CVPP
Lead Veterinarian and Director of Hospice and Palliative Care, Caring Pathways, Virginia Beach, Virginia, USA

JASON DOLL, DVM, MPH, CVHEP
Associate Veterinarian, Lap of Love Veterinary Hospice, Lutz, Florida, USA

REBECCA K. FRANK, DVM, CVHEP, CT (Certified in Thanatology: Death, Dying, Loss, and Bereavement)
Associate Veterinarian, Lap of Love Veterinary Hospice, Member of IAAHPC, Reading, Pennsylvania, USA

ERIC D. GARCIA
Founder and CEO, Tapir, Animal Health Digital Strategist, Tampa, Florida, USA

MARY GARDNER, DVM, ACPEV
CEO and Co-Founder, Lap of Love Veterinary Hospice, North Palm Beach, Florida, USA

HEIDI B. LOBPRISE, DVM
Diplomate of the American Veterinary Dental College; Veterinary Dental Specialist, Cibolo Creek Veterinary Hospital, Boerne, Texas, USA

SARA LYNCH, DVM, MPH
Veterinarian, Lap of Love Veterinary Hospice, Memphis, Tennessee, USA; Lap of Love Veterinary Hospice, Lutz, Florida, USA

KIMBERLY MOEN, DVM, CPEV
Veterinarian, Early Career Veterinary Programs Manager, Lap of Love Veterinary Hospice & In-Home Euthanasia, Lutz, Florida, USA

MICHAEL C. PETTY, DVM
Consultant, Dogtor Consulting, LLC, Plymouth, Michigan, USA

MARY BETH SPITZNAGEL, PhD
Professor, Department of Psychological Sciences, Kent State University, Kent, Ohio, USA

MONICA TARANTINO, DVM, MBA
Co-Founder, Senior Dog Veterinary Society, Pet Loss Community, Alexandria, Virginia, USA

RACHEL WELCH, DVM
Associate Veterinarian, Lap of Love Veterinary Hospice, Lutz, Florida, USA

Contents

VETERINARY CLINICS OF NORTH AMERICA: SMALL ANIMAL PRACTICE

FORTHCOMING ISSUES

May 2026
Gastroenterology
M. Katherine Tolbert and Sara Jablonski, *Editors*

July 2026
Respiratory Medicine
Jonathan D. Dear, *Editor*

September 2026
Artificial Intelligence in Small Animal Veterinary Medicine
Casey Cazer, *Editor*

RECENT ISSUES

January 2026
Advances in Fluid, Electrolyte, and Acid-Base Disorders
Helio Autran de Morais, Kate Hopper and Stephen P. DiBartola, *Editors*

November 2025
Integrative Veterinary Medicine
Laurie Dohmen, *Editor*

September 2025
Neonatology and Pediatrics
Sophie A. Grundy and Autumn P. Davidson, *Editors*

SERIES OF RELATED INTEREST

Veterinary Clinics: Exotic Animal Practice
https://www.vetexotic.theclinics.com/
Advances in Small Animal Care
https://www.advancesinsmallanimalcare.com/

Erratum

In the January 2026 *Veterinary Clinics: Small Animal Practice*, Volume 56 Issue 1, article, "Fluid and Electrolyte Therapy in the Patient with Cardiac Disease" (https://doi.org/10.1016/j.cvsm.2025.09.020)

In Table 4, row 3 in the 'Administration Guidelines for Hypovolemia' for Hypertonic saline in dogs, the measuring units were incorrect for this statement

"Administer 4–6 L/kg over 10–15 min then reassess perfusion parameters. Ideally follow this with a10–25 L/kg administration of an isotonic crystalloid to minimize risks of dehydration. May repeat administration"

The correct statement would be:

"Administer 4–6 mL/kg over 10–15 min then reassess perfusion parameters. Ideally follow this with a 10–25 mL/kg administration of an isotonic crystalloid to minimize risks of dehydration. May repeat administration"

Vet Clin Small Anim 56 (2026) xi
https://doi.org/10.1016/j.cvsm.2025.12.001 vetsmall.theclinics.com
0195-5616/25/

Preface

Where Medicine Meets Meaning: The Privilege of Caring for Aging Pets

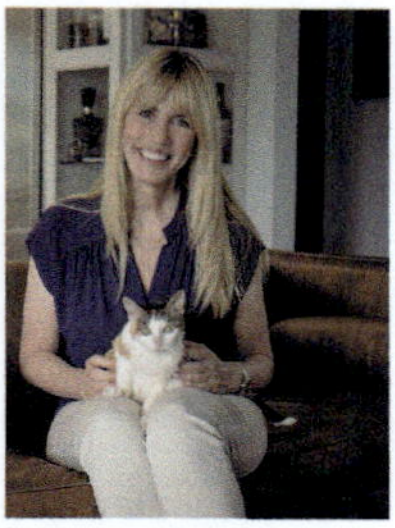

Mary Gardner, DVM, ACPEV
Editor

Geriatric medicine invites us to pause, reflect, and reimagine what it means to provide care through the final seasons of a pet's life. Our patients are living longer than ever, and with that gift comes new layers of complexity. Aging is not a disease but a state of increasing fragility that requires a different lens—a shift from cure to comfort, from extending life to enriching it.

This issue of *Veterinary Clinics of North America: Small Animal Practice* is devoted entirely to that stage of life when experience, compassion, and clinical skill intersect most deeply. Each article was chosen to help build a comprehensive, practical, and thoughtful guide to caring for senior and geriatric patients.

From redefining what "geriatric" truly means to addressing chronic pain, mobility, and sensory decline, this series explores the subtle but significant changes that shape an older pet's daily experience. It covers the physical, cognitive, and emotional aspects of aging while offering tools for managing comorbidities, guiding client education, and creating care plans that align with a family's values and resources.

The collection also recognizes that quality of life is not defined by days lived, but by comfort, connection, and meaning. Topics such as hospice, end-of-life decision making, and euthanasia are presented with honesty and respect, along with strategies for supporting the caregivers who walk this path alongside us.

Finally, we include perspectives that remind us that love and loss are not limited to dogs and cats alone. Every species, every bond, deserves the same level of dignity and understanding.

My hope is that this issue serves as both a reference and a reflection—a reminder that geriatric care is not the conclusion of medicine, but its highest expression. In

Vet Clin Small Anim 56 (2026) xiii–xiv
https://doi.org/10.1016/j.cvsm.2025.11.004
0195-5616/26/© 2025 Published by Elsevier Inc.

helping pets age with grace, we honor the trust they place in us and the love that lead every decision we make.

Mary Gardner, DVM, ACPEV
Lap of Love Veterinary Hospice
North Palm Beach, FL, USA

E-mail address:
marygardnerdvm@gmail.com

Senior Versus Geriatric: Unpacking the Frailty of Aging

Lauren Adelman, DVM[a,1,*], Monica Tarantino, DVM, MBA[a,2]

KEYWORDS

• Frailty • Geriatric dogs • Functional aging • Caregiver burden • Quality of life
• Aging in dogs

KEY POINTS

- Veterinary geriatrics requires more than age-based classification—it demands a functional, frailty-informed lens on aging that integrates medical, behavioral, and quality-of-life factors.
- Frailty assessment tools (eg, CFI, VetMetrica health-related quality of life, and North Carolina State University [NCSU] screening models) are emerging as valuable predictors of decline and can guide early intervention.
- Functional aging recognizes that a *medically stable* patient may still suffer from significant impairment in mobility, cognition, or social function.
- Caregivers are essential partners in geriatric care. Their observations—when captured through structured tools—enhance early detection and strengthen decision-making.
- Proactive, personalized aging care is possible when veterinarians use tools that blend clinical science with empathy, communication, and support for both pet and person.

INTRODUCTION

As companion animals live longer, veterinary teams are increasingly tasked with managing the complexities of aging in dogs. However, unlike in human medicine—where geriatrics is a distinct and well-established discipline—veterinary geriatrics remains underdefined and underrepresented in both clinical training and practice. Most veterinary care for older patients still relies on age thresholds to signal change, rather than functional assessments that reflect how well a patient is actually coping with the biological and behavioral impacts of aging. This gap has critical implications for care planning, client communication, and quality of life (QOL).

[a] Senior Dog Veterinary Society, Alexandria, VA, USA
[1] Present address: 380 East 16 Avenue, Vancouver, BC, Canada.
[2] Present address: 900 Peele Pl, Alexandra, VA 22304.
* Corresponding author. Senior Dog Veterinary Society, PO Box 3022, Alexandria, VA 22302.
E-mail address: lauren@seniordogvets.com

Vet Clin Small Anim 56 (2026) 331–344
https://doi.org/10.1016/j.cvsm.2025.09.022 vetsmall.theclinics.com
0195-5616/26/

Abbreviations	
CFI	canine frailty index
CGS	canine geriatric syndrome
CSOM	client specific outcome measure
DAP	dog aging project
FIDo	frailty instrument for dogs
QOL	quality of life
ZBI	Zarit burden interview

Emerging models from human geriatrics offer a roadmap for advancing veterinary aging care. Concepts like frailty, functional versus medical aging, and caregiver burden provide a more nuanced lens to assess and support senior pets. This article explores these evolving frameworks in the context of canine health, drawing from both veterinary literature and adapted human geroscience. By shifting focus from chronologic age to physiologic resilience, and from disease control to lived experience, clinicians can offer more personalized, proactive care that aligns with both the patient's and the caregiver's needs.

DEFINING THE TERMS: SENIOR VERSUS GERIATRIC

Age is a sensitive subject—one that often stirs discomfort, denial, or humor. Think of how we respond to the question, *How old are you*? or the compliment, *You must have great genes*! We tend to carry these same sentiments into our relationships with our pets. What we call our older companions—*seniors*, *geriatrics*, or the ever-affectionate *gray muzzles*—is not just wordplay. These labels shape how we think about aging and influence the way we support pets in their final life stages.

In veterinary medicine, the term senior has traditionally been used as a chronologic milestone. The American Animal Hospital Association proposes that dogs be considered senior when they reach the last 25% of their expected lifespan, with breed and size being key variables.[1] More specifically, based on lifespan estimation charts, pets are typically classified as senior when they reach the following thresholds[2,3]:

- 10 year old for dogs ≤20 pounds
- 9 year old for dogs 21 to 50 pounds
- 8 year old for dogs 51 to 90 pounds
- 7 year old for dogs greater than 90 pounds

Geriatric, on the other hand, implies more than age. It suggests functional decline, comorbidities, or reduced physiologic reserve—an inflection point where even minor stressors can result in disproportionate impacts. An 8-year-old Labrador retriever who runs 5 km daily may be senior by age but not geriatric by function; whereas a 13-year-old with mobility issues, cognitive decline, and chronic pain clearly qualifies as geriatric, regardless of their blood work.

However, there remains no strict, universally accepted definition for when a dog becomes geriatric. In many cases, senior and geriatric are used interchangeably, even though they can describe vastly different life stages and care needs.

In contrast, human medicine draws clearer lines. The American Association of Retired Persons begins outreach at age 50, while *senior* is typically defined at 65 and older.[4] The term *geriatric*, however, carries functional implications—it refers to individuals who may be experiencing declines in strength, cognition, mobility, or independence, regardless of their numerical age.[5]

Veterinary medicine is increasingly turning to the concept of frailty—a measurable decline in physiologic reserve that reflects cumulative aging rather than any single disease.[6] This concept, adapted from human geriatrics, offers a more functional lens for assessing older pets. Human physicians routinely evaluate frailty using tools that assess grip strength, gait speed, and ability to perform activities of daily living. Similar efforts are now emerging in veterinary practice, as clinicians seek to identify early signs of vulnerability before a crisis occurs.

Ultimately, reframing aging through a functional and frailty-based lens enables more tailored, proactive care for pets and more meaningful conversations with families. Aging is not a diagnosis, but a context—and one that deserves nuance, sensitivity, and strategy.

In the sections that follow, we explore how concepts such as frailty, caregiver perception, and medical versus functional aging can inform a more individualized and compassionate approach to geriatric veterinary care.

FRAILTY—UNPACKING THE FRAGILITY

In human geriatric medicine, *frailty* is recognized as a multidimensional syndrome defined by reduced physiologic reserve, diminished resilience to stress, and an increased vulnerability to adverse outcomes.[7] Frailty is not synonymous with disease—it is a holistic measure of biological aging that reflects the cumulative impact of life on the body and mind. Tools that quantify frailty, such as the Frailty Phenotype or the Frailty Index, are now routinely used to predict hospitalization risk, surgical outcomes, institutionalization, and mortality in older adults.[8–10]

Veterinary medicine is beginning to incorporate the concept of frailty, recognizing that chronologic age alone is an inadequate guide for clinical decision-making in older pets. The first canine frailty index (CFI) was developed by Banzato and colleagues (2019), who applied a deficit-accumulation model similar to that used in human geriatrics.[11] In a cohort of over 400 dogs, higher frailty scores strongly predicted 6-month mortality, while chronologic age added little predictive value once frailty was accounted for. This work provided the first demonstration that frailty, rather than age, more accurately reflects biological vulnerability in dogs.

More recently, Chen and colleagues (2023) conducted a large, multi-center U.S. study of 451 dogs to evaluate the CFI alongside an owner-reported QOL instrument (VetMetrica health-related quality of life [HRQL]).[12,13] As expected, frailty scores increased with age and were inversely correlated with HRQL scores, confirming that both measures captured age-related decline from complementary perspectives. While this cross-sectional study did not assess survival outcomes, it established the practicality of combining veterinarian- and caregiver-based tools in general and specialty practice.

Further support comes from the Exceptional Aging in Rottweilers Study (Waters and colleagues, 2024), which applied a 34-item frailty index to exceptionally long-lived dogs.[14] Higher frailty scores were associated with significantly shorter survival, with an estimated frailty limit consistent with human centenarian data. Taken together, these studies suggest that frailty indices offer a more nuanced and clinically relevant framework than chronologic age for assessing vulnerability, guiding care, and counseling families of geriatric canine patients.

In addition to deficit-based models, researchers have explored phenotypic approaches to canine frailty—focusing on observable characteristics such as exhaustion, reduced mobility, undernutrition, and low physical activity. A 2024 study by Blanchard and colleagues applied a 5-domain frailty phenotype model to 88 healthy senior dogs, finding a frailty prevalence of 42%.[15] Notably, frailty was associated not only with older age and lower physical health scores but also with factors like diminished owner attachment and mismatched dog–owner personality traits, suggesting complex biopsychosocial interplay.

At North Carolina State University, a simplified frailty screening tool was developed to support use in primary practice.[16] This tool evaluates five domains—body and muscle condition, appetite and nutrition, energy level, mobility, and social activity. Dogs identified as impaired in 3 or more domains had nearly twice the 6-month mortality risk compared to nonfrail dogs, regardless of breed, age, or weight. The tool is designed to be completed by either the clinician or the owner and offers a practical, scalable way to identify at-risk patients.

Finally, the Dog Aging Project (DAP) has proposed the development of a standardized Frailty Instrument for Dogs (FIDo), inspired by human frailty tools.[17] This instrument aims to use a combination of caregiver observations and clinical data to screen for phenotypic frailty in a variety of settings—from general practice to research environments. Though not yet widely deployed, the FIDo tool holds promise for large-scale application and may eventually serve as a benchmark for canine frailty screening (**Table 1**).

Together, these emerging tools reflect a fundamental shift away from age as the primary marker of geriatric status and toward functional and physiologic vulnerability as a more meaningful measure.

The concept of frailty challenges the assumption that a patient is *doing fine* if their diagnostics are normal. Frailty is not just the presence of disease—it is the *loss of resilience*, even in the face of stable medical metrics. Frailty tools offer clinically actionable

Table 1
Comparative overview of canine frailty assessment tools

Tool/Model	Type	Key Features	Outcome Measures
Chen et al. CFI (2023)	Deficit accumulation	Validated in 451 dogs using routine clinical data; correlates with HRQL scores	Differentiates frailty severity; predicts reduced QOL
VetMetrica HRQL	Owner-reported domains	Measures vitality, comfort, and emotional well- being	Correlates with CFI; reflects perceived QOL
Banzato's frailty index	Deficit accumulation	Clinical/lab-based score (0–1)	Correlates with age and mortality
EARS-FI	Deficit accumulation	34-item owner survey	Predicts mortality risk in centenarian dogs
Frailty phenotype (Blanchard)	Observable domains	5 criteria (activity, mobility, etc)	~42% frail prevalence; influenced by owner/dog factors
NCSU screening tool	Owner + physical examination	5 domains via questionnaire + body condition score and muscle condition score (BCS/MCS)	2 × risk of 6-mo mortality
DAP FIDo (proposed)	Phenotypic screening	Multidomain survey and routine data	Designed for broad clinical usage

insights. They can help inform anesthetic decisions, guide frequency of monitoring, prompt early intervention for declining patients, and support end-of-life care planning.

As these instruments become more refined and better validated, their role in routine veterinary care will likely expand. Frailty assessment may soon be as commonplace as body condition scoring or mobility scoring—offering a quick, structured snapshot of aging that can prompt deeper conversations and more personalized care plans. Identifying frailty is not just about recognizing decline—it's about intervening early, setting realistic expectations, and improving health span (the length of time an individual remains healthy, functional, and free from significant disease or disability[18]) alongside lifespan.

MEDICAL VERSUS FUNCTIONAL AGING

In veterinary care, it's common to label a senior pet as *medically stable* based on routine diagnostics. Yet, clinical stability doesn't always equate to functional well-being. A dog may have well-controlled chronic conditions—say, manageable osteoarthritis or early-stage heart disease—but still struggle with daily tasks like rising, navigating stairs, or engaging with family. This contrast between medical stability and functional decline underscores why a functional-aging lens is essential for high-quality geriatric care.

Consider a 12-year-old Labrador Retriever with a history of hypothyroidism and osteoarthritis. On paper, her laboratory work is normal, her thyroid levels are stable on medication, and her radiographs are unchanged. Yet the owner reports she no longer greets them at the door, avoids slick floors, and hesitates before jumping into the car. These changes don't register on a complete blood count (CBC) or chemistry panel—but they are clinically meaningful. They may signal untreated pain, loss of confidence, or fear of mobility-associated discomfort. Without assessing and addressing these changes, we risk declaring her *stable* while her daily life quietly deteriorates.

Emerging research highlights the nuances of functional aging. A study from North Carolina State University found that gait speed in senior dogs was significantly associated with cognitive decline, mirroring human data where slower walking predicts increased dementia risk.[19] Another study examined postural stability, showing that older dogs rely more heavily on visual input to maintain balance—indicating a loss of multisensory integration with age.[20] These metrics point to declining adaptability in dogs that may otherwise appear healthy on physical examination or laboratory work.

Veterinary medicine is beginning to recognize that function deserves measurement. One tool that holds promise is the Client Specific Outcome Measure (CSOM), which allows pet owners to identify 3 specific activities their pet struggles with (eg, climbing stairs, chasing a ball, and getting in the car).[21] These tasks are then scored regularly over time, giving both the owner and veterinarian a functional data point to monitor response to interventions. CSOMs are particularly helpful in chronic pain management and rehabilitation but have potential applications in broader geriatric care.

Functional decline is often the driver behind changes in the human–animal bond. Dogs who can no longer participate in their families' routines—going for walks, greeting guests, or sleeping through the night—may become more isolated or anxious. Owners, too, may feel increasing burden, frustration, or grief. While these elements are sometimes dismissed as *part of getting old*, they are often modifiable with environmental adaptation, medical treatment, or supportive care.

Recognizing and tracking function over time allows clinicians to move from reactive to proactive care. Functional aging assessments, especially when repeated, create a framework for early intervention, caregiver education, and more compassionate decision-making. In doing so, they help shift the focus from test results to what matters most: a pet's ability to live comfortably, meaningfully, and with dignity.

This growing recognition of the limitations of disease-centric models is a driving force behind the formation of the Senior Dog Veterinary Society (*seniordogvets.com*), a professional community cofounded by the authors and dedicated to reshaping veterinary geriatrics. The Society's work centers on elevating awareness of functional aging, advocating for tools and strategies that go beyond blood work and radiographs to assess what truly matters: how dogs live, move, interact, and enjoy their lives. Through education, collaboration, and clinical innovation, the Society helps veterinarians support aging patients with personalized, proactive care that honors both longevity and QOL.

WHY FUNCTIONAL AGING MATTERS

- Bridges the gap between disease control and lived experience—a normal chemistry panel means little if the pet can't get up to greet their family.
- Enables early, tailored intervention—subtle declines in gait, posture, or engagement can inform when to begin supportive care.
- Guides client communication and planning—focusing on function clarifies expectations and helps navigate quality-of-life decisions.
- Supports proactive aging strategies—from therapeutic exercise to environment modification, maintaining function should be a central goal.

THE ROLE OF CAREGIVER PERCEPTION

Caregiver perception plays a pivotal role in recognizing and responding to aging in pets. Subtle changes—like pacing at night, unusual vocalization, or intermittent difficulty rising—can signal significant functional decline. Yet these early signs are often overlooked or dismissed as *just old age*, both by owners and, occasionally, by veterinarians. When subtle signs become normalized, the opportunity for early intervention may be lost.

Surveys from the United Kingdom and North America highlight this disconnect. In 1 study of over 600 dog owners and 300 veterinary professionals, more than 80% of dogs whose owners believed they were *perfectly fine* were found by veterinarians to have at least one undetected health issue. Owners most commonly reported slowing on walks, difficulty rising, or withdrawal from play—but often did not seek veterinary advice for these signs unless they worsened dramatically.[22] This is not due to lack of care or interest, but to mismatched understanding of what is *normal* aging versus what is clinically meaningful.

Caregivers are often the first to notice changes, but they may underreport behaviors they view as age-appropriate or inevitable. For example, panting, nighttime restlessness, clinginess, or house-soiling may be viewed as expected parts of aging rather than signs of pain, cognitive decline, or anxiety. Cultural factors and emotional bias can further influence perception. Some owners may over-pathologize aging behaviors out of worry, while others underreport due to fear of bad news or guilt about *missing something*. In either case, emotional investment runs deep—and it affects communication, care decisions, and outcomes.

The emotional toll of caregiving for aging pets is real and increasingly recognized. Studies have shown that pet owners caring for older animals with chronic conditions experience symptoms of anticipatory grief, guilt, and caregiver fatigue—paralleling findings in human eldercare. One study found that caregiver burden in veterinary clients correlated with anxiety, depression, and financial strain.[23] Importantly, higher burden was associated with reduced adherence to treatment plans, reinforcing the need for compassionate, 2-way communication between veterinary teams and pet families.

One of the most effective strategies for improving caregiver communication is the use of previsit questionnaires and checklists. While individually validated tools such as the CADES,[24] CCDR,[25] and DISHAA[26] provide validated assessments for cognitive dysfunction, they can feel overwhelming or overly clinical for some families. When used without context, these forms may generate anxiety or confusion rather than clarity.

To address this, the Senior Dog Veterinary Society has created a 1-page preexamination questionnaire that consolidates the key domains of senior and geriatric health into a simple, approachable format. This tool invites owners to reflect on and report changes in

- Chronic pain
- Mentation (cognitive function)
- Mobility
- Sensory changes (vision and hearing)
- Incontinence
- Overall QOL
- Anticipatory grief (**Fig. 1**)

By streamlining the assessment into a single form, the questionnaire helps focus the visit on areas of greatest concern to the caregiver and patient. It also validates the client's emotional experience—especially around topics like grief or uncertainty—which can otherwise go unspoken. Completed before the examination, the tool encourages collaborative conversation and ensures that subtle signs are not missed amid more urgent medical findings.

KEY TAKEAWAYS: CAREGIVER PERCEPTION IN GERIATRIC PETS

- Owners often underreport or misinterpret behavior changes as inevitable aging; this contributes to delayed diagnosis and care.
- Consolidated, structured tools like the Senior Dog Veterinary Society's one-page questionnaire can help focus appointments and empower caregivers.
- Addressing caregiver emotional context—with sensitivity to their perception of burden, bonding, or guilt—is as critical as understanding the pet's physical signs.

ARE WE BORROWING TOO MUCH (OR NOT ENOUGH) FROM HUMAN GERIATRICS?

Veterinary medicine is still in the infancy of geroscience. Despite the increasing number of aging pets seen in clinical practice, most veterinarians receive no dedicated training in geriatrics during veterinary school—not even a single required course in many curricula. As a result, veterinary geriatric care lacks the structured, interdisciplinary frameworks that define human geriatric medicine. We are only beginning to recognize aging as a process that requires proactive assessment, not just reactive disease management.

In contrast, human medicine has spent decades building tools and care models to support aging adults—tools that prioritize function, resilience, and independence. Structured frameworks like frailty indices, health span tracking, and caregiver burden assessments are integral to clinical decision-making. Veterinary medicine remains behind in this regard, but recent developments show promise in adapting and translating these tools for companion animals.

Patient Name: ______________________ Date: ______________

Senior Wellness Pre-Visit Screening Checklist

As they get older, senior and geriatric dogs are prone to more diseases and risks like chronic pain, dementia and cancer. Screening helps us identify issues and intervene and monitor areas that may impact their happiness as they age.

History

- ☐ Change in Appetite
- ☐ Increased Drinking or Urination
- ☐ Vomiting/Diarrhea
- ☐ Coughing/Breathing changes
- ☐ Changes in housing or environment
- ☐ Social or family change

Chronic Pain Screening

Older dogs are prone to having chronic pain that they can easily hide. Have you noticed any of the following?

Dental Pain:
- ☐ Smelly or foul odor from mouth
- ☐ Brown, gray or red coloring on teeth
- ☐ Loose or wiggly teeth
- ☐ Dropping food or hesitancy with eating

Joint Pain:
- ☐ Limping after exercise
- ☐ Slow to rise
- ☐ Stiffness or 'warms up' as the day goes on
- ☐ Lagging behind on walks

Functional Screening

The risk of cognitive and functional decline increases every year as a dog ages. Have you noticed any of the following?

Mentation:
- ☐ Disorientation
- ☐ Getting stuck in corners
- ☐ Changes in sleep pattern
- ☐ More anxious or restless
- ☐ Less social or less interest in pets

Mobility:
- ☐ Falls or slips more easily
- ☐ Difficulty with stairs or jumps
- ☐ Difficulty posturing to potty
- ☐ Needs assistance at times

Senses:
- ☐ Decrease in vision (ex: hesitation on stairs, bumping into things, reluctance to go out at night etc.)
- ☐ Decrease in hearing (ex startles more easily, less responsive etc.)

Elimination: ☐ Frequent messes in house ☐ Unable to hold bowels or bladder

Quality of Life Screening

Does your pet seem to enjoy their life? ☐ Yes ☐ Maybe ☐ No ☐ Not sure

Other

Are you interested in learning how to 'senior dog proof' your home?	☐ Yes	☐ No
Do you experience caretaker exhaustion at times?	☐ Yes	☐ No
Are there any other concerns we haven't asked about?	☐ Yes	☐ No

Fig. 1. Senior dog veterinary society screening questionnaire. (Senior dog veterinary Society 2025; Monica Tarantino, DVM.)

A key difference lies in the goals of care. In human medicine, the overarching aim is often to extend life—with preserved function whenever possible. In veterinary medicine, most families prioritize comfort and QOL, even when that means a shorter lifespan. Still, who wouldn't want more time—more walks, more belly rubs, and more joy—if it meant good time? This duality speaks to the power of adapting human geriatrics in thoughtful, compassionate ways: not just to prolong life but to enhance living.

Veterinary medicine has already begun to benefit from human geriatric frameworks. The development of canine frailty tools like the Canine Frailty Index, VetMetrica HRQL, and phenotype-based screening models are all rooted in human methodologies. The

DAP's FIDo[17] directly reflects this translational approach—recognizing frailty's predictive value across species.

Similarly, the concept of caregiver burden, long studied in human caregiving, is gaining traction in veterinary medicine. Spitznagel and colleagues adapted the Zarit Burden Interview (ZBI) for pet caregivers and demonstrated that owners of chronically or terminally ill pets report significant emotional, financial, and logistical stress.[23] Caregiver burden impacts treatment adherence, appointment follow-through, and overall patient welfare.

Despite these advances, veterinary geriatrics cannot simply transplant human frameworks. The pet–owner relationship is emotionally rich but medically unique: animals cannot report symptoms, and their care often includes the ethical complexity of euthanasia. While human geriatrics tends to pursue longevity and autonomy, veterinary care must account for the emotional, logistical, and financial realities of pet guardianship.

Frameworks like Canine Geriatric Syndrome (CGS) proposed by McKenzie and colleagues[17] attempt to bridge this divide. CGS includes physical decline, behavioral changes, metabolic shifts, and caregiver factors to create a more holistic model of aging in dogs—designed to support not just survival but health span. Importantly, CGS recognizes that aging is not just a medical process, but a lived experience shared between pet and owner.

The veterinary profession benefits by borrowing wisely from human geriatrics—adapting what works, discarding what doesn't, and filling in the gaps with species-specific solutions. This means

- Customizing frailty models to reflect canine behaviors, physiologies, and breed-specific aging patterns.
- Developing pet-focused caregiver support tools that reflect the emotional realities of guardianship, including grief, guilt, and anticipatory loss.
- Prioritizing QOL over survival time, while still appreciating that functional aging tools can help preserve both.
- Accounting for access and choice, recognizing that veterinary medicine must balance ideal care plans with what families can emotionally and financially manage (**Table 2**).

These adaptations are already underway. The Senior Dog Veterinary Society, for example, exists specifically to close the gap between emerging geroscience and everyday veterinary practice—integrating functional aging, caregiver perception, and anticipatory care into a unified model for companion animals.

Table 2
Key Lessons from human geriatrics for veterinary care

Takeaway	Veterinary Adaptation
Use of frailty indices for proactive aging assessment	Tools like CFI, VetMetrica, FIDo adapted to species-specific behaviors
Recognition of caregiver burden as a core factor in decision-making	Pet-focused assessments (eg, adapted ZBI) and interventions for burden support
Focus on functional aging and health span, not just disease and lifespan	Frameworks like CGS embrace quality alongside quantity
Value of multidisciplinary support—therapists, social workers, and caregivers	Growing interest in veterinary social work, enriched communication tools, and anticipatory grief support

Veterinary geriatrics doesn't need to reinvent the wheel—but it does need its own steering system. By integrating the best of human models while designing around the unique needs of aging animals and their families, we can shape a future of veterinary care that is not only longer, but better.

PREDICTING DECLINE

One of the most difficult challenges in geriatric veterinary medicine is predicting *when*—when decline becomes irreversible, when QOL is meaningfully compromised, or when an owner should begin preparing for end-of-life decisions. These questions rarely have straightforward answers. Unlike human medicine, where outcome forecasting is more formalized, veterinary medicine often relies on clinician intuition, caregiver observation, and a mix of functional, behavioral, and emotional cues.

In human geriatrics, the use of frailty as a predictive model has transformed how clinicians anticipate outcomes. Frailty assessments—whether phenotype-based or index-based—are used to forecast a wide range of health events, including hospitalization, prolonged recovery from surgery and mortality.[9,27–29] Tools like the Clinical Frailty Scale or Timed Up and Go test are part of routine screening in older adults.[30,31] These allow physicians to guide patients and families through complex decisions based on data, not guesswork.

Veterinary medicine needs similar tools. Recent research in dogs shows that frailty scores and functional assessments—such as the CFI, the NCSU frailty screen, and VetMetrica HRQL—can predict outcomes more effectively than age alone.[11,13,16] In Chen and colleagues' 2023 study, dogs with higher frailty scores and lower caregiver-perceived QOL had a significantly higher risk of mortality within 6 months, even in the absence of overt disease progression.[13] This kind of stratification can help veterinarians guide discussions about prognosis, lifestyle modifications, and palliative planning much earlier than we typically do today.

But predicting decline in pets requires a different kind of sensitivity. Most veterinary patients do not die in hospitals or long-term care facilities. They are cared for at home by owners who must make the decision to end suffering through euthanasia—often with little medical certainty about timing. This makes the role of functional aging and caregiver perception even more critical in guiding when to shift from curative to comfort-focused care.

QOL scoring systems are essential tools in evaluating the lived experience of aging pets. Several structured frameworks exist—from the (Hurt, Hunger, Hydration, Hygiene, Happiness, Mobility, More Good Days than Bad [HHHHHMM]) scale[32] to multidomain assessment tools like VetMetrica[12] and Dr Gardner's QOL scoring method[33]—each aiming to capture changes in comfort, engagement, and daily function over time. These tools can guide discussions between veterinarians and caregivers, helping to identify trends that may indicate declining well-being. Regardless of the specific tool used, QOL assessments should be revisited regularly—not just at the end of life, but throughout the aging process—to support earlier planning, emotional preparedness, and compassionate decision-making.

Anticipating decline isn't just about knowing when a pet might die—it's about helping families recognize the transition from treatable condition to progressive syndrome. Tools like the CGS model[34] support this shift, integrating frailty, behavioral changes, metabolic markers, and caregiver strain into a unified aging profile. Similarly, the 1-page preexamination questionnaire from Senior Dog Veterinary Society helps surface signs of decline across multiple domains—giving clinicians a framework to plan ahead with families, rather than catching up during crisis.

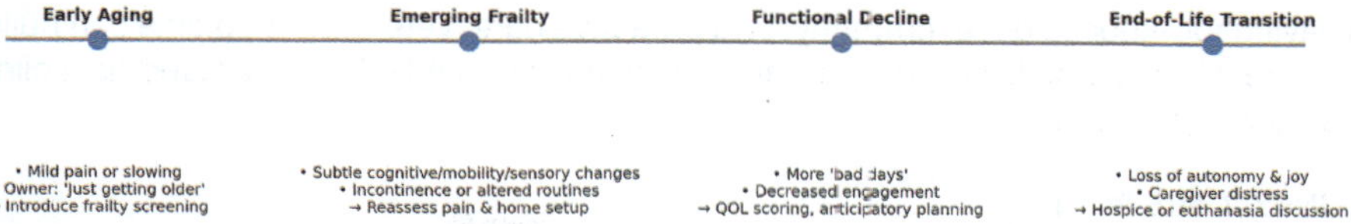

Fig. 2. Aging trajectory and decision inflection points.

When used consistently, these tools build a story—not just of decline, but of care. They allow veterinarians to measure change over time, identify meaningful trends, and communicate clearly with families about the likely road ahead. In doing so, they transform ambiguity into guidance, and give both pets and people the grace of a well-prepared goodbye (**Fig. 2**).

SUMMARY

As veterinary professionals, we are increasingly called upon to guide patients and families through the complexities of aging—but our understanding of what it means to grow old is still evolving. Traditionally, aging in pets has been approached through a chronologic lens, with age-based classifications like *senior* and *geriatric* used to signal shifting expectations. But age alone is not enough. A more meaningful approach to veterinary geriatrics centers on function, frailty, and QOL —all of which offer a more individualized, proactive, and compassionate model of care.

This article has explored how veterinary medicine can adopt and adapt key concepts from human geriatrics—such as frailty scoring, caregiver burden assessment, and functional status evaluations—to better serve aging pets and their families. While tools like the Canine Frailty Index, the NCSU screening model, and caregiver questionnaires are still in their early stages, they offer powerful insights that go beyond traditional diagnostics. These frameworks allow veterinarians to identify risk earlier, plan care more intentionally, and communicate more clearly with caregivers navigating uncertainty.

Throughout the article, we have emphasized that functional aging often diverges from medical stability. A dog may have excellent laboratory results and radiographs but suffer from mobility limitations, pain, cognitive decline, or withdrawal. Recognizing these disconnects empowers veterinarians to intervene earlier, communicate more effectively with caregivers, and maintain a focus on well-being rather than disease alone.

We also explored how caregiver perception influences care-seeking behavior, treatment adherence, and end-of-life decisions. The emotional toll of caregiving—particularly when combined with anticipatory grief or decision paralysis—can overwhelm families. Structured tools, like previsit screening forms, not only validate these experiences but also guide collaborative conversations around care planning, prognosis, and QOL.

Ultimately, geriatrics is not a diagnosis—it is a lens. It asks us to look beyond age, beyond laboratory work, and beyond symptoms. It invites us to see the whole patient, their function, their comfort, and their role in a family. It also challenges us to create systems of care that recognize aging not as a period of decline, but as a time of increased vulnerability and increased opportunity—opportunity to provide comfort, prevent crisis, and preserve dignity.

In veterinary medicine, we are working to help bridge the gap between emerging geroscience and practical application—developing tools, educational resources, and frameworks that help general practitioners incorporate aging care into daily practice. The ultimate goal is not just to add years to a pet's life, but life to their years. By weaving together science, empathy, and proactive care, veterinary medicine can build a future where aging is no longer treated as an afterthought—but embraced as a clinical focus in its own right.

CLINICS CARE POINTS

- *Functional age matters more than chronologic age* when it comes to planning care for senior and geriatric patients. Tools that assess mobility, cognitive function, and social engagement provide a more complete picture than age alone.
- *Frailty is a valuable predictor of risk*—Incorporating frailty screening into routine wellness care can support earlier intervention and may improve outcomes.
- *Caregiver perception often drives veterinary visits and decisions.* Structured tools like previsit questionnaires and quality-of-life (QOL) scoring systems help focus appointments and align care with owner priorities.
- QOL *is dynamic and multidimensional.* Repeated assessment over time can help guide treatment, palliative care, or end-of-life planning.
- *Veterinary geriatrics is an evolving discipline.* Organizations like the Senior Dog Veterinary Society are helping clinicians translate emerging research on aging, frailty, and health span into practical, compassionate care.

DISCLOSURE

The authors have no disclosures to report.

REFERENCES

1. American Animal Hospital Association. Defining the senior patient. In: 2019 AAHA Canine Life Stage Guidelines. Lakewood, CO: American Animal Hospital Association. 2019. Available at: https://www.aaha.org/resources/2023-aaha-senior-care-guidelines-for-dogs-and-cats/defining-the-senior-patient/. Accessed August 23, 2025.
2. Lobprise H. Geriatrics. In: Ettinger SJ, Feldman EC, Côté E, editors. Textbook of veterinary internal medicine. 9th edition. St Louis (MO): Elsevier; 2020.
3. American Veterinary Medical Association. Senior pets. Available at: https://www.avma.org/resources/pet-owners/petcare/senior-pets. Accessed August 22, 2025.
4. American Association of Retired Persons (AARP). Membership eligibility and mission focus. Available at: https://www.aarp.org/membership/age-requirement/. Accessed August 23, 2025.
5. Geriatric Syndrome—An overview. ScienceDirect topics. Elsevier. 2025. Available at: https://www.sciencedirect.com/topics/medicine-and-dentistry/geriatric-syndrome. Accessed August 22, 2025.
6. Xue QL. The frailty syndrome: definition and natural history. Clin Geriatr Med 2011;27(1):1–15.
7. Wleklik M, Uchmanowicz I, Jankowska-Polańska B, et al. Multidimensional approach to frailty. Front Psychol 2020;11:564.
8. Heikkilä E, Hätönen H, Andersson J, et al. Association of frailty and hospitalization outcomes in older adults: a population-based study. BMC Geriatr 2021;21(1):431.
9. Stuck AE, Limacher A, Feller A, et al. Frailty phenotype and deficit accumulation frailty index in predicting outcomes of hospitalized older patients. J Frailty Aging 2022;11(4):377–84.

10. Joseph B, Pandit V, Zangbar B, et al. Superiority of frailty over age in predicting outcomes among geriatric trauma patients: a prospective analysis. JAMA Surg 2014;149(8):766–72.
11. Banzato T, Franzo G, Di Maggio R, et al. A Frailty Index based on clinical data to quantify mortality risk in dogs. Sci Rep 2019;9(1):16749.
12. NewMetrica Ltd. VetMetrica HRQL. Available at: https://www.newmetrica.com/vetmetrica-hrql/. Accessed August 22, 2025.
13. Chen FL, Ullal TV, Graves JL, et al. Evaluating instruments for assessing healthspan: a multi-center cross-sectional study on health-related quality of life (HRQL) and frailty in the companion dog. Geroscience 2023;45(4):2089–108.
14. Waters DJ, Maras AH, Fu R, et al. Frailty and mortality risk among dogs with extreme longevity: development and predictive validity of a clinical frailty index in the Exceptional Aging in Rottweilers Study. Animals (Basel) 2024;14(24):3651.
15. Blanchard T, Mugnier A, Déjean S, et al. Exploring frailty in apparently healthy senior dogs: a cross-sectional study. BMC Vet Res 2024;20(1):436.
16. Russell KJ, Mondino A, Fefer G, et al. Establishing a clinically applicable frailty phenotype screening tool for aging dogs. Front Vet Sci 2024;11:1335463.
17. Melvin RL, Ruple A, Pearson EB, et al. A review of frailty instruments in human medicine and proposal of a frailty instrument for dogs. Front Vet Sci 2023;10:1139308.
18. Mayo Clinic. Lifespan vs healthspan. Mayo Clinic News Network. 2024. Available at: https://newsnetwork.mayoclinic.org/discussion/mayo-clinic-q-and-a-lifespan-vs-healthspan/. Accessed August 23, 2025.
19. Mondino A, Khan M, Case B, et al. Winning the race with aging: age-related changes in gait speed and its association with cognitive performance in dogs. Front Vet Sci 2023;10:1150590.
20. Lutonsky C, Peham C, Affenzeller N, et al. Impact of aging and visual input on postural stability in dogs: insights from center-of-pressure analysis. Sensors (Basel) 2025;25(5):1300.
21. Lascelles BD, Hansen BD, Roe S, et al. Evaluation of client-specific outcome measures and activity monitoring to measure pain relief in geriatric arthritic dogs. J Vet Intern Med 2007;21(2):410–9.
22. Wallis LJ, Radford AD, Belshaw Z, et al. Cross-sectional United Kingdom surveys demonstrate that owners and veterinary professionals differ in their perceptions of preventive and treatment healthcare needs in ageing dogs. Front Vet Sci 2024 11:1358480.
23. Spitznagel MB, Cox MD, Mehaffey C, et al. Caregiver burden in owners of a sick companion animal: a cross-sectional observational study. Vet Rec 2019;185(22):686.
24. Madari A, Farbakova J, Katina S, et al. Assessment of severity and progression of canine cognitive dysfunction syndrome using the CAnine DEmentia Scale (CADES). Appl Anim Behav Sci 2015;171:138–45.
25. Salvin HE, McGreevy PD, Sachdev PS, et al. The canine cognitive dysfunction rating scale (CCDR): a data-driven and ecologically relevant assessment tool. Vet J 2011;188(3):331–6.
26. Purina Institute. Cognitive dysfunction syndrome. Purina Institute CentreSquare—Advancing brain health. Available at: https://www.purinainstitute.com/science-of-nutrition/advancing-brain-health/cognitive-dysfunction-syndrome. Accessed August 22, 2025.
27. Wen YC, Chen LK, Hsiao FY. Predicting mortality and hospitalization of older adults by the multimorbidity frailty index. PLoS One 2017;12(11):e0187825.

28. Hao Q, Zhou L, Dong B, et al. Frailty assessed by a 36-item Frailty Index predicts 3-year mortality and hospital readmission in older inpatients. Sci Rep 2019;9(1).
29. Aceto P, Schipa C, Luca E, et al. Diagnosis of frailty and implications on surgical process and postoperative outcomes in older patients. Eur J Anaesthesiol Intensive Care 2023;6.
30. Mendiratta P. *Clinical frailty scale*, . StatPearls. Treasure Island (FL): StatPearls Publishing; 2023.
31. Zasadzka E, Borowicz AM, Roszak M, et al. Assessment of the risk of falling with the use of timed up and go test. BioMed Res Int 2015;2015:919637.
32. Villalobos AE. Quality of life scale for dogs: the HHHHHMM scale. PetMD. 2023. Available at: https://www.petmd.com/cat/general-health/cat-euthanasia-when-put-cat-down. Accessed August 22, 2025.
33. Gardner M. Quality of life assessment. In: Gardner M, McVety D, editors. Treatment and care of the veterinary geriatric patient. Hoboken (NJ): Wiley-Blackwell; 2017. p. 299–309.
34. McKenzie B, Coe J, Niel L. Canine geriatric syndrome: proposal for a new paradigm. J Am Vet Med Assoc 2021;258(2):123–30.

Chronic Pain

Effective Relief Strategies for Geriatric Pets

Michael C. Petty, DVM

KEYWORDS

• Geriatric • Pain • Chronic pain • Canine • Dog • Feline • Cat

KEY POINTS

- Considerations must be given when treating geriatric dogs and cats because of the increased likelihood of preexisting comorbidities that would affect the choice of certain pharmaceuticals and physical modalities.
- Untreated chronic pain will often lead to premature decisions on the part of the caregivers to unnecessarily euthanize their pets.
- It is important to enlist the caregiver as a team player when making decisions about what modalities (pharmaceutical, interventional, or physical) when preparing a treatment plan for their pet.
- It is important to consider referral for the geriatric patient when the primary care veterinarian does not have the equipment or skill set to perform those treatments that would be beneficial for their patient. For example, photobiomodulation therapy, acupuncture, and rehabilitation therapy, to name a few.

INTRODUCTION

Veterinary medicine and nutrition have made many advances over the past several decades, and as a result, our patients are living longer. As these animals age, they are increasingly affected by a range of age-related conditions, many of which are associated with acute or chronic pain. Common sources include degenerative joint disease such as osteoarthritis (OA).[1] Additionally, the need for anesthesia and surgical pain management has increased as well, following procedures like tumor excision or other surgical interventions. Managing pain in geriatric patients presents unique challenges, as these animals, including those that seem healthy and robust, may not be suitable candidates for certain pharmacologic or interventional treatments due to comorbidities, altered pharmacokinetics, or diminished organ function. This article explores multimodal approaches to pain management in the geriatric population, with an emphasis on individualized care, modified pharmaceutical dosing protocols, and evidence-based nonpharmacologic therapies to optimize comfort and quality of life.

Dogtor Consulting, LLC, Plymouth, MI, USA
E-mail address: paindocmike@gmail.com

Vet Clin Small Anim 56 (2026) 345–360
https://doi.org/10.1016/j.cvsm.2025.09.027 vetsmall.theclinics.com

Abbreviations	
CBD	Cannabidiol
COX	Cyclooxygenase
FDA	Food and Drug Administration
MPS	myofascial pain syndrome
NGF	nerve growth factor
NMDA	N-methyl-D-aspartate
NSAID	nonsteroidal anti-inflammatory drugs
PBMT	photobiomodulation therapy

PHARMACEUTICAL CONSIDERATIONS FOR CHRONIC PAIN

Nonsteroidal Anti-inflammatory Drugs

Nonsteroidal anti-inflammatory drugs (NSAIDs) have long been regarded as the cornerstone of both acute and chronic pain management in veterinary medicine, going back to the introduction of carprofen for canine use in the United States in 1997. This was subsequently followed by the development and approval of other NSAIDs, including NSAIDs formulated for feline patients. These drugs exert both central and peripheral analgesic effects in dogs and cats, making them useful in a broad application of pain cases.

Despite their efficacy, NSAIDs are associated with a risk of adverse effects, the most common of which are gastrointestinal in nature—gastric ulceration being the most frequently reported. Geriatric patients, particularly those with concurrent hepatic, renal, or cardiovascular disease, are at increased risk for NSAID-associated complications due to reduced physiologic reserve and concurrent comorbidities.

A variety of NSAIDs are approved for veterinary use, yet no product has demonstrated clinical superiority or safety[2] over others. In the United States, NSAIDs are not approved for chronic use in cats; however, both meloxicam and robenacoxib are authorized for long-term administration in feline patients within the European Union.

Some clinicians advocate for titration to the lowest effective dose to minimize risk, but there is currently no robust evidence that dose reduction mitigates adverse effects. On the contrary, underdosing may lead to inadequate analgesia. It is imperative to thoroughly review the full prescribing information for any NSAID and adhere closely to the manufacturer's guidelines to ensure safe and effective use. See **Box 1** for some recommendations to minimize NSAID use risk.

Box 1
Minimizing NSAID risk in geriatric dogs

1. Do not use concurrently with certain drugs, including other NSAIDs, corticosteroids, any herbal supplements that have NSAID-like activity or may interact with NSAIDs, such as gingko, ginseng, and Arnica, to name a few.
2. Caution is indicated in patients who are hypovolemic/dehydrated and have renal, hepatic, or cardiac dysfunction
3. Emphasize to caregivers, preferably in writing, that any unusual behavior following the start of NSAID therapy should prompt them to stop the NSAID and call the veterinarian. This is especially true of dogs and cats that exhibit any gastrointestinal signs.
4. Dosage should be based on lean body mass.
5. Laboratory monitoring should be utilized both prior to starting an animal on an NSAID, 2 to 3 weeks later, and at any point that you suspect an adverse event.

A Word About Grapiprant

While the U.S. Food and Drug Administration (FDA) classifies grapiprant as a NSAID, the World Health Organization (WHO) more accurately categorizes it as a piprant receptor antagonist.[3] This distinction is clinically significant, especially for geriatric patients with comorbidities that preclude the use of traditional NSAIDs.

Mechanism of Action

Grapiprant is a selective EP4 receptor antagonist. Rather than inhibiting cyclooxygenase (COX) enzymes like conventional NSAIDs, it blocks the EP4 prostaglandin receptor, a key mediator of pain and inflammation associated with OA in dogs. This targeted action may reduce the risk of adverse effects traditionally associated with COX inhibition.

Clinical Relevance in Geriatric Patients

Many older patients with renal, hepatic, or cardiovascular compromise cannot tolerate COX-inhibiting NSAIDs due to the potential for exacerbated organ dysfunction. Grapiprant, by bypassing COX pathways, offers a potentially safer alternative—although caution is still warranted.

Adverse Events

It is important to recognize that while grapiprant's mechanism differs from traditional NSAIDs, its adverse event profile is still similar in many respects—primarily gastrointestinal in nature (eg, vomiting, diarrhea, inappetence). However, individual responses may vary, and some patients intolerant to NSAIDs may tolerate grapiprant better. The reader should not assume that grapiprant is devoid of risk. Monitor geriatric patients closely, especially during the initial stages of therapy, and perform routine follow-up bloodwork to assess for subclinical effects.

Anti-nerve Growth Factor Monoclonal Antibodies

The introduction of antinerve growth factor (anti-NGF) monoclonal antibodies—bedinvetmab[4] for dogs and frunevetmab for cats[5]—has expanded the therapeutic options for managing osteoarthritic pain, particularly in patients who cannot tolerate NSAIDs due to adverse effects, have comorbidities or inadequate analgesic response.

Nerve growth factor (NGF) plays a crucial role in the development and differentiation of peripheral nerves in young animals and in the regeneration of injured peripheral nerves. However, in animals with OA, NGF accumulates within affected joints where it contributes to pain, neuronal sensitization, and neurogenic inflammation. Anti-NGF monoclonal antibodies bind to NGF within the joints, preventing its interaction with chemical signaling to nociceptors and reducing both peripheral sensitization and neurogenic inflammatory pain.

Although generally well tolerated, anti-NGF monoclonal antibodies are associated with specific adverse events. Unlike NSAIDs, however, there is no well-defined subset of geriatric patients predisposed to these reactions. Refer to **Table 1** (dogs) and **Table 2** (cats) for a summary of FDA-reported adverse events and warnings associated with this drug class. But keep in mind this statement from the FDA regarding **Table 1**: *The following adverse events are based on post-approval adverse drug experience reporting for LIBRELA. Not all adverse events are reported to FDA/CVM. It is not always possible to reliably estimate the adverse event frequency or establish a causal relationship to product exposure using these data.* For example, if a drug is widely used to treat certain conditions, there may be more adverse drug event (ADE)s for

Table 1
Summary of FDA-reported adverse events and warnings associated with NSAIDs drug class for dogs

Adverse Reaction	Librela	Placebo
Urinary tract infection	11.1%	8.0%
Bacterial skin infection	8.1%	6.6%
Dermatitis	7.4%	5.8%
Dermal mass	5.9%	3.6%
Erythema	4.4%	3.6%
Dermal cyst	3.0%	1.5%
Pain on injection	3.0%	1.5%
Inappropriate urination	3.0%	0.7%
Histiocytoma	2.2%	0.0%

Post approval experiences include neurologic signs, anorexia, lethargy, pu/pd, vomiting and diarrhea, muscle weakness and tremors, and lameness. Death including euthanasia has been reported as an outcome of the adverse events listed above.

Table 2
Summary of FDA-reported adverse events and warnings associated with NSAIDs drug class for cats

Adverse Reaction	Solensia	Placebo
Vomiting	13.2%	10.8%
Injection site pain	10.9%	14.0%
Diarrhea	6.6%	5.4%
Behavioral disorders	6.6%	5.4%
Renal insufficiency	6.6%	4.3%
Anorexia	6.6%	4.3%
Lethargy	6.0%	3.2%
Dermatitis	6.0%	1.1%
Alopecia	5.5%	2.2%
Dehydration	4.4%	0.0%
Lameness	4.4%	2.2%
Pruritis	3.8%	0.0%
Weight loss	3.3%	5.4%
Scabbing on head/neck	3.3%	1.1%
Gingival disorder	2.7%	0.0%
Bacterial skin infection	2.2%	1.1%
Otitis externa	2.2%	0/0%

that drug than for another product that is not used as often. This would not mean that the first drug was more unsafe than the second. The number of reports simply represents the number of ADEs received for a particular drug and should not be used for any type of comparison purposes. Additionally, as with all drugs, reported events are just that without implying any causal link between the drug and the reported event.

One of the more frequently observed concerns in canine patients is the emergence of neuropathic signs. While a direct causal link to the administration of anti-NGF therapy has not been definitively established, it is plausible that some signs reflect pre-existing neurologic conditions unmasked by improved mobility along with changes in clinical presentation. This includes dogs with early onset of Geriatric Onset Laryngeal Paralysis Polyneuropathy, which might go unnoticed in a dog that is sedentary because of chronic OA pain but become obvious with increased activity as the OA pain lessens. In dogs with OA, signs such as limb weakness, paw dragging, or general unsteadiness may be misinterpreted as joint pain when, in fact, they could stem from previously undiagnosed neurologic deficits such as proprioceptive loss. Keep in mind that 5% of all dogs have signs of neurologic disease and that can rise to 12% of senior dogs.[6]

Clinical Recommendation

Prior to initiating anti-NGF therapy, a comprehensive neurologic examination is advised for all canine patients. Additionally, just as with NSAID use, a baseline blood panel should be performed to screen for systemic or metabolic disorders that might be confused with a drug interaction.

Future Anti-nerve Growth Factor Monoclonal Antibodies

In late 2025 The Committee for Veterinary Medicinal Products (CVMP) of the European Medicines Agency (EMA), which is the European equivalent of the FDA, adopted a positive opinion recommending the granting of two new injectable long-term Anti-NGF monoclonal antibodies for dogs (izenivetmab/Lenivia) and cats (relfovetmab/Portela). Both products have novel binding properties that will provide three months of action to reduce the pain of osteoarthritis. This will provide a convenient option for those caregivers that find it difficult to return every 28 days for injections of either bedinvetmab or frunevetmab. Both products have demonstrated a safety profile, including cats that need treatment for OA but also have IRIS stage 1, 2 or 3 kidney disease.

Although a positive opinion is not an absolute guarantee of product approval, it is expected that this will be available in the European Union in 2026. Regulatory approval for a long-acting mAb for both dogs and cats for the control of OA pain is being sought in additional global markets as well.

Adjunctive Analgesic Drugs

Adjunctive analgesics are agents administered to enhance the efficacy of primary analgesic therapies, particularly in complex or refractory cases of pain. These drugs are not intended for use as monotherapy, but rather as components of a multimodal pain management strategy.

Many adjunctive analgesics act via mechanisms that complement those of traditional agents such as NSAIDs or opioids, including modulation of neuropathic pain pathways, attenuation of central sensitization, or reduction of muscle spasm and anxiety. Common examples include gabapentinoids (eg, gabapentin, pregabalin), tricyclic antidepressants, N-methyl-D-aspartate (NMDA) receptor antagonists (eg, amantadine), and certain anticonvulsants.

However, it is important to note that robust, species-specific evidence for the efficacy, optimal dosing, and safety of many adjunctive agents in veterinary patients is limited. Most data are extrapolated from human medicine or based on small-scale or anecdotal studies. As such, their use requires clinical judgment, careful patient selection, and close monitoring for adverse effects or drug interactions. Common dosing regimens have been suggested for the adjunctive agents in this section.

Amantadine

Originally developed as an antiviral agent for the treatment of type A influenza in humans, amantadine has since gained clinical relevance in veterinary medicine as an adjunctive analgesic, particularly in the management of chronic or refractory pain. In dogs and cats, amantadine exerts its analgesic effects primarily through inhibition of the NMDA receptor, a critical component of central pain pathways.[7] The NMDA receptor plays a significant role in the development of central sensitization, a process in which prolonged or inadequately managed pain leads to an amplified and persistent pain response. By blocking NMDA receptor activity, amantadine helps suppress pain signal transmission from the periphery to the central nervous system, thereby reducing hyperalgesia and allodynia associated with chronic pain conditions, such as OA or neuropathic pain.

Other NMDA antagonists, including ketamine and methadone, share similar mechanisms of action but are more commonly used in acute or perioperative settings due to their administration routes and sedative effects. Amantadine, in contrast, is favored for long-term outpatient use because it is administered orally and is generally well tolerated with a low incidence of adverse effects. Amantadine should never be used as a stand-alone analgesic; rather, it is most effective when used in conjunction with NSAIDs or other primary pain control agents as part of a multimodal analgesic plan.

The World Small Animal Veterinary Association Pain Guidelines recommend a dose of 2 to 5 mg/kg per os every 12 to 24 hours in both dogs and cats.

Amitriptyline

Amitriptyline is a tricyclic antidepressant that exerts its pharmacologic effects primarily by inhibiting the reuptake of norepinephrine and serotonin, neurotransmitters involved in both mood regulation and pain modulation.[8] In veterinary medicine, it may serve an adjunctive role in the management of chronic pain, particularly in cases where neuropathic mechanisms are suspected.

While the analgesic effects of amitriptyline in dogs and cats are not as robust as those seen in humans, its ability to modulate descending inhibitory pain pathways can provide ancillary benefits, especially when used as part of a multimodal analgesic regimen. Common side effects include sedation (which may diminish over time with chronic use), weight gain, and poor hair coat quality.

Risk of Serotonin Syndrome. Amitriptyline, like other drugs that enhance serotonergic activity, carries a risk of serotonin syndrome when combined with other serotonergic agents such as tramadol, imipramine, or duloxetine. This potentially life-threatening condition is characterized by.

- Neuromuscular hyperactivity (eg, tremors, hyperreflexia),
- Hyperthermia,
- Tachycardia,
- Tachypnea,
- Agitation or restlessness.

Serotonin syndrome is a medical emergency, and treatment options are limited and often unsuccessful if not initiated promptly. For this reason, concomitant use of multiple serotonergic agents should be avoided entirely by understanding the mode of action of each drug the patient is receiving.

The World Small Animal Veterinary Association pain guidelines recommend that dogs receive 1 to 4 mg/kg every 12 to 24 hours. Cats should receive 2.5 to 12.5 mg *per cat*, not based on body weight. This drug is extremely unpalatable and that should be taken into consideration prior to prescribing, especially with cats.

Gabapentin and Pregabalin

Gabapentin and pregabalin are structurally related anticonvulsants that are increasingly used in veterinary medicine as adjunctive analgesics, particularly in cases involving neuropathic pain. While their precise mechanism of action remains incompletely understood, both drugs are believed to modulate pain by binding to the $\alpha 2\delta$ subunit of voltage-gated calcium channels, thereby reducing excitatory neurotransmitter release—specifically glutamate and substance P—within the dorsal horn of the spinal cord.

Indications. These agents are most effective for chronic pain with a neuropathic component,[9] including

- OA, especially when neuropathic sensitization is suspected
- Cancer-associated pain
- Diabetic neuropathy
- Pelvic or spinal trauma
- Limb amputation, including declaw procedures in cats
- Intervertebral disc disease

Important clinical note: Gabapentin and pregabalin are *not* effective for acute pain, general non-neuropathic chronic pain, or routine postsurgical analgesia, and should not be relied upon as sole agents in such contexts.

Contraindications and adverse effects

- Renal impairment: Both drugs are renally excreted, and impaired renal clearance can lead to drug accumulation, resulting in marked sedation and ataxia.
- In patients with normal renal function, transient sedation or ataxia may still occur—especially during the initiation phase—but these effects typically diminish over time with continued administration.

Dosing guidelines

Gabapentin dogs: 10 to 20 mg/kg per os every 8 hours. Cats: 5 mg/kg per os twice daily.

Pregabalin dogs: 3 to 4 mg/kg every 8 to 12 hours. Cats: 1 to 2 mg/kg per os twice daily.

Close monitoring and dose adjustment are recommended in geriatric patients or those with suspected or confirmed renal dysfunction.

Tramadol

Tramadol is a centrally acting analgesic with a dual mechanism of action, functioning as both a weak μ-opioid receptor agonist and an *inhibitor of serotonin and norepinephrine reuptake*. These combined effects contribute to its analgesic potential, though species-specific responses vary significantly.

Indications

- Cats: Tramadol may be used for the treatment of chronic pain via oral administration, typically in combination with other analgesics as part of a multimodal approach. Feline patients appear more responsive to the drug's opioid and monoaminergic effects compared to canines.
- Dogs: The efficacy of tramadol in dogs is considered low, largely due to limited biotransformation into its active metabolite, O-desmethyltramadol (M1), which is responsible for opioid activity in humans.[10] Consequently, tramadol should only be used as an adjunctive analgesic in dogs, and primarily in scenarios where access to more effective medications is restricted. Any potential benefit in dogs may stem from its monoaminergic (serotonin reuptake inhibition) properties, though this effect is modest and inconsistently observed.

Clinical considerations

- Tramadol's serotonergic properties mean it carries a risk for serotonin syndrome, particularly if used concurrently with other serotonergic agents (eg, amitriptyline, duloxetine, SSRIs). See section on Serotonin Syndrome under the amitriptyline section for further details.
- Formulation and palatability may be limiting factors, particularly in cats, who often reject oral preparations unless compounded appropriately.

Dosing for chronic and acute pain in cats: 2 to 4 mg/kg every 8 to 12 hours.

Cannabidiol

Cannabidiol (CBD) is a nonpsychoactive compound part of a family of compounds named "cannabinoids." Cannabinoids, typically derived from hemp, can be separated and concentrated for pharmaceutical/nutraceutical use. CBD-specific concentrates contain negligible levels of other cannabinoids, such as tetrahydrocannabinol. Its analgesic (and maybe some evidence for anti-inflammatory) effects are believed to occur primarily through modulation of the endocannabinoid system, which plays a role in pain perception, immune response, and homeostasis.

Therapeutic Use in Osteoarthritis. Emerging research supports the use of CBD for managing chronic pain associated with OA in dogs and, to a lesser extent, in cats. Several randomized, blinded, placebo-controlled studies have demonstrated significant improvements in mobility and comfort. One notable study reported clinical improvement in 92% of dogs treated with CBD, highlighting its potential as part of a multimodal pain management plan.

Side Effects and Safety. CBD is generally well tolerated in both dogs and cats. Reported side effects include:

- Mild sedation, typically dose-dependent and transient
- Elevations in alkaline phosphatase on bloodwork, which do not appear to correlate with clinical hepatic dysfunction

Because of its favorable safety profile, CBD may be particularly useful in geriatric patients, including those with concurrent hepatic, renal, or cardiovascular comorbidities where other analgesics (eg, NSAIDs) may be contraindicated.

Considerations for Use. Palatability can be a challenge, especially in cats, as they do not seem to like the taste or smell of whole hemp extracts. The CBD market is currently unregulated, raising serious concerns regarding purity (eg, contamination with heavy metals such as lead or arsenic, or pesticide residues), potency (inconsistent concentrations between batches), residual solvents used in processing and label accuracy. Veterinarians are strongly advised to request certificates of analysis from independent laboratories for any CBD product being considered. These should include information on cannabinoid profile, contaminant testing (eg, mycotoxins, pesticides, heavy metals), and microbial screening. Hopefully, the CBD industry will be regulated in the future, minimizing these concerns.

Doses for OA management in dogs vary by study, but 2 mg/kg once daily is commonly cited as effective for providing analgesia without inducing sedation. More research is needed to establish standardized dosing in cats, though anecdotal reports and small-scale studies suggest cautious use with close monitoring.

Nonpharmaceutical Considerations for Chronic Pain

There are several modalities that can be considered as nonpharmaceutical treatments for chronic pain. Some of these modalities have a low learning curve or are easy to accomplish, such as laser (photobiomodulation therapy, PBMT) and environmental modifications. Other modalities are also important but require a steeper learning curve, like acupuncture or rehabilitation therapy. There is no claim being made as to which one is "better." They can all serve a purpose in reducing pain and returning the patient to normal function.

PHOTOBIOMODULATION THERAPY IN PAIN MANAGEMENT

Mechanism of Action

PBMT utilizes low-level red or near-infrared light to stimulate biological processes at the cellular level. It is used therapeutically to promote tissue repair and healing, reduce inflammation and edema and finally, to alleviate pain, particularly in conditions such as OA, neurologic injury, postsurgical pain, and trauma. PBMT facilitates mitochondrial activity, enhancing ATP production, nitric oxide release, and the modulation of inflammatory mediators, all of which contribute to pain relief and improved tissue recovery. The effect of PBMT on chronic pain issues will be discussed here.

Pain relief via PBMT is closely tied to its anti-inflammatory action. Following tissue insult—whether surgical, traumatic, or disease-related—immune cells such as macrophages, mast cells, and neutrophils release proinflammatory cytokines and mediators. These bind to nociceptors, amplifying pain through sensitization. PBMT modulates this response by reducing the infiltration and activation of inflammatory cells and downregulating inflammatory cytokines. These effects make PBMT a viable nonpharmacological alternative to anti-inflammatory medications in appropriate cases.

Photobiomodulation Therapy in Osteoarthritis Management

OA management often requires polytherapy to address the multifactorial nature of chronic pain. PBMT is safe and effective[11] to use in conjunction with all conventional pain medications, including NSAIDs, anti-NGF monoclonal antibodies, and adjunctive analgesics. Effective PBMT requires appropriate dose and energy delivery, typically 10 to 20 J/cm^2 per joint, depending on severity and depth. Higher doses may be needed for dense or deeper joints (eg, elbows). Devices with integrated software help standardize dosing, but clinicians should verify that protocols are current and evidence-based.

Research demonstrates that PBMT-treated patients may exhibit faster and more sustained improvements in pain and mobility than NSAID-treated controls. One controlled study showed that dogs treated with PBMT had superior pain reduction and range of motion improvements compared to dogs receiving meloxicam over 3 weeks. These benefits persisted longer posttreatment in the PBMT group.

Photobiomodulation Therapy in Neuropathic Pain

Neuropathic pain is challenging to diagnose definitively in veterinary patients, but clinical indicators may include.

- Lameness without orthopedic cause
- Pain following intervertebral disc disease
- Prolonged discomfort following nerve or spinal injury
- Suspected central sensitization in chronic OA cases

PBMT has demonstrated efficacy in managing neuropathic pain, potentially by interrupting nociceptive signaling at the dorsal root and spinal cord, modulating glial cell activation and enhancing axon regeneration.

Dose Considerations

Neuropathic pain often requires higher irradiance levels than those used in OA. Consider $\geq$270 mW/cm^2 at the site of the nerve. Adequate depth and tissue penetration are critical for the efficacy of treatment.

Environmental Modification

It would be difficult if not possible to discuss every possible environmental modification: chronic pain issues are greatly varied, and every living environment is different. The physical and time capabilities of the pet's caregiver also must be taken into consideration. Prior to discussing environmental modifications with the caregiver, have a conversation about what difficulties their pet is encountering at home, which will lead to some possible solutions. Modifications are recommended by the Canine Osteoarthritis Staging Tool group.[12]

Steps and stairs are one of the largest obstacles for animals with OA. Depending on the limbs affected, an animal may have difficulty maneuvering up and/or down to go outside, or in the case of litter-trained pets, to a different level of the house, for elimination purposes, or to join family members for reasons of socialization. For any size animal, a harness designed to assist with mobility can make a huge difference. For large dogs, especially where the owner is physically not capable of helping them, they may find using a ramp a lot easier than steps. However, for most dogs, training on how to safely use the ramp must be involved.

Vehicles also present problems for many dogs with OA. The same solutions as for using steps can work here as well, but usually with ramps or steps that are designed to assist large dogs to get into vehicles.

Litter box issues are often related to OA in cats. The problem can be 2-fold (assuming the litter box is not out of reach due to other obstacles like stairs): some litter boxes have high sides, making it difficult for cats with chronic pain to jump into the box. The other issue involves the litter itself, as some litters are difficult to walk on. Provide the cats with at least one low side to enter the litter box. Make sure there are obstacles in the way that could make it difficult to reach and recommend geriatric litters that are easier to walk on.

Floors with slippery surfaces are not only hard for many animals with OA to walk on, but they can also be distressing as well, with the animal choosing not to walk on it until necessary. This can lead to social isolation as well as slips and falls, leading to injury. Consider the use of nonslip runner rugs or yoga mats to help animals navigate through rooms with slippery floors. Another solution for slippery floors is assistive devices such as nonslip socks, rubber nail caps, and products that temporarily adhere to the pad to make them slip-resistant.

Weight Loss

Discussing weight loss can be difficult for both the caregiver and the veterinary professional. However, the importance of losing weight in an animal with OA is important. The increased weight puts additional stress on arthritic joints, exacerbating the pain. One study in dogs showed that losing even a minimal amount of weight can have beneficial pain-reducing effects like those seen with NSAID use.

The following are some tools for discussion of body weight and implementing a weight loss program.

1. Enlist the help of the caregiver as you look at a Body Condition Score (BCS) chart. If you choose an obesity score together, the caregiver will be more likely to "be on board" with the weight loss program
2. If your geriatric patient requires a prescription diet, this is a good time to set up some strict feeding guidelines
3. Pet food labels can be very misleading, with implications that it is good for adult or geriatric pets, when it is not. Ask the caregiver to look for the AAFCO statement on the side of the bag: if it says, 'For all life stages,' then the food is designed for those pets with the highest caloric needs, namely kittens and puppies and lactating mothers.
4. Schedule regular weigh-in rechecks

Acupuncture

The reason that acupuncture is an effective treatment modality is complex and beyond the scope of this article. In a nutshell, acupuncture encourages the body's own capacity for healing itself. This is done by many routes including the stimulation of neural pathways, release of hormones and other substances, activation of something called the parasympathetic nervous system, and the local action of the acupuncture needle to cause micro trauma, with the resulting influx of anti-inflammatories and healing substances to the area. The following are pain conditions I most commonly treat in geriatric animals.

Osteoarthritis[13] is a common issue among most geriatric animals. The point selection is straightforward for these cases, and most of them are relatively painless. Most patients see relief within 3 treatments given at 1-week intervals. However, for many patients, acupuncture alone is not enough. It is common to give many of the pharmaceutical treatments mentioned earlier in this article.

Spondylosis is a condition that has a foot in both the OA world and the neurologic world. It not only affects the functionality of the movement of the spine but can also interfere with the nerve roots as they come out between the vertebrae from the spinal cord to innervate different areas of the body. The subsequent compression results in pain and dysfunction of these nerves. Acupuncture can both restore the functionality of those nerves and reduce the pain and inflammation.

Myofascial Pain Syndrome

Myofascial pain syndrome (MPS) is a painful condition associated with the presence of myofascial trigger points in the skeletal muscles. MPS is a poorly understood and unknown problem in veterinary medicine, and like the section on acupuncture, it is beyond the scope of this article to describe it in its entirety.

Animals with chronic OA pain are commonly affected by MPS. Briefly, in the limb with pain, animals have submaximal muscle contractions to reduce the weight on that limb. This compensatory stance changes the muscle activity and small muscle fiber activity within that muscle. At the same time, additional weight is shifted to another limb, putting increased stress on that limb. Both the affected and supporting limbs are at risk of developing MPS. Untreated MPS can lead to unsatisfactory outcomes in OA.[14] Ultimately, the myosin–actin bond becomes fixed in place secondary to resulting local hypoxia and disruption in the mitochondrial energy metabolism, resulting in reduced ATP formation. The clinical approach to treatment is to bypass the ATP pathway and induce a spinal reflex. This is easily accomplished by using one of several treatments, including dry needling, therapeutic laser, extracorporeal shockwave therapy, thermal therapy, and manual therapy.

Although technically not difficult to treat, it does take some hands-on instruction to become proficient at it. Most rehabilitation centers and acupuncturists are skilled in treating MPS, and referrals should be considered for refractory OA cases.

Rehabilitation Therapy

Rehabilitation therapy in animals (called physical therapy or physiotherapy in human medicine) is a wide and diverse collection of treatments meant to decrease pain, improve muscle and limb function, and treat neurologic issues. The practitioner who wants to practice rehabilitation therapy needs to complete months-long courses to become certified, or years-long training to become boarded in Sports Medicine and Rehabilitation.

Rehabilitation therapy is a useful treatment adjunct for geriatric patients suffering from OA or other chronic pain conditions. The reader should establish a relationship with a facility that provides this service.

Radiosynoviorthesis

Radioactive tin-117m is marketed under the name Synovetin OA and is used to treat OA in joints in dogs, especially those that are refractory to many other treatments such as elbow OA. There is recent evidence that this treatment is useful in cats as well.[15] The tin is in a suspension, which can be injected into the joint space. These particles are absorbed and retained by macrophages, synoviocytes, and other phagocytic cells in the joint, resulting in apoptosis and reduction of inflammatory cells. Reduction of the pro-inflammatory cells and associated cytokines helps reduce the drivers of inflammation, pain, and progression of OA. This procedure is termed radiosynoviorthesis: restoration of the synovium using a radioisotope.

When administered, the beneficial effects can last up to 1 year. The only recorded side effect is postinjection pain that can last for about 3 days. Special licensing is needed to store and handle radioactive tin.

Platelet-Rich Plasma

Like radiosynoviorthesis, this is another joint injection. The platelet-rich plasma that is injected is harvested from a blood sample from the patient being treated. Unlike the radiosynoviorthesis, this can be administered to both dogs[16] and cats.[17]

A blood sample is drawn and treated to concentrate that fraction of plasma that has a high concentration of platelets. It is felt that the action of these platelets helps clean up dead and injured cells while also releasing growth factors; proteins that are responsible for tissue regeneration. Therapeutic effects generally last from 6 to 12 months.

The technique is simple, only requiring a knowledge of how to tap a joint. Special equipment is needed to both treat the blood sample and centrifuge properly to access the platelets.

Botanicals

Many caregivers express interest in using botanicals to manage their pet's pain, often due to concerns about the side effects of long-term pharmaceutical use and a desire for more natural treatment options. While some botanicals may provide benefit, it is essential to recognize that certain herbs can be toxic, and robust scientific evidence supporting their efficacy is limited.

Veterinarians must ensure that only high-quality, contaminant-free products are used, adhere to appropriate dosing guidelines, and monitor for side effects or potential interactions with concurrent medications. Gradual introduction is recommended, as gastrointestinal upset is a common adverse effect. Herbal treatments should be incorporated as part of a multimodal pain management plan to optimize safety and effectiveness. Commonly used botanicals are reviewed below.

Boswellia (Boswellia serrata)

Also known as Indian frankincense, Boswellia is a resin extract from the *Boswellia serrata* tree, native to India, North Africa, and parts of the Middle East. The active compounds, primarily boswellic acids, support anti-inflammatory pathways by inhibiting 5-lipoxygenase (5-LOX) and leukotriene synthesis. This leads to reduced production of pro-inflammatory cytokines, decreased cartilage degradation, and improved cartilage regeneration.

The most notable active constituents are 11-keto-β-boswellic acid and acetyl-11-keto-β-boswellic acid. These compounds have shown anti-inflammatory effects in various inflammatory diseases, including OA.

Turmeric (Curcuma longa)

Curcuminoids, the active constituents of turmeric, exert anti-inflammatory, antioxidant, and anticancer effects. However, curcuminoids exhibit poor bioavailability due to limited absorption, rapid metabolism, and systemic elimination. Products with enhanced bioavailability (eg, those combined with black pepper extract or formulated as nanoparticles or liposomes) are recommended.

Curcuminoids may act synergistically with NSAIDs to boost anti-inflammatory effects without increasing the risk of side effects.

Devil's Claw (Harpagophytum procumbens)

Devil's claw contains bioactive compounds such as harpagoside and harpagide, which contribute to its anti-inflammatory properties. These effects are believed to be mediated by COX-2 inhibition and suppression of inducible nitric oxide synthase

Note: Devil's claw is contraindicated in patients with gastric ulcers.

White Willow Bark

The primary active compound in white willow bark is salicin, a precursor to salicylic acid (the basis of aspirin). It is a nonselective COX-1 and COX-2 inhibitor. Although limited animal studies exist, it is assumed that its side effect profile may resemble that of NSAIDs.

Caution: Do not administer white willow bark concurrently with anticoagulants (eg, warfarin), NSAIDs, beta blockers, diuretics, methotrexate, or phenytoin due to potential drug interactions.

Corydalis (Yan Hu Suo)

Corydalis is frequently used in traditional Chinese pain-relief formulas. Its analgesic and sedative effects are attributed to tetrahydropalmatine, which acts on dopamine receptors. Corydalis may be effective for both acute and chronic inflammatory pain.

Nutritional Supplements

Nutritional supplements, sometimes referred to as Nutraceuticals, are another area of potential treatment for chronic pain. Like botanicals, many caregivers are looking for nonpharmaceutical means of treatment, often because they either want to avoid pharmaceuticals, their pet has not responded to pharmaceutical intervention for OA, or because their pet cannot tolerate pharmaceuticals for various reasons, including comorbidities. Also, like botanicals, many of these supplements have not undergone rigorous studies for efficacy, as well as safety. Additionally, this industry can be self-regulating unless they submit their product to outside organizations such as USP (US Pharmacopeia) for evaluations of purity. An approval from USP is not to be confused with an endorsement of efficacy. The following four nutritional supplements are the ones with the most robust evidence for efficacy.

Undenatured Type II Collagen

This supplement has had a lot of robust studies to look at efficacy in treating OA.[18] The mechanism of action is reducing inflammation at the arthritic joint, through a complex interaction involving the gastrointestinal tract. Although some studies suggest pain relief in as early as 2 weeks, in the author's experience, it is usually closer to 4 weeks.

Giving undenatured type II collagen concurrently with glucosamine and chondroitin sulfate may reduce its efficacy.

Green-Lipped Mussel (Perna canaliculus)

Green-lipped mussels contain glucosamine, chondroitin, and omega-3 fatty acids. Their efficacy for treating OA has been primarily investigated through clinical studies.

Omega-3 Fatty Acids

Omega-3 fatty acids that contain eicosapentaenoic acid (EPA) and docosahexaenoic acid (DHA) from fish oil have shown efficacy in improving joint health in animals with OA. The most efficacious proportions of DHA and EPA differ in dogs and cats. For dogs, a 1:1 ratio is considered adequate. For cats, there should be more DHA than EPA, about a 1.5:1 ratio.

It should be noted that dogs are unable to convert flaxseed into omega-3 fatty acids, and such supplements are of no benefit.

Glucosamine and Chondroitin Sulfate

I have included this supplement, although their effectiveness in treating OA is a topic of ongoing debate. Research shows that they may provide mild benefits in the treatment of pain from OA.

SUMMARY

Effectively managing chronic pain in geriatric dogs and cats often requires a comprehensive approach that combines pharmaceutical and nonpharmaceutical treatments, along with thoughtful environmental modifications. Success depends on careful consideration of the type of pain, the presence of comorbidities, and the caregiver's ability to implement a realistic and sustainable plan. By addressing these factors, veterinarians can not only alleviate suffering but also enhance mobility, preserve the human–animal bond, and significantly improve quality of life in our aging patients.

CLINICS CARE POINTS

- Pearls: When administering pharmaceuticals, start low and go slow as decreased hepatic and renal clearance can make even a routine procedure risky.
- The majority of geriatric patients have osteoarthritis. Proceed as such unless proven otherwise.
- Multi-modal treatments combining physical modalities and nutraceuticals to any pharmaceutical regimen can reduce the side effects of a single-burden drug.
- Adjusting the animal's home environment to accommodate the patient's issues is a necessary part of any treatment program.
- Caregivers must be on board with any treatment plan you provide them: financially, emotionally, physically and having the time to implement their part of the treatment.
- Animals fear pain. But they don't ponder death. Impress on your caregivers that quality of life trumps the length of life.
- Pitfalls: Do not overlook potential drug interactions when using polypharmacy.
- Do not ignore the potential for caregiver emotional fatigue. Talk to them about how they feel about their animal's issues and what else they may have happening in their lives that make it hard to help their aging pets.
- Monitor known health issues often by making recheck appointments before the caregiver leaves the clinic.
- Avoid overzealous treatments and council the caregivers when they are looking to add treatments with little or no benefit to their animals.
- Pain often causes social isolation if it is difficult to the animal to follow the owner from room to room and activity to activity. Social isolation can speed up a geriatric animal's demise.

DISCLOSURE

M.C. Petty: Occasionally lecture for Zoetis and Enovis.

REFERENCES

1. Anderson KL, Zulch H, O'Neill DG, et al. Risk factors for canine osteoarthritis and its predisposing arthropathies: a systematic review. Front Vet Sci 2020;7:220.
2. Monteiro-Steagall BP, M Steagall PV, Lascelles BDX. B.D.X lascelles systemic review of nonsteroidal anti-inflammatory drug-induced adverse effects in dogs. J Vet Intern Med 2013. https://doi.org/10.1111/jvim.12127.
3. Sartini I, Giorgi M. Grapiprant: a snapshot of the current knowledge. J Vet Pharmacol Therapeut 2021;44(5):679–88. Epub 2021 May 31. PMID: 34057218; PMCID: PMC8518515.
4. Available at: https://www.fda.gov/animal-veterinary/cvm-updates/fda-approves-first-monoclonal-antibody-dogs-osteoarthritis-pain (Accessed 05 May 2023).
5. Gruen ME, Myers JAE, Tena JS, et al. Frunevetmab, a felinized anti-nerve growth factor monoclonal antibody, for the treatment of pain from osteoarthritis in cats. J Vet Intern Med 2021;35(6):2752–62. Epub 2021 Nov 1. PMID: 34724255; PMCID: PMC8692178.
6. Nam Y, White M, Karlsson EK, et al, Dog Aging Project Consortium. Dog size and patterns of disease history across the canine age spectrum: results from the dog aging project. PLoS One 2024;19(1):e0295840. https://doi.org/10.1371/journal.pone.0295840. PMID: 38232117; PMCID: PMC10793924.

7. Lascelles BD, Gaynor JS, Smith ES, et al. Amantadine in a multimodal analgesic regimen for alleviation of refractory osteoarthritis pain in dogs. J Vet Intern Med 2008;22(1):53–9. PMID: 18289289.
8. Cashmore RG, Harcourt-Brown TR, Freeman PM, et al. Clinical diagnosis and treatment of suspected neuropathic pain in three dogs. Aust Vet J 2009;87(1): 45–50. PMID: 19178477.
9. Ruel HLM, Watanabe R, Evangelista MC, et al. Pain burden, sensory profile and inflammatory cytokines of dogs with naturally-occurring neuropathic pain treated with gabapentin alone or with meloxicam. PLoS One 2020;15(11):e0237121. https://doi.org/10.1371/journal.pone.0237121. PMID: 33253197; PMCID: PMC 7703878.
10. Budsberg SC, Torres BT, Kleine SA, et al. Lack of effectiveness of tramadol hydrochlorids for the treatment of pain and joint dysfunction in dogs with chronic osteoarthritis. JAVMA 2018;252(4):L427–32.
11. Looney AL, Huntingford JL, Blaeser LL, et al. A randomized blind placebo-controlled trial investigating the effects of photobiomodulation therapy (PBMT) on canine elbow osteoarthritis. Can Vet J 2018;59(9):959–66. PMID: 30197438; PMCID: PMC6091142.
12. Cachon T, Frykman O, Innes JF, et al. COAST development Group's international consensus guidelines for the treatment of canine osteoarthritis. Front Vet Sci 2023;10:1137888. https://doi.org/10.3389/fvets.2023.1137888. PMID: 37601753; PMCID: PMC10436090.
13. Pye C, Clark N, Bruniges N, et al. Current evidence for non-pharmaceutical, non-surgical treatments of canine osteoarthritis. J Small Anim Pract 2024;65(1):3–23. Epub 2023 Sep 29. PMID: 37776028.
14. Petty MC, Monteiro BP, A S. Robertson myofascial pain syndrome in small animal practice. J Small Anim Pract 2024;1–6. https://doi.org/10.1111/jsap.13795.
15. Bendele A, Doerr CA, Gonzales GR, et al. Evidence of osteoarthritis disease modification with a Sn-117m microparticle device: a review and validation in mammalian models. Front Vet Sci 2025;12:1621296. https://doi.org/10.3389/fvets.2025.1621296. PMID: 40717911; PMCID: PMC12290414.
16. Carr BJ, Miller AV, Colbath AC, et al. Literature review details and supports the application of platelet-rich plasma products in canine medicine, particularly as an orthobiologic agent for osteoarthritis. J Am Vet Med Assoc 2024;262(S1): S8–15. PMID: 38382202.
17. Huntingford J, Looney A, Johnson J, et al. The use of platelet rich plasma in the treatment of degenerative joint disease in cats: an exploratory case series. Front Vet Sci 2024;11:1394055. https://doi.org/10.3389/fvets.2024.1394055. PMID: 38863451; PMCID: PMC11165359.
18. Gencoglu H, Orhan C, Sahin E, et al. Undenatured type II collagen (UC-II) in joint health and disease: a review on the current knowledge of companion animals. Animals (Basel) 2020;10(4):697. PMID: 32316397; PMCID: PMC7222752.

Movement Is Medicine

How Rehabilitation Revitalizes Aging Pets

Leilani X. Alvarez, DVM

KEYWORDS

- Benefits of exercise • Movement medicine • Rehabilitation • Functional mobility
- Longevity • Therapeutic exercise • Strengthening • Balance/coordination

KEY POINTS

- Exercise improves cardiovascular, musculoskeletal, and mental health.
- Exercise reduces pain and improves and functional mobility.
- Regular movement is essential for joint nutrition and general health.
- Routine moderate level exercise promotes longevity.
- Exercise plans should always be customized to the patient's needs.

Video content accompanies this article at http://www.vetsmall.theclinics.com.

INTRODUCTION/BACKGROUND

The benefits of mobility extend far beyond joint health. Regular exercise reduces pain, elevates mood, promotes cardiovascular fitness, extends quality of life and longevity, and even reduces the risk of chronic illness, including certain cancers.[1] Regular moderate levels of exercise improve all aspects of health in humans and is well accepted as a preventative and therapeutic strategy for combating various chronic illnesses.[2] Advances in therapeutics and specialty veterinary medicine have significantly increased the lifespan of companion animals, with owners identifying approximately 33% of dogs as senior (over the age of 8 years old), constituting nearly 30 million dogs in the United States.[3] As dogs continue to live longer, there is a rising need to improve their functional mobility and quality of life as they age.

Regular physical activity, prescribed by veterinarians, appears to mutually benefit humans and dogs, promoting decreased hypertension, reducing body weight and improving health indices.[4] In addition, joint outdoor exercise with humans and their companion dogs improves quality of life, body condition, and the human-animal bond.[5]

Physical rehabilitation is a relatively novel area of veterinary medicine that is rising in popularity. The American College of Veterinary Sports Medicine and Rehabilitation

Department of Integrative & Rehabilitative Medicine, Schwarzman Animal Medical Center, 510 E 62nd Street, New York, NY 10065, USA
E-mail address: Leilani.Alvarez@amcny.org

Vet Clin Small Anim 56 (2026) 361–373
https://doi.org/10.1016/j.cvsm.2025.09.032 vetsmall.theclinics.com
0195-5616/26/

Abbreviations	
ACVSMR	American College of Veterinary Sports Medicine and Rehabilitation
ADL	Activities of Daily Living
AVMA	American Veterinary Medical Association
BADIM	Basic Activity for Daily Independent Mobility
c-MMT	canine Manual Muscle Test
DACVSMR	Diplomate American College of Veterinary Sports Medicine and Rehabilitation
IADQOL	Instrumental Activity for Daily Quality of Life

(ACVSMR) is the most newly recognized specialty by the American Veterinary Medical Association (AVMA). The practice of veterinary rehabilitation focuses on reducing pain and improving functional mobility in companion animals.[6] The benefits of rehabilitation in dogs are wide ranging from improving surgical recovery and healing of tissues, increasing muscle mass and strength, reducing lameness, improving neuroadaptation, and enhancing return to function.[7,8] The application of thoughtful and customized exercise programs to senior dogs is essential not only for maintaining and improving mobility but also to revitalize their health and well-being.

OBJECTIVES

- Understand how physiologic changes of aging impact mobility
- Review how movement improves musculoskeletal and general health
- Learn how to develop customized exercise plans
- Learn specific exercises to improve strength, balance and coordination, endurance and specific functional tasks

PHYSIOLOGIC CHANGES OF AGING THAT REDUCE MOBILITY

Aging changes in dogs range from physical alterations to internal system failures that significantly impact mobility and quality of life.[9] Understanding these changes is crucial for providing appropriate care. Notable changes include:

- Brain atrophy (especially of the hippocampus)
- Slower nerve conduction and reaction times
- Decreased production of neurotransmitters
- Decreased lung capacity
- Decreased cardiac output, heart contractility, and valvular degeneration
- Generalized and disuse muscle atrophy
- Loss of muscle-tendon coordination
- Increased body fat
- Decreased hearing and vision

These physiologic changes lead to *lower exercise tolerance, decreased proprioception, and increased risk of slipping/falling*.

Other physiologic changes that can increase frailty and have secondary impacts on mobility include:

- Kidney atrophy and reduced renal function
- Increased protein catabolism and decreased protein synthesis
- Decreased hepatic function
- Reduced immune function
- Increased risk of cancer
- Cachexia

Age-related changes that contribute to a spectrum of *common age-related conditions in dogs*:

- Osteoarthritis
- Sarcopenia
- Diabetes
- Geriatric-onset laryngeal paralysis and polyneuropathy
- Hypothyroidism
- Degenerative myelopathy
- Cognitive decline

By recognizing these changes and conditions, veterinarians and care givers can tailor strategies to meet the unique needs of aging dogs, improving quality of life, and longevity.

PHYSIOLOGIC CHANGES TO THE MUSCULOSKELETAL SYSTEM

As dogs age, a significant loss of skeletal muscle mass and function occurs in the absence of disease, known as *sarcopenia*. Factors contributing to sarcopenia include physical inactivity, changes in muscle fiber types, reduced protein production, increased anti-muscle cytokine generation, insulin resistance, and decreased levels of anabolic hormones.[10] Muscle mass in humans can decrease by up to 30% between the ages of 30 and 80, highlighting the profound impact of sarcopenia on muscle strength, immunity, and overall frailty, significantly raising the risk of disability, poor quality of life, and mortality.[11] Although less researched in dogs, canine sarcopenia shares similar pathologic mechanisms with humans and leads to comparable negative impacts.[10,12,13] Routine exercise, including aerobic and resistance activities, is shown to combat sarcopenia in humans.[14] Aging dogs show a shift toward retaining more adipose tissue and loosing lean muscle mass due to decreased metabolic rate, inactivity, and decreased protein synthesis.[15] Studies in overweight dogs have demonstrated that exercise mitigates the shift from muscle accumulation to fat by helping to preserve lean muscle mass.[16]

CACHEXIA

Cachexia is a disease-associated syndrome marked by accelerated muscle loss, distinct from sarcopenia, and commonly linked to chronic illnesses in senior dogs such as cancer, heart failure, or kidney disease.[12] It leads to severe muscle depletion, weakness, and increased caregiving demands, while driving inflammation, immune dysfunction, impaired healing, higher infection risk and reduced treatment efficacy, lifespan, and quality of life.[12]

Unlike healthy senior dogs, weight loss in cachexia primarily reflects muscle rather than fat loss, with disrupted protein, carbohydrate, and fat metabolism and frequent inappetence further worsening the condition.[10]

Management requires addressing the underlying disease while preventing muscle wasting through nutrition and exercise. Senior dogs should receive higher protein (>75 g/1000 kcal) to support protein synthesis and healthy muscle mass.[17] Tailored aerobic and resistance activities, even moderate ones such as walking, can help preserve muscle mass, highlighting the essential role of physical activity in mitigating cachexia and supporting healthy aging.[10] Dogs with hip dysplasia who exercise regularly (at least 60 minutes or more per day) demonstrate reduced lameness scores compared with dogs who exercise 20 minutes or less per day,[18] further supporting the notion that exercise mitigates disease and helps maintain muscle mass and function.

NEUROLOGIC CHANGES

Gray and white matter brain tissue atrophies in aging dogs and people, resulting in increased ventricular volume.[19–22] Cognitive dysfunction in aging dogs, shares similarities with Alzheimer's disease and dementia in humans, demonstrating accumulation of beta-amyloid plaques and tau proteins.[20,23–25] Evidence demonstrates that physical activity and exercise protect against cognitive decline in both species.[26,27] A cross-sectional study in over 11,000 companion dogs aged 6 to 18 years demonstrated robust association between regular physical activity and improved cognitive function.[28] Exercise may also promote neurogenesis, improve neuromuscular conduction and reduce age-related brain atrophy.[29]

IMPACT OF AGING ON MOBILITY

Aging leads to physiologic changes and diseases that can directly and indirectly impact mobility. Reduced mobility and a sedentary lifestyle in older dogs are closely linked to a lower quality of life and an increased risk of mortality.[15] Therefore, enhancing functional movement is an effective strategy for improving the health of geriatric dogs. Lack of physical activity diminishes overall well-being and increases susceptibility to secondary conditions such as decubital ulcers, skin infections, urinary and respiratory tract infections.[15]

Implementing a balanced exercise program helps to mitigate these secondary comorbidities associated with aging. Exercise programs that include resistance and endurance training are particularly effective for improving aerobic capacity, maintaining and enhancing muscle mass, and delivering comprehensive physical and cognitive health benefits for aging dogs.[30]

EVIDENCE THAT EXERCISE REDUCES OA PAIN AND IMPROVES MOBILITY

Exercise offers many benefits to patients suffering from osteoarthritis (OA) and aging. Evidence in both human and canine literature has demonstrated ample evidence of exercise improving mobility and reducing pain. In a recent systematic review, the highest quality practice guidelines consistently recommend exercise for managing patients with knee and hip osteoarthritis.[31] In addition, systematic review level of evidence supports that strengthening and aerobic exercise utilizing both land-based, and aquatic programs reduce pain, improve physical function, and quality of life in humans with knee osteoarthritis.[32] In dogs with hip dysplasia, exercising at least 60 minutes or more per day (regardless of low or high impact activities), reduces lameness more than controls who exercised 20 minutes or less.[18]

EXERCISE PLANS FOR SENIOR DOGS

In general, senior dogs are weaker and have a lower cardiovascular and respiratory tolerance; therefore, exercise plans should begin with short duration, lower intensity but higher frequency.

When designing exercise programs for geriatric dogs, account for a dog's unique health needs including any chronic illnesses, neurologic or orthopedic disease, and other risk factors.

Key considerations include:

- Coexisting diseases (diabetes, cancer, chronic kidney disease [CKD], heart disease)
- Delayed reaction times

- Reduced cardiovascular and pulmonary tolerance
- Level of frailty
- Higher risk of injury

Differentiating between functional decline due to aging from age-related diseases is vital for providing appropriate care. Addressing comorbidities and distinguishing between primary mobility disorders and diminished mobility due to other illnesses is essential for formulating a tailored rehabilitative care program.[15] This approach allows for a more targeted intervention that accounts for the dog's specific limitations and functional needs.

Ultimately, mitigating the effects of aging on a dog's health, quality of life, and longevity involves a comprehensive strategy encompassing tailored exercises and environmental modifications.

CUSTOMIZATION OF AN EXERCISE PROGRAM FOR SENIOR DOGS

- Thorough examination by a board-certified sports medicine and rehabilitation specialist or experienced rehabilitation certified therapist or experienced practitioner in geriatric medicine
- Identify comorbidities and risk factors
- Begin at level of fitness appropriate for the dog
- Always use traction flooring during exercise
- Begin with warm-up (5–10 minutes leash walk)

BUILDING A SUCCESSFUL EXERCISE PROGRAM

Developing a successful exercise program involves 4 key elements: (1) patient cooperation and trainability, (2) following correct form, (3) incorporating multiple types of exercise, and (4) progressing the program according to patient progress.

Patient Cooperation and Trainability

Therapeutic exercises rely on the patient's ability to perform foundational behaviors and movements. The following postures or motions are essential building blocks for more advanced exercises:

- Sit
- Down
- Stand
- Stay/Wait
- Target (touch)
- Shake (bilaterally)
- Heel (walking without pulling on a leash)

If a patient cannot perform these behaviors, care givers should integrate basic training into the rehabilitation plan, potentially collaborating with trainers. When a dog can reliably perform these behaviors, exercise programs can more easily be adapted and progressed to meet the patient's needs.

Ensure Correct Form

Proper form during any exercise is critical to the success of any therapeutic rehabilitation program. Incorrect movements reinforce maladaptive patterns and can exacerbate underlying conditions. Therapists must closely monitor form, especially during repetitions, and intervene when fatigue or improper mechanics appear. Correct form should be emphasized over the number of repetitions or sets. Always reward and reinforce accurate performance to build motor memory and neuromuscular control.

Incorporate a Variety of Exercise Forms

A comprehensive rehabilitation plan should incorporate a variety of exercise strategies that improve function in multiple areas that are essential for activities of daily living and specific for the dog's needs. Exercise programs should not focus on any one form of exercise, otherwise they will be limited in progress and will be at higher risk for injury.

A comprehensive therapeutic exercise and rehabilitation plan should include the following elements:[6]

- *Strength*: Exercises targeted for limb strengthening improve functional tasks (see Videos 1–6) and core strengthening improves posture, reduces risk of falls, and improves general mobility (see Videos 7–9).
- *Endurance*: Improves cardiovascular and pulmonary capacity, improves circulation and enhances joint mobility. Examples include leash walking, treading underwater, and swimming.
- *Balance & coordination*: These exercises are essential for maintaining and improving proprioception and protecting against slips and falls[33,34] (see Videos 5, 7, 8; Videos 10 and 11).
- *Flexibility and range of motion*: Improve muscle function and circulation, promote joint health and function (see Video 7; Videos 12–14).
- *Specific Skills:* Dogs have essential tasks that allow them to complete activities of daily living (ADL) such as the ability to rise, the ability to squat to urinate, and the ability to sit and stand (see Videos 1 and 2).

Progression of Exercises

Progression should ensure *accurate and error-free completion* of tasks before advancing.

In general, senior dogs are weaker and have a lower cardiovascular and respiratory tolerance; therefore, exercise plans should begin with short duration, lower intensity but higher frequency (**Table 1**). As the patient begins to improve, strength exercises can increase in hold times (suggested start is 5-second hold) and increase every 5 to 7 days as the patient progresses. Dynamic exercises can begin with 5 repetitions and a maximum of 3 sets and progress every 5 to 7 days as tolerated. Resistance training is particularly effective for muscle strengthening in aging dogs (see Video 6). This can be implemented with resistance bands (eg, square standing with lateral pull with the resistance band), as well as hydrotherapy.

Hydrotherapy provides resistance due to hydrostatic pressures of the water against the moving limbs. Senior dogs should begin with a warm-up walk on the underwater treadmill for a few minutes. The suggested time to start is half the amount of time that the dog can walk on land (eg, if the dog is walking 10 min on leash, the dog should walk no more than 5 minutes in the underwater treadmill). After warm-up walking, the dog can swim for very short intervals (suggested 1–2 minutes at a time followed a by 3–5-minute rest period). Exercises in senior dogs should be focused on activities that are essential for function (activities of daily living), like being able to squat for urination/defecation, being able to rise, being able to sit (see Video 1), being able to stand while eating or drinking (**Fig. 1**).

MODIFICATIONS TO IMPROVE SAFETY AND EFFICACY OF EXERCISE

- Provide traction flooring (yoga mat, gym mat, grass, cement, carpet)

Table 1
Stepwise guide for senior dog therapeutic exercises

Step	Focus	Actions/Examples
Assessment	Health status and risks	Specialist examination; ID comorbidities (DMVD, CKD, cancer, ortho/neuro); assess frailty and tolerance
Foundations	Trainability and cooperation	Ensure dog can reliably sit, down, stand, stay, target, heel, shake
Safety setup	Prevent injury	Traction flooring, trimmed nails, assistive devices, orthopedic bedding, elevated food bowls, warm-up (5–10 min leash walk)
Initial program	Start safe	Low intensity, short duration, higher frequency; emphasize correct form over repetitions
Exercise variation	Comprehensive approach	Strength (sit-to-stand, resistance bands); endurance (walks, underwater treadmill); balance/coordination (cavalettis, backward walking; flexibility (cookie stretches, downward dog); specific skills
Implementation	Early loading	Isometrics: 5 s holds, ↑every 5–7 d; Dynamics: 5 reps, ≤3 sets, progress q 5–7 d
Progression	Gradual and safe	Increase duration before intensity; add resistance bands/hydrotherapy; hydro start with ½ land walk time, swim 1–2 min bouts
Reassessment	Ongoing monitoring	Evaluate form, strength, endurance, gait; watch for fatigue, pain, intolerance
Long-Term	Functional independence	Maintain ADLs: rise, squat, sit, stand while eating; adjust as health changes

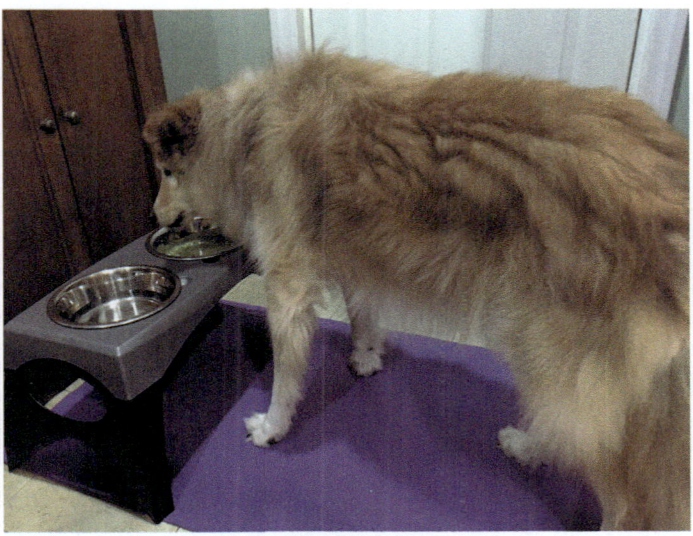

Fig. 1. Feeding with traction flooring and elevated food bowl.

- Always keep paw hair and nails trim
- Use assistive devices as needed (toe grips, harness, booties, cart)
- Provide firm orthopedic bedding without a lip (enables easier rising and decreases falls)
- Elevate food bowls to improve standing while eating (see **Fig. 1**)

ASSESSMENT

Before initiating any new forms of exercise, it is essential to make a thorough assessment of a senior dog to determine their capability and readiness to engage in the activity. Ideally, patients should have a complete musculoskeletal and neurologic evaluation with a specialist (diplomate of ACVSMR, American College of Veterinary Surgeons [ACVS], or American College of Veterinary Internal Medicine [ACVIM]-Neurology); however, any veterinarian with advanced training in rehabilitation or geriatric medicine could also be qualified. There are multiple ways to assess a patient. Perhaps the most important is a *functional assessment*. This involves determining the basic tasks that a dog can perform. They consider mobility during a functional task (such a rising from a down position; see Video 2). Functional outcomes remain the primary outcome measure in most human physical therapy studies.[35,36] Although supporting veterinary literature is less robust, several practical tests have been developed in dogs to functionally evaluate parameters including strength, range of motion, endurance, and proprioception.

STRENGTH TESTING

The 5-point canine manual muscle test (c-MMT) is a reliable outcome measure in dogs; however, significance was not reached to validate the test.[37] As described, c-MMT tests isometric strength in dogs and may be a useful tool in progression of strength exercises (**Fig. 2**).

CANINE MANUAL MUSCLE TEST PROTOCOL

Dogs should be evaluated in static, square standing, position on nonslippery surface.[37] Contralateral limb should be elevated for 15 seconds duration with no incline

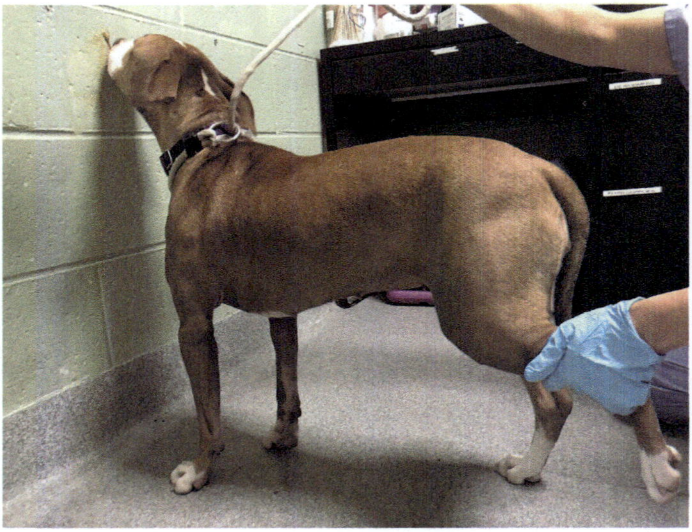

Fig. 2. Dog performing c-MMT demonstrating score of 3/5.

(grades 1–3), and with limbs elevated on box to elbow height (grades 4–5). There should be a 30-second rest period before introducing the incline to avoid exhaustion. Compensation is defined as breaking isometric hold (moving tested or other limbs) or trembling. Failure to stand is defined as limb collapse during test.

Equipment required: Stable box or platform at elbow height.

Score Interpretation (**Table 2**):

Higher scores indicate greater strength.

- ≥2: necessary to begin strengthening exercises
- ≥ 3: required to progress strengthening exercises

Benefits: Easy to perform, minimal equipment, inter-rater and intra-rater reliability.

Limitations: May be a test of concentration and ability to focus more than strength of the dog. Failed to meet validity in healthy dogs.[37]

Tip: Train the dog first and acclimate to the equipment prior to starting the c-MMT.

Activities of Daily Living are lists of tasks that are used to evaluate physical, cognitive, and motivational abilities.[15] As independent function declines and a patient's ability to perform these tasks diminishes, there is a higher risk for hospitalization and death.[15]

These tasks fall into 2 primary categories according to degree of complexity (**Table 3**):

- *Basic Activity for Daily Independent Mobility (BADIM):* includes basic tasks such as the ability to stand to eat and squat to urinate
- *Instrumental Activity for Daily Quality of Life (IADQOL):* includes more complex tasks such climbing stairs and interactive play

The *Canine Geriatric Functional Score*[15] test has been adapted from human functional assessment systems to evaluate mobility in geriatric patients. This test consists

Table 2
Canine manual muscle test scoring[37]

Numerical Score	Qualitative Score	Description
5	Normal	Able to maintain standing position against gravity on tested limb on an incline with contralateral limb elevated
4	Good	Able to maintain standing position on an incline, but shows compensation with contralateral limb elevated
3	Fair	Able to maintain standing position without compensation when contralateral limb is elevated on neutral ground (see **Fig. 2**)
2	Poor	Able to maintain tested limb in standing position when contralateral limb is elevated on neutral ground, but shows compensation
1	Trace	Failure to stand against gravity when contralateral limb is elevated on neutral
0	Zero	Nonweight bearing on tested limb on neutral ground

From Alvarez, LX, Repac, J, Zink C, et al. Reliability and validation of the canine manual muscle test (c-MMT) as a measure for hindlimb strength in dogs. Vet Comp Orthop Traumatol Open 2023;06(S 01):A1–11. https://doi.org/10.1055/s-0043-1768882.

Table 3
Basic activity for daily independent mobility (BADIM) and instrumental activity for daily quality of life (IADQOL) adapted for dogs[15]

Basic Activity for Daily Independent Mobility (BADIM)	Instrumental Activity for Daily Quality of Life (IADQOL)
• Rising from a down position • Ambulating in and out of home • Posturing to eliminate • Posturing to eat and drink	• Ascending/descending flight of stairs • Moving in and out of a vehicle • Walking short distances outside • Exploring the home environment • Interactive play (fetch, tug of war, etc) • Navigating rest place (bed, couch, etc) • Controlling urine/defecation for 6–8 h

From Frye C, Carr BJ, Lenfest M, et al. Canine geriatric rehabilitation: considerations and strategies for assessment, functional scoring, and follow-up. Front Vet Sci 2022;9:842458. https://doi.org/10.3389/fvets.2022.842458.

of 4 tasks scored on a 0 to 4 scale. The "timed up and go" test was reported to be the most objective and reliable.[38]

The 4 tasks include[38]:

1. Timed up and go: stand up from down position and walk a straight distance of 10 body lengths on neutral ground
2. Cavaletti: walk on leash over 2 rails spared body length apart (nose to rump) at hock height once in each direction for a total of 2 passes (4 rails)
3. Figure 8: walk on leash in a figure 8 pattern around cones spaced body length apart for 4 repetitions
4. Down: Move from sternal to rise position as many times as possible in a 60-second period

Equipment:

- 2 cavaletti rails
- Yoga mat or other traction surface
- 2 cones

Score interpretation:

Lower scores indicate worse performance.

- Poor (0–4)
- Fair (5–8)
- Good (9–12)
- Excellent (13–16)

Benefits: easy to perform, minimal equipment required, strong interrater reliability[38]

Limitations: can be difficult to perform in patients who are not trained with basic commands or unmotivated

IMPLEMENTATION AND PROGRESSION

Keeping in mind a thorough assessment utilizing functional outcomes measures as described, one can choose appropriate exercises for the senior dog (**Fig. 3**). Continuous monitoring and reassessment are crucial to determine progression and adjustment to the plan (see **Fig. 3**, **Table 1**). Caregivers should notice improvement in strength and coordination approximately 4 to 6 weeks after implementation of a customized exercise program; however, more geriatric dogs are less likely to show

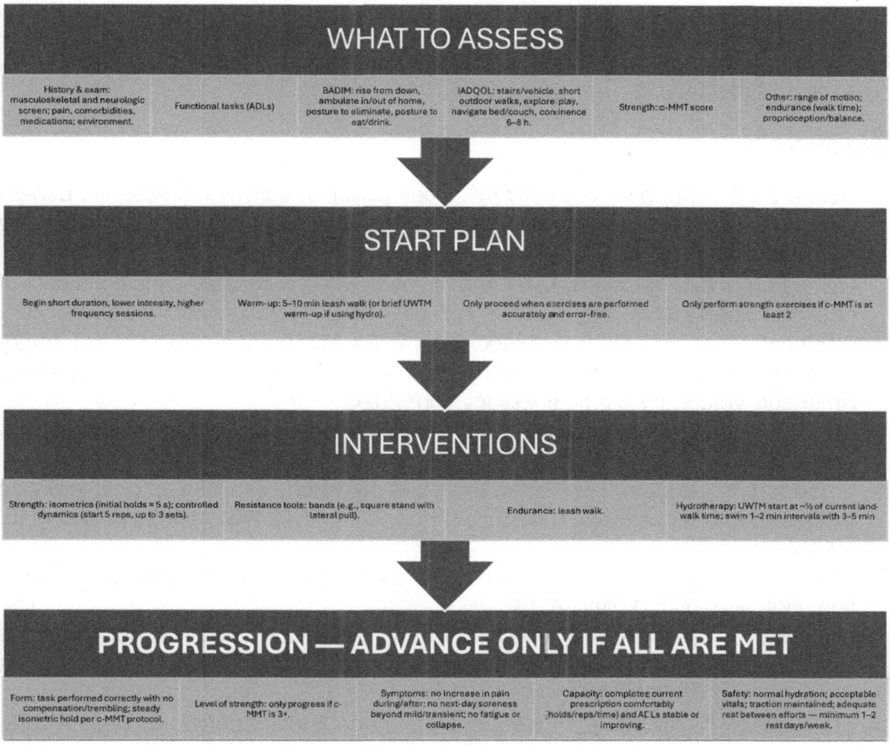

Fig. 3. Flow-chart of assessment and progression of an exercise program.

significant improvement. In more fragile pets, maintenance of mobility is a reasonable expectation.

CLINICS CARE POINTS

- Exercise is essential for maintaining mobility and quality of life in senior dogs.
- Aim for at least 60 minutes of daily walking (break up into 3–6 segments).
- Develop tailored exercise programs that include strength, endurance, balance/coordination, flexibility/ROM, and specific tasks.
- Always provide traction flooring and assistance as needed.
- Stop exercise if patient declines.

DECLARATION OF AI AND AI-ASSISTED TECHNOLOGIES

During the preparation of this work, the author used ChatGPT in order to improve readability. After using this tool/service, the author reviewed and edited the content as needed and takes full responsibility for the content of the publication.

DISCLOSURE

The author declares no commercial or financial conflicts of interests.

SUPPLEMENTARY DATA

Supplementary data related to this article can be found online at https://doi.org/10.1016/j.cvsm.2025.09.032.

REFERENCES

1. Reimers CD, Knapp G, Reimers AK. Does physical activity increase life expectancy? A review of the literature. J Aging Res 2012;2012:243958. https://doi.org/10.1155/2012/243958.
2. Qiu Y, Fernández-García B, Lehmann HI, et al. Exercise sustains the hallmarks of health. J Sport Health Sci 2023;12(1):8–35.
3. American Veterinary Medical Association. 2024 AVMA pet ownership and demographics sourcebook. Schaumburg (IL): Center for Information Management, American Veterinary Medical Association; 2024.
4. Duncan C, Carswell A, Nelson T, et al. Veterinary-prescribed physical activity promotes walking in healthy dogs and people. BMC Vet Res 2020;16(1):468.
5. Smedberg K, Lundbeck E, Roman E, et al. A pilot study of a joint outdoor exercise program for dog owners and dogs. Sci Rep 2024;14(1):14321. https://doi.org/10.1038/s41598-024-65033-0.
6. Zink C, Van Dyke JB, editors. Canine sports medicine and rehabilitation. 2nd edition. Hoboken (NJ): Wiley; 2018.
7. Alvarez LX, Repac JA, Kirkby Shaw K, et al. Systematic review of postoperative rehabilitation interventions after cranial cruciate ligament surgery in dogs. Vet Surg 2022;51(2):233–43.
8. Kirkby Shaw K, Alvarez L, Foster SA, et al. Fundamental principles of rehabilitation and musculoskeletal tissue healing. Vet Surg 2020;49(1):22–32.
9. Bellows J, Colitz CM, Daristotle L, et al. Common physical and functional changes associated with aging in dogs. J Am Vet Med Assoc 2015;246(1):67–75.
10. Freeman LM. Cachexia and sarcopenia: emerging syndromes of importance in dogs and cats. J Vet Intern Med 2012;26(1):3–17.
11. Santilli V, Bernetti A, Mangone M, et al. Clinical definition of sarcopenia. Clinical Cases in Mineral and Bone Metabolism 2014;11(3):177–80.
12. Freeman LM. Cachexia and sarcopenia in companion animals: an under-utilized natural animal model of human disease. JCSM Rapid Commun 2018;1:1–17.
13. Pagano TB, Wojcik S, Costagliola A, et al. Age related skeletal muscle atrophy and upregulation of autophagy in dogs. Vet J 2015;206(1):54–60.
14. Yoo SZ, No MH, Heo JW, et al. Role of exercise in age-related sarcopenia. J Exercise Rehabilitation 2018;14(4):551–8.
15. Frye C, Carr BJ, Lenfest M, et al. Canine geriatric rehabilitation: considerations and strategies for assessment, functional scoring, and follow-up. Front Vet Sci 2022;9:842458. https://doi.org/10.3389/fvets.2022.842458.
16. Vitger AD, Stallknecht BM, Nielsen DH, et al. Integration of a physical training program in a weight loss plan for overweight pet dogs. J Am Vet Med Assoc 2016;248(2):174–82.
17. Shmalberg J, Wakshlag JJ. Nutrition for working and service dogs. Vet Clin N Am Small Anim Pract 2014;44(4):719–vi.
18. Greene LM, Marcellin-Little DJ, Lascelles BDX. Associations among exercise duration, lameness severity, and hip joint range of motion in Labrador Retrievers with hip dysplasia. J Am Vet Med Assoc 2013;242(11):1528–33.
19. Borràs D, Ferrer I, Pumarola M. Age-related changes in the brain of the dog. Veterinary Pathology 1999;36:202–11.

20. Tapp PD, Siwak CT, Gao FQ, et al. Frontal lobe volume, function, and beta-amyloid pathology in a canine model of aging. J Neurosci 2014;24(38):8205–13.
21. West MJ, Kawas CH, Martin LJ, et al. The CA1 region of the human hippocampus is a hot spot in Alzheimer's disease. Ann N Y Acad Sci 2000;908:255–9.
22. Prpar Mihevc S, Majdič G. Canine cognitive dysfunction and Alzheimer's disease—two facets of the same disease? Front Neurosci 2019;13:604.
23. Smolek T, Madari A, Farbakova J, et al. Tau hyperphosphorylation in synaptosomes and neuroinflammation are associated with canine cognitive impairment. J Comp Neurol 2016;524(4):874–95.
24. Smith GK, Paster ER, Powers MY, et al. Lifelong diet restriction and radiographic evidence of osteoarthritis of the hip joint in dogs. J Am Vet Med Assoc 2006;229(5):690–3.
25. Abey A, Davies D, Goldsbury C, et al. Distribution of tau hyperphosphorylation in canine dementia resembles early Alzheimer's disease and other tauopathies. Brain Pathol 2020. https://doi.org/10.1111/bpa.12893.
26. Etnier JL, Drollette ES, Slutsky A. Physical activity and cognition: a narrative review of the evidence for older adults. Psychol Sport Exerc 2019;42:156–66.
27. Meng Q, Lin MS, Tzeng IS. Relationship between exercise and Alzheimer's disease: a narrative literature review. Front Neurosci 2020;14:131.
28. Bray EE, Raichlen DA, Forsyth KK, et al. Dog aging project consortium. Associations between physical activity and cognitive dysfunction in older companion dogs: results from the dog aging project. GeroScience 2023;45(2):645–61.
29. McKenzie BA, Chen FL, Gruen ME, et al. Canine geriatric syndrome: a framework for advancing research in veterinary geroscience. Front Vet Sci 2022;9:853743
30. Perkins Johnson T. Mobility issues. In: Gardner M, McVety D, editors. Treatment and care of the veterinary geriatric patient. Hoboken (NJ): John Wiley & Sons; 2017. p. 145–76.
31. Gibbs AJ, Gray B, Wallis JA, et al. Recommendations for the management of hip and knee osteoarthritis: a systematic review of clinical practice guidelines. Osteoarthr Cartil 2023;31(10):1280–92.
32. Raposo F, Ramos M, Cruz AL. Effects of exercise on knee osteoarthritis: a systematic review. Muscoskel Care 2021;19(4):399–435.
33. McArdle WD, Katch FI, Katch VL. Exercise physiology: nutrition, energy and human performance. 9th edition. Philadelphia (PA): Lippincott Williams & Wilkins; 2023.
34. Hübscher M, Zech A, Pfeifer K, et al. Neuromuscular training for sports injury prevention: a systematic review. Med Sci Sports Exerc 2010;42(3):413–21.
35. Jette DU, Hunter SJ, Burkett L, et al, American Physical Therapy Association. Physical therapist management of total knee arthroplasty. Phys Ther 2020;100(9):1603–31.
36. Michener LA, Heitzman J, Abbruzzese LD, et al. Physical therapist management of glenohumeral joint osteoarthritis: a clinical practice guideline from the American physical therapy association. Phys Ther 2023;103(6):pzad041.
37. Alvarez LX, Repac J, Zink C, et al. Reliability and validation of the canine manual muscle test (c-MMT) as a measure for hindlimb strength in dogs. Veterinary and Comparative Orthopaedics and Traumatology Open 2023;06(S 01):A1–11.
38. McMullin KM, Carney PC, Juran IG, et al. Timed up and go demonstrates strong interrater agreement and criterion validity as a functional test in geriatric dogs. Am J Vet Res 2024;85(8). https://doi.org/10.2460/ajvr.24.03.0062. ajvr.24.03.0062.

Sensory Decline

Real-World Tactics for Managing Vision and Hearing Loss

Monica Tarantino, DVM, MBA[a,*], Lauren Adelman, DVM[b]

KEYWORDS

• Sensory decline • Vision loss • Hearing loss • Canine cognitive dysfunction • Senior pets • Geriatric dogs and cats • Quality of life • Presbycusis

KEY POINTS

- Vision and hearing loss are highly prevalent in aging dogs and cats yet frequently underrecognized.
- Owner observations often mimic signs of cognitive dysfunction and must be carefully distinguished.
- Simple screening tools and structured questionnaires can aid early detection in general practice.
- Practical management strategies can improve quality of life and reduce caregiver stress.
- Sensory decline is linked with cognitive dysfunction and frailty, emphasizing the need for proactive care.

Video content accompanies this article at http://www.vetsmall.theclinics.com.

INTRODUCTION

As pets age, a gradual decline in sensory function, particularly vision and hearing, is both common and underrecognized. While musculoskeletal and systemic health issues dominate geriatric care discussions, sensory impairments can significantly impact a senior pet's behavior and meaningful interactions within their environment. It further complicates diagnosis by mimicking or exacerbating comorbidities like cognitive dysfunction, anxiety, mobility, and chronic pain.[1–3] Currently, there are no standardized protocols for screening, diagnosing, or managing sensory impairment, and limited research exists on how to best support pets experiencing it.

The goal of this review is to provide a practical, evidence-based overview of age-related sensory decline in dogs and cats and guide clinicians to a proactive shift in how we diagnose, approach, and manage this impactful process in aging pets. It

[a] Senior Dog Veterinary Society and Pet Loss Community; [b] Canada West Veterinary Specialists and Senior Dog Veterinary Society

* Corresponding author. Senior Dog Veterinary Society, PO Box 3022, Alexandria, VA 22304.
E-mail address: monica@seniordogvets.com

Vet Clin Small Anim 56 (2026) 375–389
https://doi.org/10.1016/j.cvsm.2025.09.028 vetsmall.theclinics.com

Abbreviations	
BAER	brainstem auditory-evoked response
DHA	docosahexaenoic acid
ERG	electroretinography

also seeks to highlight areas for advancement in our understanding of these conditions and emerging connections between canine cognitive dysfunction syndrome and sensory impairment.

AGE-RELATED HEARING LOSS

While bilateral age-related hearing loss (presbycusis) is nearly universal in senior dogs, it is often underrecognized until advanced because changes are gradual and pets adapt behaviorally. Despite this, hearing impairment in senior dogs does affect quality of life, communication, family bond, and even safety.[3,4] In this section, we outline the expected age-related changes in auditory function, common clinical findings, and diagnostics that help distinguish normal aging from treatable contributors to hearing loss.

Background

Deafness in pets has many causes, including congenital abnormalities, chronic otitis externa/media, noise-induced trauma, and ototoxic drug exposure.[5] Among seniors, however, presbycusis is the predominant etiology. Presbycusis typically begins around 8 to 10 years of age, with loss of mid-to-high frequency hearing (8–32 kHz) occurring first, followed by broader impairment.[5–7] Owners often report that pets appear "stubborn," fail to respond to commands, or startle when approached. These signs can mimic anxiety or cognitive dysfunction, both of which commonly coexist in senior dogs.[2,8] Because canine baseline hearing exceeds human sensitivity, deficits often go unnoticed until lower frequencies are affected, making decline seem sudden.[5]

Age-related cochlear degeneration is the most common cause of presbycusis in senior dogs, paralleling changes seen in humans.[9] Pathologic studies in aging dogs show progressive degeneration of cochlear hair cells, stria vascularis, and spiral ganglion neurons, with changes detectable as early as 5 years, and severity increasing as dogs age.[5,9] While most research has emphasized these peripheral changes, emerging evidence indicates that central auditory pathways may also be affected, even without severe peripheral loss. In one study of 23 dogs, animals aged over 10 years showed degenerative changes within the cochlear nucleus of the brainstem.[9] More recent MRI study in elderly dogs with intact peripheral hearing demonstrated age-related white matter changes within the central auditory system mirroring findings of both peripheral and central components to hearing loss as seen in human presbycusis.[10]

Noise Sensitivity and Aging

Noise sensitivity, defined as anxious or fearful responses to noise, occurs in dogs of all ages and can manifest as shaking, panting, trembling, or escape behaviors. Common clinical triggers include thunder or fireworks, though even benign human sounds (eg, a sneeze, cough, or clattering dishes) may provoke exaggerated reactions in some older dogs.[11] Several factors are associated with noise hypersensitivity, including smaller body size, separation anxiety, and advancing age.[12,13] One large survey-based study found the risk of noise hypersensitivity increased by approximately 3.4% with each additional year of age.[13] Clinicians may also hear clients describe older dogs suddenly reacting to noises they have tolerated for years, for example, bolting out of a room at the sound of an ice maker or a sneeze.[14]

The apparent paradox of increasing noise sensitivity despite concurrent hearing loss has also been noted in humans, where evidence suggests it may reflect a combination of reduced peripheral input and exaggerated central auditory "gain" mechanisms.[11,15] Importantly, a recent small study suggested a potential link between noise sensitivity and pain, underscoring the need for clinicians to evaluate underlying discomfort when managing these cases.[14] Taken together, these findings highlight that noise sensitivity in older dogs is multifactorial and can meaningfully impact quality of life and owner–pet relationships.

HISTORICAL AND CLINICAL EXAMINATION FINDINGS

Otoscopic examination findings will vary depending on cause of hearing loss. For dogs with chronic otitis, signs of lichenification, stenosis, erythema, and ruptured tympanic membrane may be found. However, many otic examinations will be normal.

Brainstem auditory-evoked response (BAER) testing demonstrates that senior dogs develop elevated thresholds, particularly at higher frequencies, consistent with presbycusis.[2] In some cases, owners report normal hearing even when BAER reveals marked deficits, reflecting the ability of dogs to compensate behaviorally until hearing loss is advance.[3]

DIAGNOSTIC APPROACH IN SENIOR PETS

Assessing hearing loss in senior pets' benefits from a systematic yet practical approach. A thorough history is essential, particularly regarding prior medication exposure (eg, aminoglycosides), noise exposure, and any history of chronic otitis, all of which can contribute to auditory decline. On physical examination, otoscopic assessment should be performed to identify ceruminous debris, tympanic membrane changes, or signs of otitis externa or media that may be contributing to hearing loss.

Because age-related hearing loss is gradual and frequently masked by owner adaptation, proactive screening using a senior wellness screening tool (**Fig. 1**) for auditory changes should be integrated into senior wellness visits to support earlier recognition and client education. Though BAER testing remains the gold standard for confirming sensorineural hearing loss, its use is often limited to referral settings.

Hearing-Specific Therapies

In humans, hearing aids and implantable devices improve quality of life, reduce social isolation, and may even mitigate cognitive decline.[16,17] In veterinary medicine, however, hearing rehabilitation remains limited. Reports of external hearing aid use in dogs describe mixed outcomes, largely limited by differences in residual hearing, tolerance, and training compliance, while middle ear implants (eg, Vibrant Soundbridge) remain experimental.[6] Working dogs routinely exposed to loud sounds (engines, gunfire, and explosives) and shelter dogs in chronically noisy kennels are particularly vulnerable to noise-induced hearing loss, as highlighted in previous studies [18,19] Use of canine hearing protection devices and preventative methods in at-risk populations, along with proactive management of chronic otitis and allergies, may help preserve hearing capacity in aging dogs.

FUNCTIONAL VISION DECLINE

Age-related ocular changes are nearly universal in senior dogs and cats and can significantly affect function, behavior, and quality of life. Some are expected physiologic changes, while others reflect disease processes requiring intervention.

Patient Name: ______________________________ Date: ____________________

Senior Wellness Pre-Visit Screening Checklist

As they get older, senior and geriatric dogs are prone to more diseases and risks like chronic pain, dementia and cancer. Screening helps us identify issues and intervene and monitor areas that may impact their happiness as they age.

History

- ☐ Change in Appetite
- ☐ Increased Drinking or Urination
- ☐ Vomiting/Diarrhea
- ☐ Coughing/Breathing changes
- ☐ Changes in housing or environment
- ☐ Social or family change

Chronic Pain Screening

Older dogs are prone to having chronic pain that they can easily hide. Have you noticed any of the following?

Dental Pain:

- ☐ Smelly or foul odor from mouth
- ☐ Brown, gray or red coloring on teeth
- ☐ Loose or wiggly teeth
- ☐ Dropping food or hesitancy with eating

Joint Pain:

- ☐ Limping after exercise
- ☐ Slow to rise
- ☐ Stiffness or 'warms up' as the day goes on
- ☐ Lagging behind on walks

Functional Screening

The risk of cognitive and functional decline increases every year as a dog ages. Have you noticed any of the following?

Mentation:

- ☐ Disorientation
- ☐ Getting stuck in corners
- ☐ Changes in sleep pattern
- ☐ More anxious or restless
- ☐ Less social or less interest in pets

Mobility:

- ☐ Falls or slips more easily
- ☐ Difficulty with stairs or jumps
- ☐ Difficulty posturing to potty
- ☐ Needs assistance at times

Senses:

- ☐ Decrease in vision (ex: hesitation on stairs, bumping into things, reluctance to go out at night etc.)
- ☐ Decrease in hearing (ex startles more easily, less responsive etc.)

Elimination: ☐ Frequent messes in house ☐ Unable to hold bowels or bladder

Quality of Life Screening

Does your pet seem to enjoy their life? ☐ Yes ☐ Maybe ☐ No ☐ Not sure

Other

Are you interested in learning how to 'senior dog proof' your home? ☐ Yes ☐ No

Do you experience caretaker exhaustion at times? ☐ Yes ☐ No

Are there any other concerns we haven't asked about? ☐ Yes ☐ No

Fig. 1. Senior Dog Veterinary Society Screening Questionnaire (available for download at www.seniordogvets.com). (© Senior Dog Veterinary Society 2025. Courtesy Image by Dr Monica Tarantino, DVM.)

Physiologic Age-Related Ocular Changes

Dogs and cats have lower acuity, brightness discrimination, and color perception than humans but are better adapted for motion detection and dim-light vision.[20] Despite vision being considered a "weaker" sense relative to smell and hearing, dogs continue to use vision heavily in daily life, even in older age. Studies show that when given the choice in a 2 task test for food, dogs tend to default to visual cues even when this reduces task accuracy.[21,22] A separate study also showed that vision is key to a senior dog's postural stability and motor mechanisms.[23]

Several age-related changes in visual function are important for clinicians to recognize when evaluating senior pets.

Nyctalopia (night blindness)

For aging dogs, not unlike aging humans, visual decline in low light settings (nyctalopia) occurs earlier than bright light vision loss (hemeralopia). In a study of 235 dogs, owners noted that older animals had more difficulty across lighting conditions, especially when navigating in near-darkness or during sudden light-to-dark transitions.[24] Electroretinography (ERG) measurements in a subset of these dogs (79) confirmed owner-reported difficulties were linked to decreases in retinal function.[24] Common complaints from owners of nyctalopic dogs include signs of hesitation on stairs, reluctance to go outside at night, bumping into furniture, or changes in behavior that resemble cognitive decline while not necessarily having other signs of cognitive decline on examination.[24]

Impaired light–dark adaptation

In humans with age-related macular degeneration, exposure to bright light can bleach photopigments, delaying recovery of sensitivity and making transitions to dim environments more difficult. A similar process is believed to occur in dogs: in one ERG study of 95 companion dogs, older pets showed significantly prolonged peak times and reduced amplitudes in both rod and cone-mediated responses, consistent with impaired dark adaptation.[25] Owners may report their senior dogs having difficulty adjusting between light and dark environments, which can be seen in a variety of settings such as going from inside a well-lit house to a dark yard or transitioning across bright and shadowed parts of a yard midday (Video 1). Owners should be counseled on these expected physiologic changes that may present like behavioral problems or confusion.

Refractive light changes (ametropia)

Aging companion animals also have an increased propensity for changes in depth perception as they age. Farsightedness (hyperopia), however, is more common as evidenced by a 2023 study of 99 mixed-breed dogs in which nearly half of geriatric animals (aged 8–13 years) and one-third of the seniors (aged 6–11 years) were hyperopic. These findings suggest that farsightedness becomes increasingly prevalent in older populations, although both hyperopia and myopia (nearsightedness) can occur. Canine emmetropia (20/75–20/100 vision) also declines modestly with age.[26,27] With regards to refractive states, it is worth noting that breed does appear to play a role. One larger cross-sectional study of over 1400 dogs across 90 breeds confirmed some breeds are prone to myopia (eg, German shepherd, toy poodle, and so forth) and others to hyperopia (eg, greyhound).[28]

In geriatric companion animals, hyperopia may become more pronounced due to a combination of structural and functional ocular changes associated with aging. One of the primary contributors is lenticular/nuclear sclerosis, a normal age-related process characterized by compaction of lens fibers and increased lens stiffness, which diminishes the eye's accommodative ability and mimics hyperopic shifts in refraction.[26] Unlike humans, dogs and cats possess limited accommodation to begin with, and age-related declines such as reduced function of ciliary body muscles to adjust the shape of the lens may render them increasingly unable to focus on nearby objects.[29] Other contributors include vitreal degeneration, retinal thinning and subtle alterations of the refractive index of the aging lens, or cornea shifting the focal point posterior to the retina, contributing to hyperopia.[26] These changes often manifest as reduced ability to detect near objects or decreased visual performance in low light environments.[26]

Pathologic Age-Related Ocular Disease

Beyond functional changes, several pathologic ocular conditions in seniors can directly impair vision. The most frequent include cataracts, retinal degeneration, hypertensive retinopathy in cats, corneal disease, glaucoma, and uveal tumors. Each carries different implications for function and quality of life, but together they represent the spectrum of issues clinicians should routinely screen for during geriatric examinations utilizing common diagnostics such as tonometry, Schirmer tear tests, and blood pressure monitoring. A detailed review of each condition is beyond the scope of this article, but clinicians should be aware of their presence and distinguish physiologic from pathologic changes. **Table 1** summarizes how typical owner-reported concerns (eg, cloudy eyes, reluctance on stairs, and sudden disorientation) align with examination findings and likely causes, providing a practical guide for busy practitioners.

DIAGNOSTIC APPROACH IN SENIOR PETS

Evaluation of vision in older animals requires more nuance than in younger patients. Traditional screening tools (menace, dazzle, and pupillary light responses) often yield all-or-nothing results and may miss partial decline, which is common in senior pets. Clinicians should combine screening tests (see **Fig. 1**), history, ophthalmic examination, and targeted diagnostics. Though ERG remains the gold standard for assessing rod and cone function, it is typically limited to referral settings.[25] Chromatic pupillometry, which uses red and blue light to stimulate photoreceptors and gauge retinal function via pupillary light reflex (PLR) response could be a tool explored for general practice use. A validated owner questionnaire such as the 29 question DogVLQ (the dog variable lighting questionnaire) can provide structured insights into functional vision at home.[24]

In cats and dogs aged 10 years and above, blood pressure measurement is an essential part of routine diagnostics and should be utilized for any geriatric patient with retinal detachment or hemorrhage. Ocular ultrasound or advanced imaging may aid when anterior segment or vitreal changes preclude fundic visualization. Imaging can assess for uveal masses, lens position, and subretinal changes. Together, these tools help differentiate normal aging from treatable disease and guide meaningful counseling for owners.

Supplements for Vision

Adjunctive therapies are often considered in managing the behavioral and quality-of-life consequences of sensory decline. Evidence for supplements remains mixed. Over a 6 month period, dogs maintained on a balanced control diet lacking vitamin C demonstrated ERG decline, while those receiving an antioxidant blend (lutein, zeaxanthin, β-carotene, astaxanthin, and vitamins C and E) were protected from this change.[30] Other studies on docosahexaenoic acid (DHA) supplementation have shown mixed findings; puppies raised on higher DHA diets demonstrated improved retinal function, while short-term supplementation in dogs with progressive rod-cone degeneration increased systemic DHA but failed to alter retinal content or disease progression.[31,32]

Table 1
Common owner observations, examination findings, and likely causes of vision loss in senior dogs

Owner-Reported Sign	Physical Examination Finding	Possible Cause(s)
Hesitation on stairs, reluctance to go outside at night, and bumping into furniture	Normal menace in bright light, reduced in dim light, retinal vascular attenuation, and tapetal hyperreflectivity	Early rod dysfunction, retinal degeneration (age-related vs genetic), and impaired dark adaptation
Cloudy or "hazy" eyes, but still navigates well	Lens appears gray-blue with fundic reflex still visible	Nuclear sclerosis (physiologic aging change, not blinding) and early immature cataract
Progressive vision loss, obvious cloudiness of the lens	Lens opacity obscuring fundic view, possible lens-induced uveitis; retinal vascular attenuation and tapetal hyperreflectivity	Cataract (age-related, diabetic, or secondary); monitor for uveitis; and retinal degeneration
Sudden blindness (often reported as acute disorientation indoors/ outdoors)	Dilated pupils, absent menace, and flat ERG	Sudden acquired retinal degeneration syndrome; glaucoma (primary or secondary)
Intermittent vision issues, hypertension or systemic illness present	Retinal detachment, hemorrhage on fundoscopy; abnormal PLRs	Hypertensive retinopathy (cats > dogs), systemic disease (CKD, hyperthyroidism etc.)
Red, painful eye; pawing at face; and cloudy eye	Elevated intraocular pressure (>25 mm Hg) and corneal edema	Glaucoma (primary or secondary)
Chronic ocular discharge or squinting	Corneal edema, vascularization, ulcers, and keratoconjunctivitis sicca (KCS) signs	Corneal disease (endothelial dystrophy, lipid/calcium deposits, and KCS)
Unresponsive pupils	Mydriasis, weak PLRs, and ruffled pupillary margin	Iris atrophy

SENSORY DECLINE AND COGNITIVE DYSFUNCTION

Age-related changes in vision, hearing, and olfaction have significant implications for cognitive health. In older pets, sensory decline can mimic, mask, or accelerate cognitive dysfunction.[33] Owners may describe a pet as confused or "stubborn" when the true issue is impaired hearing or vision, and conversely, cognitive decline may be underestimated if sensory loss is assumed to be the sole cause of behavioral change.[2,34]

In a recent study evaluating the relationship between sensory impairment and cognitive decline in 238 companion dogs, nearly 90% of geriatric dogs were reported by their owners to have at least one sensory deficit, most often hearing or vision loss, and these impairments were strongly associated with higher rates of cognitive dysfunction.[35] Several other studies support this link: dogs with hearing, vision, or olfactory deficits are significantly more likely to score higher on cognitive dysfunction scales, and those with dual sensory loss have nearly double the odds of cognitive impairment compared with unimpaired dogs.[2,35] Comparable findings have been reported in people: older adults with combined vision and hearing loss face up to an 8 fold greater dementia risk compared with those experiencing only one type of sensory deficit.[36] Further, separate studies have confirmed that blindness is overrepresented among dogs with canine cognitive dysfunction (CCD), suggesting that sensory loss may be both a risk factor and a confounder in diagnosis.[2,37]

Sensory decline is also a recognized component of canine frailty, a multidimensional syndrome that integrates mobility, comorbidities, and sensory loss.[38] Higher frailty scores in dogs have been linked to poorer quality of life and greater risk of cognitive impairment, suggesting that assessment of frailty provides a useful framework for understanding how sensory and cognitive decline intersect.[39,40]

CONSIDERATIONS IN CATS

Cognitive dysfunction is also recognized in aging cats, with clinical signs summarized by the acronym VISHDAAL (vocalization, interactions, sleep–wake changes, house-soiling, disorientation, activity, anxiety, learning/memory). As in dogs, concurrent vision or hearing loss can complicate diagnosis, with owners often attributing disorientation or vocalization to sensory decline rather than to cognitive impairment.[41] Feline studies remain fewer, but available data suggest that sensory decline may similarly magnify distress and exacerbate cognitive signs.

PROACTIVE MANAGEMENT OF SENSORY DECLINE

A broader challenge we face in geriatric medicine is only addressing age-related changes once they have become disruptive, rather than anticipated and managed early. In many areas of geriatrics, including sensory decline, we have opportunities to shift toward a more proactive approach. It is the authors' belief that sensory decline in the senior pet population should be a core component of geriatric care rather than just an incidental finding. This will not only improve detection and monitoring of sensory impairment but also provide families with practical strategies to support quality of life.

Three ways to do this are

- General Senior Screening tool (see **Fig. 1**) with the aid of validated scales
- Tailored diagnostics and physical examinations
- Practical management strategies and early client education

Sensory screening should be embedded into routine biannual examinations to reframe sensory decline as a core element of geriatric care. One easily accessible screening tool is the Senior Dog Veterinary Society Screening Questionnaire (see **Fig. 1**), a 1 page form for clients to fill out at wellness visits that integrates questions on sensory loss alongside domains such as chronic pain, mobility, caregiver fatigue, and behavior allowing clinicians to identify common senior pet ailments, including sensory impairment, earlier.

PRACTICAL MANAGEMENT STRATEGIES FOR SENSORY DECLINE

Practical management strategies are most effective when at home measures (eg, environmental modifications, safety measures, and communication adjustments) are combined with regular assessment of progressive decline by veterinarians during each visit. Discussing the following 7 components of sensory care with owners can help them to be an active participant in their senior pet's care.

Environmental Modifications

Consistency within the home is critical for pets adapting to vision or hearing loss. Furniture, feeding stations, and rest areas should remain in predictable and easily accessible locations to help senior animals navigate familiar paths. Clear routes to food, water, and sleeping areas should be maintained, and clutter should be minimized. Nonslip flooring, carpet runners, or textured surfaces provide tactile feedback and reduce the risk of falls and injury, while furniture with rounded edges can help prevent injuries in visually impaired pets.

Training

Training can mitigate stress and preserve function in senior pets associated with sensory decline. Lifelong training experience has been associated with better attentional control in aged dogs, while large-scale cohort data suggest that regular physical activity reduces the odds and severity of canine cognitive dysfunction.[42]

Reducing Startle Reaction

Because sensory-impaired animals no longer receive the same auditory or visual warning cues, they may be more easily startled. Owners should be encouraged to alert their pets through familiar sensory channels before approaching or touching them. Vibrations from footsteps, a gentle stomp at a distance, approaching from their direct line of vision or presenting a food treat near the nose can provide nonthreatening cues.

Pain Control

One study showed that pain was tied to fear of noises or being startled. Diseases of chronic pain tend to happen naturally in aged animals whether it be from degenerative joint disease, progressive dental disease, or unmanaged medical conditions that are uncomfortable. Pain control is, therefore, an important component of managing sensory decline in aging pets.

Lighting in Dim Areas

Loss of vision in low light conditions is often one of the earliest deficits in older pets. Nightlights with motion or light sensors are especially helpful, as they provide illumination only when needed and can be placed in hallways, near toileting areas, or along frequently used paths. Outdoors, flashlights can be used during evening walks to support orientation.

Delayed Dark Adaptation Awareness

Aged pets that are transitioning from bright light to dark areas may also struggle with temporary deficits in their vision as their eyes adjust. Alerting owners to watch for signs of this during night or very bright parts of the day may reduce anxiety and support navigation of their environment.

Safety Awareness

Interactions with other pets

Management of interactions between older dogs and pets in the home that may have food aggression or behavioral issues should be taken into consideration. Many older animals with sensory deficits cannot pick up on visual or auditory cues. An older dog, previously strong at recognizing and responding to body language and audible cues like a growl, may be inhibited from reacting appropriately due to sensory decline. This may require being present for interactions between pets or keeping pets separate when owners are not around, if there is a chance for a negative interaction.

Interactions in and outside of home environment

Sensory decline can make aged animals more prone to injury such as slipping or running into things, hit by car accidents, dog attacks, and more. In a recent trauma registry study, dogs involved in low-speed vehicular rollover incidents were older on average (median age 4 years) than dogs in traditional high-speed vehicular trauma (median age 2 years), which may indicate greater vulnerability of older dogs, potentially related to reduced mobility or sensory decline.[4]

Safety barriers such as baby gates can prevent falls on stairs. The addition of colors that are visually apparent to dogs can also be helpful for challenging zones in the home. For example, marking stairs or sliding glass doors with blue or purple colored tape can enhance visibility for dogs with impaired depth perception.

Sensory aid items

In patients with more advanced visual impairment, "halo" harnesses may reduce collisions and build confidence. Mobility aids and simple home adaptations can further support stability. Products such as Dr Buzby's ToeGrips or PawFriction pads, along with routine nail trims and trimming of fur between the paw pads can help improve traction. Adhesive floor grips such as those used for bathroom and shower surfaces can be adapted to slick flooring in the home to increase stability and reduce falls.

Communication Adjustments

As sensory decline progresses, multimodal communication strategies help bridge gaps and reduce anxiety. For dogs with hearing loss, pairing verbal commands with hand signals provides redundancy, while tactile cues, such as a double tap on the shoulder to signal "outside," can help visually impaired dogs. Ideally, pairing visual and hearing cues together should be used consistently, well before a dog is a senior. Communicating in a lower frequency baritone voice may be audible to pets with partial hearing loss. Scent cues may also be used to mark activities or transitions, though more research is needed to validate effectiveness.

In the clinical setting, tactile communication and calm, predictable handling is especially important. Focusing on steady physical cues and strategic handling to accommodate for chronic pain and reduce stress for pets who can no longer rely on their vision or hearing. Senior-specific training for staff is essential to ensure optimum care of senior pets in veterinary practices (**Table 2**).

SENSORY DECLINE AND QUALITY OF LIFE

Sensory changes alter the way senior pets interact with and perceive their environment. Dogs with vision loss may restrict exploration due to fear of colliding with obstacles or being startled. In people, presbycusis is strongly associated with social isolation and reduced quality of life, and hearing aids have been shown to improve quality-of-life scores. Similar associations are emerging in veterinary medicine. In a 2022 study of 39 dogs aged 11 years or older, deterioration in hearing was most strongly associated with reduced owner-reported scores in vitality and companionship, domains that reflect engagement with the environment and the quality of the owner–pet relationship.[3] Hearing loss was also correlated with poorer executive function and higher cognitive dysfunction ratings, suggesting that sensory decline influences both quality of life and cognitive performance.[3]

Table 2
Safety hazards and recommended modifications for senior dogs with sensory decline

Hazard	Associated Risk	Recommended Modification
Stairs	Falls, hesitation due to poor depth perception	Mark edges with blue tape; install baby gates to block access when unsupervised
Slippery floors	Slips, injuries, and reluctance to walk	Add nonslip rugs, carpet runners, shower stickies; use ToeGrips/ PawFriction; trim nails and paw hair
Glass and screen doors/ windows	Collisions due to poor visual contrast	Apply visible tape or decals at dog's eye level
Furniture/clutter	Bumping, disorientation, and injury	Keep layout consistent; clear pathways; use round-edge furniture
Other pets (housemates)	Missed warning cues (growls and postures) → conflict or bites	Supervise interactions, especially around food and toys; manage feeding separately if needed
Poor lighting/nighttime mobility	Hesitation, anxiety, and accidents during toileting	Install motion-sensor nightlights indoors/ outdoors; use headlamps or flashlights on walks
Bright → dark transitions	Distress and delayed dark adaptation	Provide gradual lighting transitions where possible; reassure owners this is normal age-related change
Driveways/parking areas	Increased risk of low-speed vehicular trauma	Keep pets on leash outdoors; monitor closely in driveways and near vehicles

FUTURE DIRECTIONS AND KNOWLEDGE GAPS

Despite the high prevalence of sensory decline in aging dogs and cats, research on its natural history, impact on quality of life, and optimal management strategies remains limited. Most available data are derived from retrospective analyses, client-reported outcomes, or small-scale studies, and significant gaps remain in both the veterinary and comparative aging literature. A few areas where sensory decline research can be most helpful are

- *Validated clinical tools for primary care settings:* Development of practical, in-clinic methods to stage functional vision and hearing loss would enable earlier detection and intervention.
- *Link with cognition:* Further clarifying the relationship between sensory impairment and cognitive dysfunction to guide prevention and treatment strategies

- *Formal evaluation of interventional strategies:* Prospective veterinary studies on health and welfare impact can help guide best practices.
- *Caregiver impact:* Owners often misinterpret sensory decline as suffering or poor quality of life signaling for euthanasia. Educational interventions, decision aids, and caregiver-focused tools may reduce distress and improve decision-making.
- *Feline-specific research:* Very limited data exist on sensory decline in cats. Studies addressing its prevalence, clinical manifestations, and interactions with comorbidities such as osteoarthritis, hyperthyroidism, and chronic kidney disease (CKD) are needed.

SUMMARY

In summary, sensory decline is a prevalent but often underrecognized aspect of aging senior pets. Vision and hearing loss may emerge insidiously and are frequently misattributed to cognitive dysfunction or normal aging. Left unaddressed, these changes can contribute to anxiety, disorientation, decreased mobility, and diminished quality of life for both pets and their caregivers. Dual sensory loss warrants special attention due to its ability to further compromise independence, social interaction, and quality of life. Veterinarians should recognize that dogs presenting with one sensory deficit are at an elevated risk of developing the other and counsel owners accordingly.

A proactive, multisystem approach is essential for evaluating senior pets presenting with behavioral or functional changes. Vision and hearing should be routinely assessed alongside pain, neurologic function, and systemic health prior to diagnosing cognitive dysfunction. The implementation of practical and proactive strategies to pets at risk of sensory decline should be employed by veterinarians to improve the day-to-day function and welfare of their senior patients.

The veterinary profession is becoming increasingly equipped to recognize and discuss sensory decline, but continued research is necessary to improve diagnostics, refine management strategies, and deepen our understanding of how these changes shape the aging experience for companion animals.

CLINICS CARE POINTS

- *Screen early:* Use senior wellness screening questionnaire and history to detect vision or hearing loss earlier.
- *Rule out pathologic causes:* Distinguish physiologic changes (eg, nuclear sclerosis and presbycusis) from pathology that requires treatment.
- *Treat as core component of geriatric care:* Include routine sensory checks and incorporate sensory support into comprehensive plans for aging pets.
- *Normalize in communication:* Proactively discuss expected sensory decline and steps to help seniors to reduce owner stress and improve support.
- *Preserve quality of life*: Discuss important steps at clinic and at home to support overall senior pet wellness (multimodal communication, safety precautions, signs to monitor for, and so forth).
- *Monitor comorbidities, pain, cognition, and frailty:* Dual sensory loss raises risk for cognitive dysfunction and frailty; pets with one deficit merit closer follow-up.

DISCLOSURE

The authors have no disclosures to report.

SUPPLEMENTARY DATA

Supplementary data related to this article can be found online at https://doi.org/10.1016/j.cvsm.2025.09.028.

REFERENCES

1. Landsberg GM, Nichol J, Araujo JA. Cognitive dysfunction syndrome: a disease of canine and feline brain aging. Vet Clin North Am Small Anim Pract 2012;42(4):749–68, vii.
2. Ozawa M, Inoue M, Uchida K, et al. Physical signs of canine cognitive dysfunction. J Vet Med Sci 2019;81(12):1829–34.
3. Fefer G, Khan MZ, Panek WK, et al. Relationship between hearing, cognitive function, and quality of life in aging companion dogs. J Vet Intern Med 2022;36(5):1708–18. Epub 2022 Aug 6. PMID: 35932193; PMCID: PMC9511086.
4. Yoon H, Brainard BM, Thevelein BAL, et al. Characteristics of low-speed vehicular rollover trauma in dogs presenting to an emergency service at a veterinary teaching hospital. J Vet Emerg Crit Care 2025;35(3):246–57.
5. Strain GM. Canine deafness. Vet Clin Small Anim Pract 2012;42(6):1209–24.
6. Haar, Gert ter. "Age-related hearing loss in dogs and treatment with vibrant soundbridge middle ear implant." *Veterinary Sciences Tomorrow 2010*, (2010).
7. Ter Haar G, Venker-van Haagen AJ, van den Brom WE, et al. Effects of aging on brainstem responses to toneburst auditory stimuli: a cross-sectional and longitudinal study in dogs. J Vet Intern Med 2008;22(4):937–45.
8. Landsberg GM, Deporter T, Araujo JA. Clinical signs and management of anxiety, sleeplessness, and cognitive dysfunction in the senior pet. Vet Clin North Am Small Anim Pract 2011;41(3):565–90. PMID: 21601747.
9. Shimada A, Ebisu M, Morita T, et al. Age-related changes in the cochlea and cochlear nuclei of dogs. J Vet Med Sci 1998;60(1):41–8.
10. Yang CC, Yap PT, Wu Y, et al. Voxelwise analysis of the central hearing pathway in senior dogs reveals changes associated with fractional lifespan. Sci Rep 2024;14:18121. https://doi.org/10.1038/s41598-024-68828-3.
11. Chin JTY, Poh SX, Fernandez EJ, et al. Turn the volume down: noise hypersensitivity in dogs. Journal of Veterinary Behavior 2025;79:75–82.
12. Martínez ÁG, Santamarina Pernas G, Diéguez Casalta FJ, et al. Risk factors associated with behavioral problems in dogs. Journal of Veterinary Behavior 2011;6(4):225–31.
13. Storengen LM, Lingaas F. Noise sensitivity in 17 dog breeds: prevalence, breed risk and correlation with fear in other situations. Appl Anim Behav Sci 2015;171:152–60.
14. Lopes F, Luisa A, McPeake KJ, et al. Noise sensitivities in dogs: an exploration of signs in dogs with and without musculoskeletal pain using qualitative content analysis. Front Vet Sci 2018;5:17.
15. Paulin J, Andersson L, Nordin S. Characteristics of hyperacusis in the general population. Noise Health 2016;83(18):178–84.
16. Cohen SM, Labadie RF, Dietrich MS, et al. Quality of life in hearing-impaired adults: the role of cochlear implants and hearing aids. Otolaryngology-Head Neck Surg (Tokyo) 2004;131(4):413–22.

17. Kitterick PT, Melanie AF. Hearing aids and health-related quality of life in adults with hearing loss. JAMA 2018;319(21):2225–6.
18. Scheifele P, Martin D, Clark JG, et al. Effect of kennel noise on hearing in dogs. Am J Vet Res 2012;73(4):482–9. PMID: 22452494.
19. Schneider DC, Foss KD, De Risio L, et al. Noise-induced hearing loss in 3 working dogs. Top Companion Anim Med 2019;37:100362.
20. Barber ALA, Mills DS, Montealegre-Z F, et al. Functional performance of the visual system in dogs and humans: a comparative perspective. Comp Cogn Behav Rev 2020;15.
21. Szetei V, Miklósi Á, Topál J, et al. When dogs seem to lose their nose: an investigation on the use of visual and olfactory cues in communicative context between dog and owner. Appl Anim Behav Sci 2003;83(2):141–52.
22. Khan MZ, Mondino A, Russell K, et al. A novel task of canine olfaction for use in adult and senior pet dogs. Sci Rep 2023;13:2224.
23. Lutonsky C, Peham C, Affenzeller N, et al. Impact of aging and visual input on postural stability in dogs: insights from center-of-pressure analysis. Sensors 2025;25(5):1300.
24. Rogers CM, Salzman MM, Li Z, et al. Subjective vision assessment in companion dogs using dogVLQ demonstrates age-associated visual dysfunction. Front Vet Sci 2023;10:1244518.
25. Salzman MM, Merten N, Panek WK, et al. Age-associated changes in electroretinography measures in companion dogs. Doc Ophthalmol 2023;147(1):15–28.
26. Gelatt KN, Gilger BC, Kern TJ, et al, editiors. Veterinary ophthalmology. 6th edition. Wiley-Blackwell; 2021:Vol 1, Ch 5:225-244.
27. Balicka A, Zwolska J, Szadkowski M, et al. Refractive errors in mixed breed dogs of different ages. Vet Med 2023;68(1):11.
28. Kubai MA, Bentley E, Miller PE, et al. Refractive states of eyes and association between ametropia and breed in dogs. Am J Vet Res 2008;69(7):946–51. PMID: 18593249.
29. Ofri R. "Lens". Slatter's fundamentals of veterinary ophthalmology. St Louis (MO): WB Saunders; 2008. p. 258–76.
30. Wang W, Hernandez J, Moore C, et al. Antioxidant supplementation increases retinal responses and decreases refractive error changes in dogs. J Nutr Sci 2016;5:e18.
31. Zicker SC, Jewell DE, Yamka RM, et al. Evaluation of cognitive learning, memory, psychomotor, immunologic, and retinal functions in healthy puppies fed foods fortified with docosahexaenoic acid–rich fish oil from 8 to 52 weeks of age. J Am Vet Med Assoc 2012;241(5):583–94.
32. Aguirre GD, Acland GM, Maude MB, et al. Diets enriched in docosahexaenoic acid fail to correct progressive rod-cone degeneration (prcd) phenotype. Investig Ophthalmol Vis Sci 1997;38(11):2387–407.
33. Wrightson R, Albertini M, Pirrone F, et al. The relationship between signs of medical conditions and cognitive decline in senior dogs. Animals 2023;13(13):2203.
34. Salvin HE, McGreevy PD, Sachdev PS, et al. Under diagnosis of canine cognitive dysfunction: a cross-sectional survey of older companion dogs. Vet J 2010;184(3):277–81.
35. Hopper RG, Bromberg RB, Salzman MM, et al. Dual sensory impairments in companion dogs: prevalence and relationship to cognitive impairment. PLoS One 2024;19(10):e0310299.
36. Fuller-Thomson E, Nowaczynski A, MacNeil A. The association between hearing impairment, vision impairment, dual sensory impairment, and serious cognitive

impairment: findings from a population-based study of 5.4 million older adults. J Alzh Dis Rep 2022;6(1):211–22.

37. Szabó D, Miklósi Á, Kubinyi E. Owner reported sensory impairments affect behavioural signs associated with cognitive decline in dogs. Behav Process 2018;157:354–60.
38. Waters DJ, Maras AH, Fu R, et al. Frailty and mortality risk among dogs with extreme longevity: development and predictive validity of a clinical frailty index in the exceptional aging in rottweilers study. Animals 2024;14(24):3651.
39. Russell KJ, Mondino A, Fefer G, et al. Establishing a clinically applicable frailty phenotype screening tool for aging dogs. Front Vet Sci 2024;11:1335463. https://doi.org/10.3389/fvets.2024.1335463. PMID: 39391218; PMCID: PMC11465091.
40. Bellows J, Colitz CM, Daristotle L, et al. Common physical and functional changes associated with aging in dogs. J Am Vet Med Assoc 2015;246(1):67–75. PMID: 25517328.
41. Sordo L, Gunn-Moore DA. Cognitive dysfunction in cats: update on neuropathological anzsd behavioural changes plus clinical management. Vet Rec 2021;188(1):e3. https://doi.org/10.1002/vetr.3. Epub 2021 Jan 12. PMID: 34651755.
42. Chapagain D, Virányi Z, Wallis LJ, et al. Aging of attentiveness in border collies and other pet dog breeds: the protective benefits of lifelong training. Front Aging Neurosci 2017;9:100.

Dental Care in the Golden Years

Heidi B. Lobprise, DVM

KEYWORDS

- Oral • Dental • Tooth • Periodontal disease • Oral tumors • Tooth resorption • Inflammaging • Pathologic fractures

KEY POINTS

- The incidence of oral and dental disease increases in older pets, particularly in those that have not had regular care.
- The continued presence of untreated oral inflammation (not just infection) can greatly impact systemic health and the health span of pets.
- Seldom is a patient "too old" to be able to tolerate general anesthesia that is needed for optimal oral and dental care.
- The benefit in providing optimal oral and dental care often greatly outweighs the potential risks of anesthesia.
- The continuum of a lifetime of preventive dental care can help decrease the likelihood of having to deal with significant disease in older patients.

INTRODUCTION

- There is strong connection between oral/dental disease and senior or geriatric pets
  - Periodontal disease increases in prevalence as pets age[1]
    - Periodontal disease increases in prevalence in smaller dogs,[1] and smaller dogs tend to live longer lives
    - Unique periodontal manifestations such as chronic alveolitis with buccal bone expansion are typically seen in older cats[2]
  - The start of issues such as tooth resorption may occur in the mature adult cat or dog, but the prevalence can increase over time
  - Many oral tumors are found more frequently in older pets
- The systemic effects of untreated oral and dental disease
  - Beyond the transient bacteremia from microbes in the oral cavity, the presence of chronic inflammation can impact all organ systems.

1928 Oak Aly, Kerrville, TX 78028, USA
E-mail address: Heidident93@gmail.com

Vet Clin Small Anim 56 (2026) 391–404
https://doi.org/10.1016/j.cvsm.2025.09.024 vetsmall.theclinics.com

Abbreviations	
AL	attachment loss
CAA	canine acanthomatous ameloblastoma
CEJ	cementoenamel junction
CT	computed tomography
FSA	Fibrosarcoma
GA	general anesthesia
IV	Intravenous
MM	malignant melanoma
PD	periodontal disease
POF	peripheral odontogenic fibroma/ FEPLO - fibromatous epulis of periodontal ligament origin
TR	tooth resorption

- In a perfect scenario, these patients would have had excellent dental care throughout their lives, but often we see dogs and cats that have significant periodontal disease or other conditions that require extensive care under general anesthesia (GA) with patients that could potentially be at risk
- Too many times, the pet will not show symptoms of discomfort until the disease has progressed significantly. Regular professional examination and education of the caregiver to monitor their pet for possible issues can help lead to earlier detection of problems.

DEFINITIONS

- Periodontal disease: a progressive destruction of the tissues surrounding the teeth: the attached gingiva, the alveolar bone, the periodontal ligament, and the cementum covering the root (periodontium).
- Inflammaging: chronic, sterile, low-grade inflammation that develops with advanced age, in the absence of overt infection, and may contribute to clinical manifestations of other age-related pathologies.
- The term "tooth resorption" (TR) is simply defined as resorption of dental hard tissue (cementum, enamel, and dentin).
- Anesthesia-free dentistry—oral or dental care administered to an awake or sedated patient, not under GA.

Periodontal Disease

Periodontal disease (PD) is a progressive destruction of the tissues surrounding the teeth: the attached gingiva, the alveolar bone, the periodontal ligament, and the cementum covering the root (periodontium). If soft plaque on the tooth surface (supragingival) is not removed, and accumulations mineralize into calculus, then more plaque bacteria can start to populate the subgingival regions. Dysbiosis of the microbiome in the plaque and subgingival regions to destructive anaerobic gram-negative bacteria can directly destroy the periodontal tissues.[3] The host response to the bacteria can also damage its own tissue, sometimes at an unusual rate.

In theory, PD is preventable in most individuals, but once tissues are lost, for the most part, they cannot be recovered or regenerated easily. Stage 1 PD involves only gingival inflammation and no destruction of the tissues of attachment, but stages 2 to 4 reflect increasing levels of loss of the periodontium, until the tooth itself is lost.

Oral and dental care should be provided throughout the lifetime of a pet to help remove any irritants (plaque, calculus, and debris) to maintain stability in the microbiome. Adequate care can reduce the incidence or potentially the severity of oral and dental diseases that a senior or geriatric pet has to handle. It has been shown that the incidence of PD increases with age,[1] and this makes sense, as the teeth can have a progression of disease as they age, particularly if adequate preventive and wellness care of the oral cavity has not occurred. Even with regular professional cleaning and assessment, and effective home care by the caregivers, some individuals will still experience various levels of PD with chronic infection, inflammation, and even eventual tooth loss.

The incidence of PD also increases with the decreasing size of dogs, due to tooth crowding and a lower bone-to-tooth ratio for osseous support.[1] On top of that, smaller dogs tend to live longer, potentially increasing the incidence of PD in this group. Severe bone loss in advanced PD, particularly in the mandibles, can compromise the strength of the bone. Even minor traumatic forces, including extraction attempts, may result in pathologic fractures, particularly at the mandibular first molars, canine, and symphysis. Teeth with poor alveolar support due to bone loss may luxate or subluxate, causing pain and discomfort, and sometimes keeping the mouth from closing properly.

And more than just the infection or bacteremia that is often discussed, the continuing presence of a chronic inflammatory condition can impact systemic health. Bacteremia is typically transient,[4] and unless a patient is immunocompromised, this may not be of great concern. Chronic oral inflammation can contribute to a situation known as inflammaging, which is a critical factor in morbidity and mortality in human medicine.[5] In fact, the oral cavity is one distinct area where inflammation can be adequately managed (extractions), so its resolution is possibly the reason behind the amazing recovery of patients after major extractions. While it is so rewarding to see the "miraculous" response of these seniors, would it not have been better if they never had to experience the chronic disease in the first place?

Treatment

There are several goals of periodontal treatment, starting with the complete removal of all plaque, calculus, and debris (irritants). Removing these irritants is most important under the gum line, in the sulcus and pockets; anesthesia-free dentistry *cannot* provide this level of care. A second goal is to minimize the loss of attachment (the periodontal tissues) and to maintain attached gingiva if possible (2–3 mm minimum). Minimizing the pocket depth is also critical, as in the pockets, the decreased oxygen availability "supports" the microbiome shift to bacteria associated with PD. Any pocket deeper than 5 mm cannot be adequately cleaned without a gingival flap and deeper pockets cannot be adequately managed with standard home care procedures.

Complete assessment is necessary to determine appropriate therapy, and measuring/recording any root exposure (due to gingival and bone recession) and pocket depth is done with a periodontal probe. The total attachment loss (AL) is determined by adding the amount of root exposure in millimeters to the depth of the periodontal pocket. Imaging in the form of intraoral radiograph or advanced imaging (such as cone-beam computerized tomography) will allow the evaluation of the extent and pattern of bone loss at each tooth. Once the evaluation is complete, decisions are made as to the appropriate therapy needed. For teeth with stage 2 PD (less than 25% AL), a thorough dental cleaning, scaling, and irrigation help to remove all irritants and hopefully return the tissues to a quiescent state. Continued home care and professional therapy can help maintain these teeth in a stable condition. For teeth with stage 4 PD (greater than 50% AL), the decision is also straightforward—extraction with debridement of affected tissue, then gingival/mucosal closure.

The real decisions are made with teeth that have between 25% and 50% AL (stage 3 PD). The choice between periodontal therapy and extraction depends on a number of factors. First is the relative "importance" of the tooth itself; if it is a strategic tooth (canine tooth and carnassial tooth), then determine the extent of disease and loss of tissues around it. For example, moderate AL at a mandibular canine or first molar with bone loss between it and an adjacent, less-strategic tooth may be an ideal situation to provide advanced periodontal treatment at the time the adjacent tooth is extracted (see later discussion). Second, the overall health status of the patient must be taken into consideration. If such a tooth were a reasonable candidate for periodontal therapy, but the patient has systemic health issues (cardiac, renal, and so forth) and is at higher risk during a longer anesthetic procedure, extraction may be the best option for that patient. Permanently removing that source of chronic infection is never a bad idea, and yes, they will still be able to eat. Third, the caregiver's situation should also be taken into account. It can be satisfying to salvage a strategic tooth, but the additional initial anesthetic time, more frequent anesthetic procedures for follow-up care and expectations for optimal home care may put too much of a burden on the client.

Periodontal Therapy—Beyond Scaling

Nonsurgical

Teeth with stage 2 to 3 PD need more than just removing calculus from the crowns. Subgingival therapy and pocket management are critical aspects for optimal outcomes. Even simple closed root planing of pockets up to 5 mm in depth can help decrease pocket depth as the inflammation and edema resolves, and the tissues stabilize. Additionally, the use of subgingival medications, some with antibiotic and anticollagenase properties, as well as a perioceutic using hyaluronic acid can help promote healing of the soft tissues.

Surgical

Simple reduction of chronically thickened gingival margins (gingivoplasty with a 12 fluted bur) can immediately reduce the depth of the pocket, though root exposure may become more apparent, if present. Appropriate management of soft tissues can greatly impact intradental pocket depths between adjacent teeth. As discussed earlier, when a smaller adjacent tooth next to a strategic tooth is to be extracted, this should involve removing diseased or even redundant soft tissue between the teeth. The following example involves a mandibular canine and incisors, but the concepts can be applied to other sites. Any releasing incisions for a gingival flap should be made "away" from the tooth that will remain, combined with an effort to remove diseased soft tissue in the pocket. Simply plucking out a mandibular incisor (or if they have been lost in the past), can leave inflamed, redundant tissue creating a pocket at the canine. With tissue management/removal or at the time of extraction of the adjacent tooth, this allows for better access to the canine. In addition to debriding the diseased soft tissue away, the tooth can be thoroughly cleaned with open root planing using a curette. The surrounding bone can be evaluated for any vertical bone loss or infrabony pocket that may be an ideal site for bone graft material placement. There may even be ridges of rough alveolar bone or spicules and would benefit from a gentle alveoloplasty with a diamond bur. Once the region is treated, closure with monofilament suture (poliglecaprone) helps position a complete band of attached gingiva around the canine.[6]

Providing this additional effort of advanced periodontal therapy must be accompanied by effective home care and reassessment and treatment every 6 to 9 months to maintain periodontal health. This is why the considerations of patient and client are important prior to therapy. However, providing this care, even in earlier stages of bone loss, can help stabilize the mandible at sites that are prone to pathologic fracture.

Pathologic Mandibular Fracture Secondary to Periodontal Bone Loss

Untreated bone loss at the mandibular first molar or canine can result in compromise to the strength of the osseous structures at the site. This most commonly occurs in small, older dogs that experience orofacial trauma, sometimes just by jumping off the bed and hitting their face. Once fractured, options for repairing the fractured mandible(s) may be limited. Standard concepts of mandibular fracture repair need sufficient bone with an adequate supply of osteoblastic cells to bridge the site once it is stabilized surgically. Due to the loss of bone and general decrease in the ability to heal, successful stabilization and compete osseous may not be possible for some individuals (**Fig. 1**). Advanced procedures using implant graft materials and miniplate stabilization are possible. Maintaining the teeth in the fracture site is another principle that is more applicable in acute fractures with relatively healthy bone and teeth. In these chronic PD cases, the alveoli and even pulpal health of the teeth can further compromise the potential for healing. Any complicated cases should be referred to a dental or oral surgical specialist.

One palliative method can be the removal of the portion of the mandible rostral to the fracture site, to the mandibular symphysis, which can often have bone loss as well. Incisions are made buccally and lingually, and soft tissue elevated off the mandibular bone, with ligation of mental foramen vessels (**Fig. 2**). Once the symphysis is separated rostrally, further blunt tissue dissection of muscle and other tissues off the mandible progress to the site of fracture. If intact, the mandibular neurovascular bundle is identified, ligated and cut. Soft tissue is then closed. This modified mandibulectomy can even be done bilaterally, with appropriate excision of excessive lip/chin tissue.

Chronic Alveolitis with Buccal Bone Expansion—Assessment and Treatment

In older cats, a variation of chronic periodontal inflammation can affect the canine teeth, particularly the maxillary canines. There will be expansion of the buccal bone

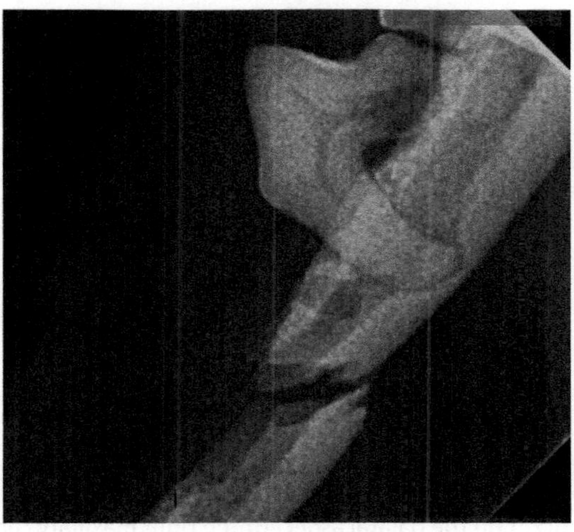

Fig. 1. Radiograph of a pathologic fracture of the left mandible in an older, small dog. The remaining bone is compromised and thin.

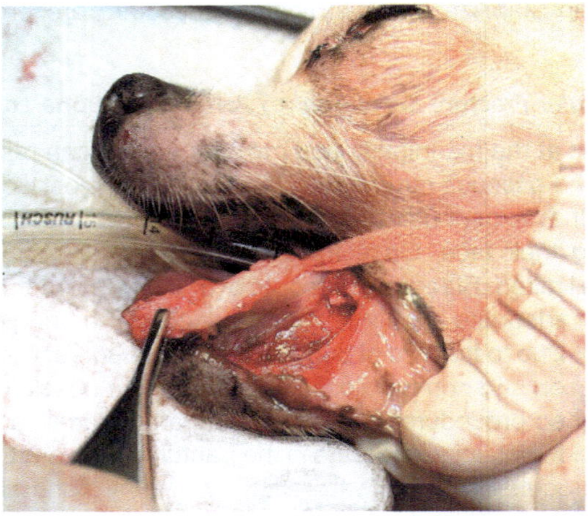

Fig. 2. Removal of the left mandible from the fracture rostrally (rostral partial mandibulectomy) as palliative treatment of the pathologic fracture.

and TR will often be present.[7] The teeth may "supererupt" with partial extrusion of the tooth, giving them an elongated appearance with some root exposure. Periodontal pockets may be present, and in advanced stages, teeth may become mobile (**Fig. 3**). Extraction is often necessary, though the gingiva covering the buccal bone expansion is usually very thin, so a typical gingival flap may be challenging to elevate,

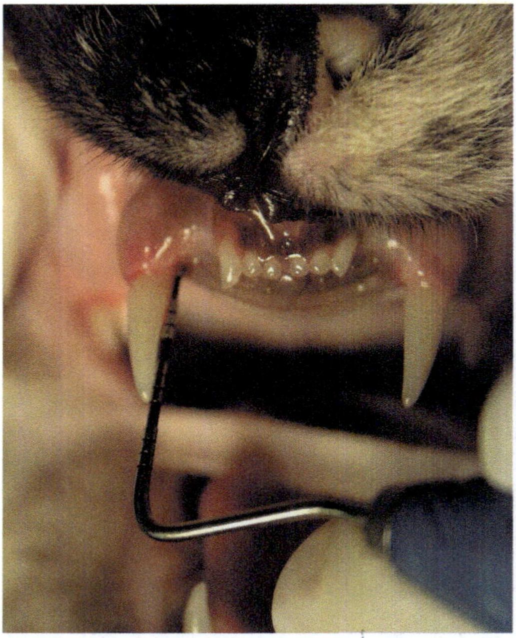

Fig. 3. Periodontal pocket on the palatal aspect of the right maxillary canine on an older cat with moderate alveolitis and buccal bone expansion. The tooth had tooth resorption and some mobility, so it was extracted.

and very challenging to close postextraction. One hint, if a maxillary canine is extracted, use a white stone bur to gently blunt the opposing mandibular canine to minimize contact lip trauma and lip entrapment.

Tooth Resorption

The term "tooth resorption" is simply defined as resorption of dental hard tissue (cementum, enamel, and dentin), as is now the primary designation for a wide range of presentations. It can cover different species (cat and dog), external or internal, categorized by the radiographic appearance (inflammatory, replacement [odontoclastic]) and staged by degree of involvement.[8] In most cases, the term feline odontoclastic resorptive lesions might spring to mind, but that is just one permutation. While these can be found in younger animals, due to their progressive nature, the incidence/prevalence tends to increase in older pets.

Prevalence

Overall, the traditional concept of feline TR has been the focus of practitioners, with a reported prevalence from 28.5% to 67%,[9] and quite commonly in older cats.[10] Clinical studies have also shown radiographic signs of TR in 53.6% of dogs, with a higher frequency in older and larger patients.[11] Just over 11% of all teeth were affected in this study with the great majority being external replacement lesions.

Treatment

Type 2 tooth resorption: replacement/odontoclastic. Appropriate management of TR is directly associated with the type and extent of resorption. From human literature, and clinical observation/experience, when the replacement resorption (Type 2) is confined to the root structure, there tends to be minimal discomfort.[12] When that lesion advances into the crown, with exposure to the environment, clinical symptoms may be experienced. Hyperplastic gingiva may "grow into" the lesions, and palpation with a dental explorer will often elicit a painful reaction, even under GA. Eventually, the lesion will progress through the crown until it is lost, and the gingiva will heal over the site, but intervention with extraction is optimal, as soon as the lesion is identified in the crown structure. Radiographic appearance of the tooth will show a narrowing or disappearance of the periodontal ligament space, with decreased radiopacity of part of the tooth, as root is being replaced with bone.[8] If there is no evidence of endodontic disease (periapical bone loss), then a modified extraction technique with the removal of the crown and closing the gingiva is often sufficient (crown amputation).[13] Approximately 95% of feline TR lesions are type 2.[2]

Type 2 with external replacement resorption is the most common form found in dogs, and in the author's clinical experience, it affects the midroot region of premolars, especially mandibular premolars, in older dogs (**Fig. 4**). If the resorption is confined to the midroot region, these teeth can be monitored on a regular basis with annual dental procedures and radiography. If the lesion has any coronal extension, then extraction is necessary. For most dogs that have no periapical bone loss, a modified extraction may also be utilized, with close monitoring of any retained root structure. To date, there is no study on leaving these roots. If there is any apical bone loss indicative of pulpal involvement, the midroot section may be "bypassed" by creating a groove or ditch on that portion in able to access the apical portion that typically has intact periodontal ligament for eventual elevation.

Type 1 tooth resorption: inflammatory. When the radiographic appearance of the tooth show a focal or multifocal radiolucency (typically near the cementoenamel

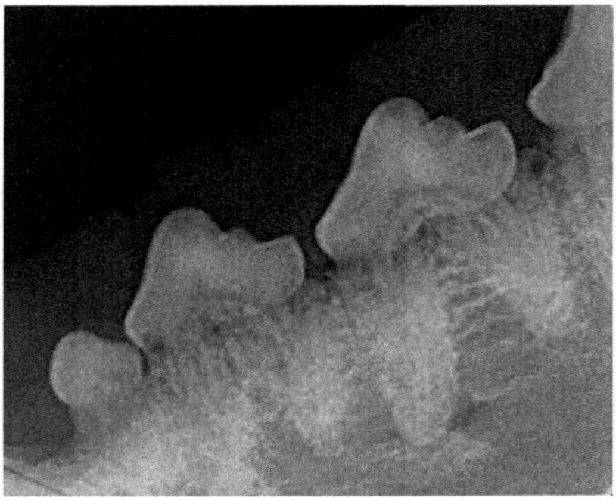

Fig. 4. Radiograph of type 2 replacement resorption in the left mandibular premolars of an older dog. Since the root resorption has extended into the crowns, extraction was necessary.

junction [CEJ] or neck), with otherwise normal periodontal ligament space and radiopacity, an inflammatory lesion is diagnosed. This resorption typically is present when PD or other inflammatory processes have caused loss of alveolar bone and gingiva, exposing the root to the environment (**Fig. 5**). While less common than the type 2 TR, these teeth must be fully elevated/extracted, especially if the cat has feline chronic gingivostomatitis.

Oral and Dental Trauma

Oral and dental trauma can occur at any age, but when it happens in older patients, consideration must be given to their decreased ability to adapt and heal. Decisions may be influenced by anticipated surgery time and outcomes for treatment options, such as electing extraction over root canal therapy.

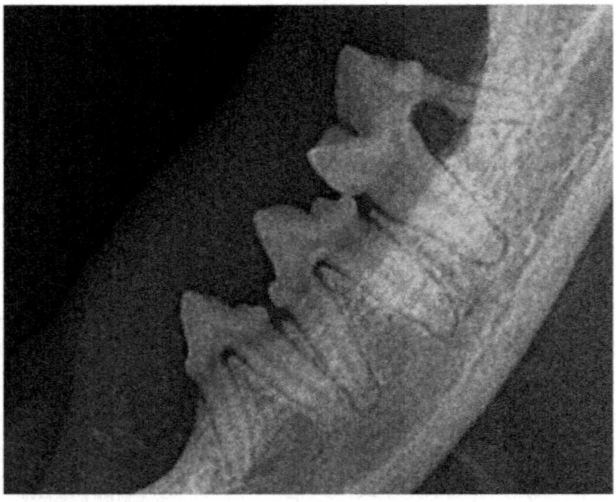

Fig. 5. Radiograph of type 1 inflammatory resorption of the distal root of the left mandibular molar (309; not an older cat). Inflammation from periodontal disease with bone and gingiva loss has exposed the furcation, where the resorption is evident. All root structures of this tooth must be extracted.

Tooth and dento-alveolar injuries (TDI): tooth and dento-alveolar injuries

One advantage senior pets have in the face of tooth wear or superficial fractures is the decreased size of the dental pulp cavity(ies) and thicker amounts of dentin in the mature tooth. Any injury that exposes the pulp or disrupts the blood supply to the apex of the tooth (luxation or pulpitis) will still need to be addressed with either extraction or endodontic therapy (root canal). The need for specialty referral and extended time to perform a root canal will often undermine the desire for this option.

Maxillofacial injuries

Injuries to the bone structure of the oral cavity can be quite extensive at times. Particularly due to the fragility of the mandible in older, smaller dogs, pathologic fractures can occur with minimal trauma forces. Full evaluation of any maxillofacial trauma is optimized with advanced imaging such as cone beam computed tomography (CT), which is often only available at specialty referral practices at this time. Decisions for surgical reduction and stabilization will depend on the remaining bone and its viability, the ability to maintain proper occlusion and the understanding that healing can be delayed in older patients. Palliative surgery to provide comfort with less invasive techniques (splinting and tape muzzles) or even removal of some of the traumatized tissues (partial mandibulectomy) may be the best choice for that patient.

Oral Tumors and Masses

While a handful of oral masses and tumors are found in younger animals (odontogenic tumors, dentigerous cysts, papilloma, feline inductive odontogenic tumor, and some fibrosarcomas [FSAs]), for the most part, there is an increased incidence of oral tumors as patients age.[14] Early detection and identification is critical for optimal outcome, but many oral tumors are not diagnosed until they are quite large. Once there is noticeable external deformation, oral pain or bleeding, the lesion may be too extensive for easy resolution. Regular oral examination and client education to encourage early detection are essential for these senior pets.

An oral tumor must be distinguished from areas of gingival enlargement (at times hyperplastic) due to familial tendencies (eg, boxers), chronic periodontitis, and even drug-related causes (diphenylhydantoin, cyclosporin, and so forth). These enlargements can cause the formation of "pseudo-pockets" that can contribute to PD, and resecting these tissues can help return these pockets to normal sulcus depth. Focal fibrous hyperplasia may also be found.

Odontogenic tumors: benign

The most common odontogenic tumors in senior pets (primarily dogs) include the peripheral odontogenic fibroma (POF—including ossified lesions) and canine acanthomatous ameloblastoma (CAA). A POF is often a firm, sessile to pedunculated, nonulcerated lesion, likely arising from periosteum or gingival ligament at the CEJ. Simple removal often results in recurrence of the mass, as the affected periodontal ligament and alveolar bone should be excised. As it is challenging to reconstruct the periodontal tissues around the tooth, extraction of the tooth in an en-bloc resection is often required to prevent recurrence.

A CAA is considered "benign" but can be locally very invasive, occasionally expansile. This is most common in the rostral mandible of larger dogs and wide resection with clean margins is the surgical goal (1–2 cm margins; **Fig. 6**). However, studies show that there tends to be no recurrence in cases with incomplete tumor excision (cells at margin).[15,16]

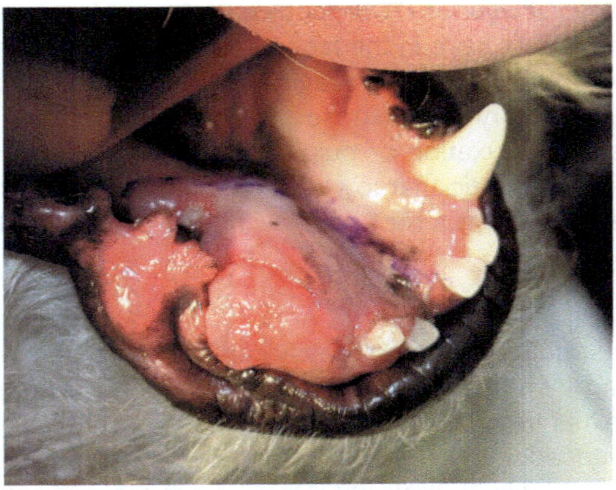

Fig. 6. Canine acanthomatous ameloblastoma (CAA) with surgical marks for aggressive rostral mandibulectomy. In this 10 year old dog, cells were found at the margin, but the lesion never recurred.

Nonodontogenic tumors: malignant

The malignant melanoma (MM) is the most common oral and maxillofacial tumors in dogs (rare in cats).[14] Pigmented tissue appear to be predisposed to MM, but amelanotic and undifferentiated types are found. These are usually black, ulcerated and friable, affecting the soft tissues with variable metastatic rates (lymph nodes and lungs). TNM (tumor-node-metastasis) staging is important to evaluate, and advanced imaging (CT) provides optimal assessment of the tumor and even the medial retropharyngeal lymph nodes. Incisional biopsies (deep and narrow) away from the tumor margins or any necrotic regions can help provide tumor identification, along with photos, for eventual treatment planning and prognosis. Wide surgical margins are essential for surgery and can be challenging to achieve if the tumor is large or the patient is small. Consultation with an oncologist or dentist is recommended.

In dogs, squamous cell carcinoma is the second most common tumor, and by far, it is the most common malignancy in cats. It can vary in appearance from a pink or red proliferative mass to just ulceration of soft tissue and loose teeth similar to PD. The gingival form in cats rapidly involves bone, and rostral tumors are thought to have lower metastatic rates, as compared to lingual and tonsillar forms. Dogs may adapt well to the radical glossectomy of a small lingual tumor (cats do not do well with this surgery) but micrometastasis may become evident later.

The second most common oral tumor in cats and the third most common in dogs, FSA is often a broad-based mass with diffuse, firm swelling. There can be forms that appear benign histopathologically but have high-grade biological characteristics (high-low FSA). It can be infiltrative, so radical surgery, along with postsurgical radiation therapy, is often the optimal treatment choice.

Other less common malignancies may include osteosarcoma, hemangiosarcoma, mast cell tumor, multilobular tumor of bone, and lymphosarcoma. Early identification, intralesional biopsies with imaging to identify the tumor type can help with treatment planning. With senior pets, it is critical to provide full information to the caregiver; while we have amazing opportunities for advanced therapy for pets, the burdens of maintaining patient comfort, evaluating state-of-the-art options, cost, and expectations may lead to the decision that palliative care is the best choice for that pet-owner combination. Quality of life can be significantly impacted by aggressive surgery, radiation therapy, and chemotherapy and must be carefully considered.

Anesthesia and Analgesia in Geriatric Pets

Utilizing GA is an essential consideration in providing oral and dental care for our senior patients, likely the most common reason for GA in this patient population. Since aging impacts everything from drug utilization to recovery and healing, personalized analgesia and anesthetic protocols for these older dogs and cats can help minimize potential risks. This section is but a brief overview of these areas; comprehensive senior anesthesia and analgesia coverage can be found elsewhere.[17,18]

The option of anesthesia-free procedures should *not* be considered, as appropriate examination, evaluation, and oral/dental care cannot be provided on an awake or sedated pet. Many publications and organizations support this viewpoint.[19]

Preoperative assessment with diagnostics and evaluation of body system diseases will include stabilization of mild-to-moderate dysfunction prior to the day of procedure. This may include updating cardiological assessment, staging renal disease, and managing diabetic concerns with appropriate delay of GA until conditions are alleviated and stabilized. Some perioperative action steps this author utilizes may include

- Prehydration of patients with renal dysfunction for 2 to 3 days prior to procedure
- Encourage any suitable use of anxiolytics (anxiety is often increased in senior pets), especially the night before and the morning of the procedure, as long as mobility is not impaired
- Maropitant can be dispensed to be given the night before the procedure (or injectable perioperatively) to decrease nausea
- Consider antiacid medication for patients that may experience regurgitation, especially brachycephalic pets. Regurgitation will not be stopped, but the contents will be less acidic; all contents are flushed and cleaned out of the oral and nasal cavities if regurgitation occurs perioperatively
- Do not withhold water at home prior to procedure
- Food should be withheld for 4 to 6 hours in healthy patients, 2 to 4 hours in patients with diabetes, and 6 to 12 hours in those patients at risk for regurgitation.[17]
  - A small meal in the morning may be given to administer medication
- Patients with diabetes—with decreased morning meal, decrease insulin injection
  - Placing a continuous glucose monitoring device at the time of the procedure will provide easy serial glucose monitoring during and after the surgery
- Most chronic medications should be given, with the exception of anticoagulants and most antitensive agents (amlodipine can be given to cats[20]).
- Adjust anesthetic medication amounts and titrate any intravenous (IV) medication to effect (eg, propofol)
- For stressed patients, alfaxalone may be given intramuscularly
- Preoxygenate all patients, especially ones with cardiopulmonary disease, if is not too stressful
- IV fluids administration may be adjusted: increased for renal patients, decreased for cardiac patients[21]
- Provide optimal analgesia—at home (nonsteroidal anti-inflammatory drug if appropriate), preanesthetic sedation/analgesia; local and regional blocks; medication for postoperative use; adjunctive methods (cool compresses, targeted pulsed electromagnetic field device, acupuncture, and so forth).

- Thermoregulation is often decreased in older patients, and dental procedures can keep them wet. Appropriate heating devices should be used (conductive blankets, warm air blankets, warm IV fluids, socks, and so forth).
- Optimal monitoring should be provided
- Continue monitoring and care (fluids and warmth) is important in the critical post-operative recovery phase, where the majority of mortality events occur[22]

This is not a comprehensive list—just some personal opinions of highlights for senior patient care. Another important concept is that of staging the procedure. Even with stable body temperature and blood pressure, being under GA for extended periods of time can be challenging for older cats and dogs, impact their recovery and healing, and can be stressful for the veterinary team as well. Become comfortable with setting time limits for procedures, maybe 2 to 2.5 hours. Splitting the entire surgery time into 2 separate procedures 2 to 4 weeks apart can be considered for several scenarios:

- You know ahead of time that there will be a significant amount of oral/dental surgery needed
- You get radiographs and assessment and diagnose several areas that need treatment but were not anticipated (and you have 3 other procedures that day)
- You get radiographs and find advanced disease that may require specialty referrals

In these cases, get full evaluation with radiographs and periodontal probing to determine the complete treatment plan. Provide phase 1 therapy—complete cleaning, some subgingival cleaning, polishing, and even simple extractions. Record what additional therapy is needed—from more advanced extractions to periodontal surgery and communicate with the owner about the benefits of providing these procedures at a later date. Not only will this decrease the anesthetic time of any one procedure, but the oral tissues will often be much healthier and easier to manipulate for the second phase of treatment. At times, the advanced treatment may be optimally provided by a dental specialist, if available.

GOALS AND CHALLENGES

To provide the best oral and dental care for your senior patients, training for all staff members is critical. Appropriate skills will translate into the best care as well as decreased anesthetic time and improved patient outcomes. Having the right equipment and instruments is also essential, from imaging to dental units and hand instruments. Proper maintenance of all tools, including sharpening and regular replacement of worn instruments can help decrease frustration with providing care.

And to help offset caregiver concerns about provided care for the senior pet, good communication and client education efforts will help build the perception of the benefits of care as compared to the risks and costs. Having a testimonial from one of those owners with a pet that "feels like a puppy again" can help others appreciate how important oral and dental care can be. We still need to be empathic about potential burdens to these caregivers, including their concerns about anesthesia, costs, and even the ability to provide home care.

SUMMARY

When we can work as a team with our staff and the pet caregiver, a lifetime of optimal oral and dental care can not only potential increase the life-span of the pet, but the health span as well!

CLINICS CARE POINTS

- Oral and dental disease is prevalent in senior dogs and cats, particularly when regular care has not been given.
- The benefits of providing oral and dental care will outweigh the potential risks of GA in many patients, with appropriate preoperative diagnostics and management to minimize those risks.
- Eliminating the source of bacteremia and chronic infection, mostly by extractions, can positively impact the systemic health and quality of life of most senior pets.

DISCLOSURE

Dr H.B. Lobprise has consulted with and/or provided sponsored lectures for: Royal Canin, France, Zomedica, Zoetis, United States, ReGum, PerioVive, Hills and Purina. These relationships do not affect the content of this material.

REFERENCES

1. Harvey CE, Shofer FS, Laster L. Association of age and body weight with periodontal disease in North American dogs. J Vet Dent 1994;11(3):94–105.
2. Reiter AM, Johnston J, Anderson JG, et al. Domestic feline oral and dental disease. In: Lobprise HB, Dodd JR, editors. Wiggs's veterinary dentistry; principles and practice. 2nd edition. Hoboken (NJ): John Wiley & Sons; 2019. p. 131–54.
3. Anderson JG, Rojas CA, Scarsella E, et al. The oral microbiome across oral sites in cats with chronic gingivostomatitis, periodontal disease, and tooth resorption compared with healthy cats. Animals (Basel) 2023;13(22):3544.
4. Blazevich M, Miles C. The presence of bacteremia in 13 dogs undergoing oral surgery without the use of antibiotic therapy. J Vet Dent 2024;41:312–23.
5. Buzoglu HD, Burus A, Bayazıt Y, et al. Stem cell and oxidative stress-inflammation cycle. Curr Stem Cell Res Ther 2023;18(5):641–52.
6. Mathis JR, Scott KI, Lobprise HB. Use of a periodontal resective procedure (proximal wedge technique) for treating gingival and periodontal pockets of mandibular canine teeth in dogs. J Small Anim Pract 2025;66(4):262–71.
7. Lewis JR, Okuda A, Shofer FS, et al. Significant association between tooth extrusion and tooth resorption in domestic cats. J Vet Dent 2008;25(2):86–95.
8. American Veterinary Dental College nomenclature. Available at: https://avdc.org/avdc-nomenclature/. Accessed August 28, 2025.
9. Gorrel C. Tooth resorption in cats: pathophysiology and treatment options. J Feline Med Surg 2015;17(1):37–43.
10. Niemiec B, Gawor J, Nemec A, et al. World small animal veterinary association global dental guidelines. J Small Anim Pract 2020;61:395–403.
11. Peralta S, Verstraete FJ, Kass PH. Radiographic evaluation of the types of tooth resorption in dogs. Am J Vet Res 2010;71(7):784–93.
12. Heboyan A, Avetisyan A, Karobari MI, et al. Tooth root resorption: a review. Sci Prog 2022;105(3):368504221109217.
13. DuPont G. Crown amputation with intentional root retention for advanced feline resorptive lesions–a clinical study. J Vet Dent 1995;12(1):9–13.
14. Goldschmidt SL, Bell CM, Hetzel S, et al. Clinical characterization of canine acanthomatous ameloblastoma (CAA) in 263 dogs and the influence of postsurgical histopathological margin on local recurrence. J Vet Dent 2017;34(4):241–7.

15. Bolek AM, Smith MM, Taney K, et al. Symphyseal-sparing mandibulectomy for canine acanthomatous ameloblastoma in dogs: 35 cases. J Vet Dent 2024;41(1):10–6.
16. Soukup J, Lewis J. Oral and maxillofacial tumors, cysts and tumor-like lesions. In: Lobprise HB, Dodd JR, editors. Wiggs's veterinary dentistry; principles and practice. 2nd edition. Hoboken, NJ.: John Wiley & Sons; 2019. p. 131–54.
17. Grubb T, Sager J, Gaynor JS, et al. AAHA anesthesia and monitoring guidelines for dogs and cats. J Am Anim Hosp Assoc 2020;56:59–82.
18. Robertson SA, Gogolski SM, Pascoe P, et al. AAFP feline anesthesia guidelines. J Feline Med Surg 2018;20(7):602–34.
19. AVDC position statement - companion animal dental scaling without anesthesia, Available at: https://avdc.org/about/ (Accesses October 28 2025).
20. Clark-Price S, Fischer JR. Physiology, pathophysiology, and anesthetic management of patients with renal disease. In: Lamont L, Grimm K, Robertson S, et al, editors. Veterinary anesthesia and analgesia. 6th ed. Hoboken (NJ): John Wiley & Sons; 2024. p. 934–9.
21. Pardo M, Spencer E, Odunayo A, et al. 2024 AAHA fluid therapy guidelines for dogs and cats. J Am Anim Hosp Assoc 2024;60(4):131–63.
22. Brodbelt DC, Blissitt KJ, Hammond RA, et al. The risk of death: the confidential enquiry into perioperative small animal fatalities. Vet Anaesth Analg 2008;35: 365–73.

FURTHER READING

Bellows J, Berg ML, Dennis S, et al. 2019 AAHA dental care guidelines for dogs and cats. J Am Anim Hosp Assoc 2019;55:49–69.

Addressing Cognitive Dysfunction

Education, Diagnosis, and Practical Care

Sara Lynch, DVM, MPH[a,b,*]

KEYWORDS

- Cognitive dysfunction syndrome • Neurobehavioral • Chronic disease • DISHAA • CADES • CCDR • Human-animal bond

KEY POINTS

- Cognitive dysfunction syndrome (CDS) is an underdiagnosed, chronic, progressive disease that affects a significant percentage of senior dogs and cats; as our pets are living longer than ever, this population will only be seen to grow requiring more options in terms of client education and symptom management.
- Clinical signs of CDS are neurobehavioral, meaning that physical and behavioral signs are often linked; recognition of these signs by clients and veterinarians alike can be difficult, but early diagnosis is important for the best treatment outcomes.
- Clinical signs of CDS most reported include disorientation, interaction alterations, sleep-wake disturbances, house soiling, activity level alterations, and anxiety—it is important to remember that many of these clinical signs can mimic those of other health concerns, making CDS a diagnosis of rule out.
- Successful management of CDS is multimodal in nature and may include medications and supplements, nutritional recommendations, environmental enrichment, and safety considerations in the home; ongoing support for both the pet and the caregivers is vital for long-term management.

INTRODUCTION

Aging pets may experience a variety of physical health concerns that are relatively easy for clients to recognize. Changes such as sudden incontinence, lameness, and gastrointestinal upset tend to be addressed with the pet's veterinarian without much delay as the clear discomfort of the pet is more apparent. However, due to often-subtle clinical signs, cognitive changes in our senior pet population can be harder to recognize as true disease and may be dismissed by the family as the pet

[a] Lap of Love Veterinary Hospice Veterinarian, Memphis, TN, USA; [b] Lap of Love Veterinary Hospice, 17804 US-41, Lutz, FL 33549, USA
* Lap of Love Veterinary Hospice, 17804 US-41, Lutz, FL 33549.
E-mail address: drsally@lapoflove.com

Vet Clin Small Anim 56 (2026) 405–418
https://doi.org/10.1016/j.cvsm.2025.09.030 **vetsmall.theclinics.com**
0195-5616/26/

Abbreviations	
AD	Alzheimer's disease
CADES	Canine Dementia Scale
CCD	canine cognitive dysfunction
CCDR	Canine Cognitive Dysfunction Rating
CDS	cognitive dysfunction syndrome
NFT	neurofibrillary tangle
SAMe	S-adenosyl methionine

simply "getting older." Because of this lack of recognition as a true health concern, cognitive changes may not be addressed with a veterinarian until clinical signs are more advanced.

Cognitive dysfunction syndrome (CDS) is a chronic, progressive neurodegenerative disease affecting senior and geriatric pets.[3] This disease is characterized by a variety of mentation and personality changes including disorientation, increased anxiety, sleep–wake disturbances, and altered interactions with family members.[3] Often compared to human Alzheimer's disease (AD), CDS can cause significant changes to a pet's quality of life as it advances (**Table 1**). While initial changes may be very mild such as the occasional house soiling or loss of previously learned commands, end-stage disease is often severely debilitating, leaving the pet unable to cope with everyday activities without human assistance.

Treatment is based on the management of clinical signs in attempts to maintain quality of life. Recommendations for treatment are often multimodal in nature and should include prescription medications, supplements for cognitive health, enriched nutrition, and environmental/lifestyle modifications for both safety and enrichment purposes. It is important that veterinary professionals remember that the chronic, progressive nature of this disease requires ongoing support for both the pet and the caregivers within the family. Investing time and knowledge into early diagnosis, client education, and a variety of disease management options tailored to the family's priorities ensures the best possible outcomes for maintaining the well-being of both the animal patient and human caregivers.

EPIDEMIOLOGY OF COGNITIVE DYSFUNCTION SYNDROME

Rates of CDS have been found to increase with age in both dogs and cats; predictably, as the age of an animal increases, so too does the likelihood of suspected diagnosis of cognitive dysfunction.[4] Considering that our pets are living longer than ever as veterinary medicine advances, it is expected that rates of CDS will continue to rise across domestic species. The estimated prevalence of canine cognitive dysfunction (CCD) ranges from 14% to 35% with the highest prevalence being found among more senior dogs.[3]

More specific prevalence statistics of CCD have been found to be approximately 8.1% in dogs ages 8 to 11 years, 18.8% in ages 11 to 13 years, 45.3% in ages 13 to 15 years, and 67.3% in ages 15 to 17 year old.[4] In a 2010 study of 154 cats aged 11 years or older, 35% were diagnosed as having suspected CDS.[5] Within the sample population showing clinical signs of CDS, 28% of the cats were aged 11 to 15 years and 50% were older than 15 years.[5] However, the true prevalence of CDS is difficult to ascertain due to limited means of early detection and suspected underrecognition and underreporting by pet owners.

Considering the prevalence and progressive nature of this neurobehavioral disease, early recognition, client education, and proactive approaches to minimize clinical signs is imperative to help ensure better long-term health outcomes for senior pets.

Table 1
The progression of AD and CDS often presents similarly when considered by stages, beginning with mild symptoms and advancing to clinical signs that cause loss of independence for patient[1,2]

Stage of Disease/ Severity of Symptoms	Alzheimer's Disease (AD)	Cognitive Dysfunction Syndrome (CDS)
Early/Mild	• Memory lapses in new information, people's names, etc • Increased difficulty managing tasks (especially more complex tasks) • Misplacing items	• Altered sleep cycles • Increased anxiety (panting, vocalizing) • Changes in social interactions
Middle/Moderate	• Increasing memory loss of personal history • Altered moods and personality changes • Increasingly severe disorientation • Increased likelihood of wandering or getting lost • Possible loss of continence	• Loss of learned behaviors, altered bathroom habits/ house soiling • Worsening confusion and disorientation • Increased wandering/ pacing • Worsening sleep disruptions decreased recognition of familiar people and objects
Late/Severe	• Loss of ability to respond to their environment • Loss of ability to communicate • Changes physical ability to walk, sit down, or swallow	• Decreased response to environment and family members • Loss of or altered senses (vision, smell) • Gait and mobility changes • Vocalizing due to confusion or anxiety • Altered appetite • Incontinence • Lethargy, decreased activity

From Alzheimer's Association. Stages of alzheimer's. Alzheimer's Disease and Dementia. Published 2025. https://www.alz.org/alzheimers-dementia/stages; and Managing Cognitive Dysfunction and Behavioral Anxiety. AAHA. Published December 9, 2024. https://www.aaha.org/resources/2023-aaha-senior-care-guidelines-for-dogs-and-cats/managing-cognitive-dysfunction-and-behavioral-anxiety/.

COGNITIVE DYSFUNCTION SYNDROME AND ALZHEIMER'S DISEASE—SUSPECTED PATHOGENESIS SIMILARITIES

Much like human Alzheimer's, cognitive dysfunction in animals is suspected to be the result of multifaceted age-related physiologic and chemical changes within the brain, causing neuroinflammation and neuronal loss.[3,6,7] Many human studies have demonstrated correlations between progression of AD and beta-amyloid plaques; the amyloid hypothesis suggests that these plaques interfere with neuronal signaling.[6,8–10] This interference in turn activates an immune response, resulting in the release of glial cells, specifically astrocytes and microglia, which subsequently trigger neuroinflammation.[8–10] While some canine studies suggest a similar relationship between beta-amyloids and CCD, others have found no significant correlation.[6]

A second vital finding in human AD studies that has some correlation to canine research, is the occurrence of tau phosphorylation [6,11,12] Hyperphosphorylation of the τ protein results in the formation of neurofibrillary tangles (NFTs); these tangles are another hallmark of AD.[6,11] The τ hypothesis states that the formation of NFTs by τ phosphorylation disrupts cytoplasmic functions and axonal transport, resulting in neuronal death.[11] Multiple studies have reported regionally and morphologically similar NFT distribution within the brains of dogs diagnosed with CCD,[12,13] though most were small in study sample size.

Other suspected origins of CDS include the age-related decrease of safeguards against oxidative damage.[6,7,14] For example, superoxide dismutase is a protective enzyme present in a healthy brain; it functions to protect the brain by neutralizing free radicals.[6,7,14] As the canine brain ages, the level of protective superoxide dismutase decreases, leaving the senior brain more vulnerable to oxidative damage, which progresses to demyelination and cytokine production.[7,14] Research into this possible cause of CDS suggests that preventing or reducing oxidative damage to the brain through enhanced nutrition and supplements may result in the slowing of disease progression and clinical signs including behavior changes.[7,14]

COMMON SYMPTOMS OF COGNITIVE DYSFUNCTION SYNDROME

Symptoms suggestive of CDS tend to be observed gradually as neurodegeneration occurs; it is suspected that, as in AD, there is likely a subclinical or preclinical stage of CDS in animals wherein physiologic changes are occurring, but no overt signs are yet seen. Most commonly, CDS signs reported by owners include altered sleep cycles, house soiling, confusion or episodes of disorientation, and increased pacing with loss of normal engagement with family members.[3,7,14,15] These clinical manifestations have been repeatedly reported in multiple studies over the years and thus have been categorized into a helpful acronym, DISHAA (Disorientation, Interactions with owner alteration, Sleep–wake disturbances, House soiling, Activity level alterations, and Anxiety).[3,7,14,15]

The DISHAA acronym can be utilized as a helpful tool in establishing a framework of what CDS is and how it may appear when talking with clients. By breaking down the categories of clinical signs and providing specific examples, veterinarians can better assist families who are experiencing confusion or uncertainty about their senior pet's behavior changes, thus enhancing the relevance of their observations pertaining to the disease. Encouraging proactive dialogs and CDS education with clients is imperative for early diagnosis, as well as successes in both the short-term and long-term outcomes of possible therapies and management recommendations.

Within the DISHAA categories are specific common signs of CDS, including pacing and compulsive wandering, memory loss, inattentiveness, and demented behavior, which often includes getting lost or disoriented in familiar environments, failure to recognize family members, and excessive vocalizations (especially at night).[3,7,14–16] Challenges to spatial awareness may be commonly observed which may appear as difficulty navigating stairs or attempting to pass through narrow spaces.[3,15] In addition to behavioral and mental symptoms, physical changes such as gait alterations and decreased senses of smell and vision have also been observed as part of the progression of CDS.[3,15]

COGNITIVE DYSFUNCTION SYNDROME DIAGNOSIS

The rather wide range of behavioral and physical signs which may appear throughout the course of CDS contributes to the challenge of accurate diagnosis; this is especially true when we consider the fact that many clinical signs may overlap, exaggerate, or mimic signs of other health concerns such as thyroid disease, diabetes, and organ dysfunction such as liver compromise, urinary tract infections, and kidney disease. It goes without saying that reliable and accurate diagnostics for CDS are important, but perhaps of more importance is the accessibility and usability of diagnostic tools for the general population of pet owners.

A thorough physical and neurologic assessment is a necessary starting place, and the importance of an accurate patient history is vital but it can often be challenging to attain, as many pet owners do not associate their pet's changing behaviors with an actual disease. For this reason, referencing the DISHAA assessment can be a helpful tool in discussing observed changes with families when CDS is suspected.

Screening for other common geriatric conditions is highly recommended through complete blood count, blood chemistry profile, urinalysis, and thyroid level assessment.[3,15,16] Because chronic pain can often mimic the signs of pacing and restlessness so often seen in pets with CDS, radiographs and ultrasound may also be valid considerations for appropriate diagnostics.[3,15,16] Ensuring that both senior dogs and cats are on appropriate pain management when needed is very important; chronic pain due to arthritis can significantly exaggerate signs of pacing, anxiety, and vocalizing. Blood pressure readings can also be essential, especially when considering senior cats reported to be demonstrating excessive vocalizations.[5] Increased vocalizations and activity level changes are common in cats with hypertension as well as being common signs of CDS.[5]

Finally, reviewing the pet's medications and dosing schedule can be an overlooked consideration, especially if owners have been adding over-the-counter medications or natural supplements into their pet's regime.[15] Interactions between multiple medications and/or supplements may cause clinical signs similar to those of CDS including disorientation, confusion, lethargy, and incontinence. Medication history is another example of how important a reliable and transparent patient history is to accurate diagnosis.

Though radiographs taken in a general practice setting may be helpful in ruling out age-related health concerns and potential comorbidities, the only imaging modality for the diagnosis of CCD is MRI.[15,16] Unfortunately, this modality can be limited by various factors, including accessibility, concerns regarding anesthesia in a geriatric animal, and cost concerns to the family.[15] While all options should be discussed, families should never be made to feel guilt or pressure to pursue advanced diagnostics that are outside of their personal budgets.

In comparisons between MR images, observed similarities between AD patients and CDS patients (specifically canine) included generalized cerebral cortical atrophy and ventricular enlargement.[15,16] It should be noted, however, that these findings may be consistent with normal aging of the brain, depending on severity[15]; while these MRI changes are suggestive of CDS, diagnostic results and clinical presentation should always be considered in tandem. Even when performed and correlated to the patient's presentation for CDS, MRI will not necessarily assist clinicians in the understanding of the patient's prognosis, which may also leave the pet parents feeling anxious and frustrated that they have limited options after such a significant investment in diagnostics.

So, while advanced imaging is the gold standard in the diagnosis of CDS, there are a variety of reasons as to why clients often decline referral for such options. Thus, when a clinician is presented with a patient who is suspected to be in decline due to CDS, and all other differentials have been excluded, the importance of an efficient, accurate assessment tool cannot be understated.

It is important to acknowledge that the following assessment tools are based on research and development within canine populations. While there is evidence that feline cognitive dysfunction presents similarly to CCD in both behavior and physical changes, research remains limited as to how presentations may vary. Canine-based tools are likely applicable to feline patients in most respects; however, variability in results may be observed based on species. It may be important to consider these differences when applying these tools in a clinical setting to ensure appropriate client expectations.

As mentioned previously, DISHAA (Disorientation, Interactions with owner alteration, Sleep-wake disturbances, House soiling, Activity level alterations, and Anxiety) was developed in 2012 as an acronym for the categories of clinical signs that were repeatedly reported in cases of CDS.[3,14] The DISHAA scoring tool is one option to consider when trying to determine the occurrence of CDS symptoms and the possible stage of the suspected disease.[14] Typically, this assessment can be completed by the pet owner in a matter of a few minutes, so it is efficient and generally user-friendly. Related to the DISHAA are 2 highly referred to and researched assessment tools, the Canine Dementia Scale (CADES) and the Canine Cognitive Dysfunction Rating Scale (CCDR).

The CADES assessment was developed in 2015 and consists of 17 items that can be assigned to 4 domains: "spatial orientation," "social interaction," "sleep–wake cycles," and "house-soiling".[17,18] Over the 17-item questionnaire, the total score ranges from 0 to 95 points and, based on the overall score, classifies dogs into 4 groups: normal aging (0–7 points), mild (8–23 points), moderate (24–44 points), or severe cognitive impairment (45–95 points).[17,18] As an added benefit, not only does this assessment account for severity of the CDS but also considers estimated progression based on initial and repeated evaluations.[18] Initial data collected in the development of the CADES assessment demonstrated that the 6 months conversion rate from mild cognitive impairment to moderate cognitive impairment was 24% in elderly dogs; the annual conversion rate reached up to 50%.[18] This evidence of the ability of the CADES assessment to predict the rate of continued cognitive decline makes it unique among CDS diagnostic tools. The CADES assessment was designed to be conducted in the clinical setting and can be completed in 20 to 30 minutes. It should be noted that during development, the assessment was conducted by a veterinarian through client interviews to ensure accurate reporting of clinical signs.[2]

Created by Salvin and colleagues in 2012, the CCDR scale was developed from data gathered from an online questionnaire completed by 957 owners of dogs aged 8 years or older; responses were gathered from over 11 countries.[17,19] Being an online questionnaire, the dogs were not examined by a veterinarian during the development phase of the assessment.[17] The CCDR consists of 13 questions regarding categories of spatial awareness, social interactions, and house soiling.[19] The first 7 questions examine the frequency of specified behaviors distinguishing dogs with or without cognitive impairment, and the last 6 questions pertain to changes in frequency of those specific behaviors over the last 6 months.[17,19] Once completed, the total questionnaire score ranges from 13 to 80 points and classifies dogs into one of the following 3 groups: No signs of CCD (0–39 pts), at risk for developing CCD (40–49 pts), and displaying signs of CCD (50+ patients).[17,19] Based on the initial data, the CCDR scale was found to yield high diagnostic accuracy at 99.3% indicating its ability to effectively distinguish advanced neurobehavioral changes associated with cognitive dysfunction from those of normal aging.[19]

When compared, the CADES and CCDR assessments were both considered as potentially useful in diagnosing CDS in canine populations.[17] Data analysis revealed that the CADES assessment classified dogs into more differentiated groups when it came to severity of CDS, thus potentially being a better evaluation for early diagnosis of mild disease and giving a more realistic evaluation of the study participants.[17] In contrast, the CCDR assessment was observed to be more accurate and appropriate for evaluating dogs with more severe clinical signs of CDS, and less accurate when determining normal aging signs from those of mild or early onset disease.[17] Based on this information, while both tools have their applications, veterinary professionals may want to consider the presentation of the patient and choose an assessment tool based on suspected progression of CDS symptoms.

Of course, diagnosis of any disease is only the first step in the process of treatment. Much like AD, treatment for CDS is based on management of clinical signs and changes in lifestyle to ensure safety and help preserve the individual's ability to function physically and mentally for as long as possible. Setting appropriate expectations for treatment results and providing education on disease progression and end-stage clinical signs are important steps following the diagnosis of CDS in veterinary patients.

TREATMENT AND PRACTICAL CARE RECOMMENDATIONS FOR PETS WITH COGNITIVE DYSFUNCTION SYNDROME

Because the physiologic causes of CDS remain unclear, treatment continues to be a challenge, especially as the disease progresses. A multimodal approach including prescription medications, dietary changes, nutraceuticals, exercise, and cognitive enrichment has generally been found to be the most successful in slowing the progression of cognitive dysfunction among both human and animal populations.

Neuroprotectants

Currently, selegiline (anipryl) is the only Food and Drug Administration (FDA)-approved drug for the treatment of CDS in canines; it is used off-label for feline patients exhibiting signs of CDS. As a type B monoamine oxidase inhibitor, selegiline is believed to improve CDS signs by contributing to neuroprotective effects on dopaminergic, noradrenergic, and cholinergic neurons, specifically at the cortex and the hippocampus.[6,7,20] In a study of 641 dogs exhibiting clinical signs of CDS, overall improvement was observed with daily dosing of selegiline hydrochloride administered at doses of 0.5 to 1.0 mg/kg once daily for 60 days.[20] On day 60 of the trial, 77.2% of the dogs showed an overall improvement, with only minor adverse effects, which included mild GI upset.[20] Response to treatment was noted to vary based on clinical signs considered; improvement rates ranged from 67.8% in activity or sleep–wake cycle to 77.8% in disorientation and interaction with family members.[20] These results are important to consider as sleep disturbances and changes in interaction with family members are 2 of the highest ranked concerns among caretakers of pets with CDS.[21]

In dogs, selegiline dosing is 0.5 to 1.0 mg/kg once daily for 30 days.[14] If, after 30 days, there is little to no improvement, the dose can be increased to the next tablet size for the next 30 days.[14] In cats, recommended dosing is 0.25 to 1.0 mg/kg once daily.[5,14] While side effects are relatively rare, it should be noted that combining selegiline with other psychoactive medications such as fluoxetine, mirtazapine, amitriptyline, and clomipramine (many of which are prescribed to animals with CDS signs, specifically nighttime disturbances) may increase the risk of serotonin syndrome, and such combinations should be considered with caution. For best effects, selegiline should be started as early into the CDS disease process as possible.[14]

In AD studies, there is promising data indicating that levetiracetam (Keppra) can be used to improve cognitive function in affected patients.[22] In human patients, levetiracetam is believed to work by reducing amyloid β accumulation and enhancing synaptic function thus improving cognitive function.[22] In animal models, levetiracetam has been observed to decrease neuronal network dysfunction and inflammation, thus alleviating cognitive decline.[22] It should be noted, however, that results have varied among canine patients with some negative behavior changes being reported; ongoing research is needed to better evaluate the benefits of levetiracetam when managing CDS in small animal patients.

Anxiolytics and Benzodiazepines

As discussed, 2 of the most concerning signs of CDS for pet owners include nighttime disturbances and increased signs of anxiety such as vocalizing; over time, these challenges may create exhaustion and tension within the household due to loss of sleep, worry about the pet's status, and resentment toward the pet or other family members. To help these CDS behaviors, adjunctive therapies including anxiolytics and benzodiazepines may be prescribed. Alprazolam, amitriptyline, clomipramine, fluoxetine, and trazadone are typically good options used to decrease anxiety and improve sleep among CDS patients.[7,15] As a reminder, these classes of medications should be used with caution or avoided in pets who are already taking selegiline for cognitive support.[7,15] An alternative to anxiolytics, gabapentin, a gabapentinoid class medication, can also be used as an antianxiety and sedative option for both dogs and cats and tends to carry a lower risk of side effects even when combined with other medications.

Diet and Nutraceuticals

The benefits of high-value nutrition and nutraceuticals have been well documented in AD research, and, as a result, have influenced similar research in the field of CDS. Overall, research has found positive outcomes when treatment protocols include omega-3 fatty acids, medium chain triglycerides, and antioxidants (vitamins C and E).[7,23,24] Systemic reviews on research regarding nutrition and CDS have found that omega-3 fatty acids, particularly eicosapentaenoic acid (EPA) and docosahexaenoic acid (DHA), have shown significant cognitive benefits in aging animals, much as they have been seen to do in humans.[7,23,24] These positive protective effects are the result of omega-3 fatty acids reducing pro-inflammatory metabolites, enhancing antioxidant defenses, and promoting neogenesis, thus improving blood circulation to the brain and protecting brain volume.[23] While antioxidants such as vitamins A, C, and D alone have not demonstrated clear efficacy, they remain essential in protecting omega-3 fatty acids from oxidation and so should be used in combination to ensure therapeutic effectiveness.[23]

Other supplements, such as S-adenosyl methionine (SAMe), medium-chain triglycerides, homotaurine, Ginko, and apoaequorin, have also shown promising cognitive benefits in aging pets and should not be overlooked when considering a multimodal approach to treatment.[23,24] Of particular interest, SAMe has been shown to significantly increase activity levels and improve cognitive awareness among test subjects.[14] SAMe is marketed for dogs and cats as Denosyl[R] (produced by Nutramax). Another option is Senilife[R] (produced by Ceva), a blend of phosphatidylserine, pyridoxine, Ginko biloba extract, and D-alpha-tocopherol.[14] These components have been shown to improve short-term memory and decrease the signs of CDS in canine study populations.[7,14]

Recommendations for diets shown to be neuroprotective include Brain Aging Care B/D Hills Prescription Diet and Bright Minds. These diets combine high levels of antioxidants, amino acids, and omega-3 fatty acids to ensure daily intake of enriched nutrition. Additionally, families may opt to seek input and recommendations from a licensed veterinary nutritionist if homemade diets rich in dense nutrients and omega-3 fatty acids are preferred.

Safety in the Home Environment

As cognitive and physical decline advance, CDS pets may begin to experience unsafe circumstances within homes that they have lived in for years. Even if the environment remains unchanged, CDS signs of worsening spatial awareness, increased pacing and wandering, and gait changes resulting in loss of balance may leave affected pets vulnerable to accidents. Falls, entrapment under or around furniture, and becoming lost and generally disoriented in the home are all valid concerns.

Maintaining a quiet, comfortable, safe place for any senior pet can be beneficial to their overall health, as can a consistent daily routine.[7] This is especially true for pets with CDS.[7] Providing a quiet and safe area for retreat from the daily hustle and bustle of the home is often necessary for wellness and safety. It is important to remember that as CDS progresses, clinical signs often leave pets less able to cope with everyday stresses or sudden sensory challenges. Therefore, reminding families to be cognizant of how much or how fast changes in the home are made can be important to avoiding exaggerated signs of CDS.

Environmental modifications, including baby gates to create safety boundaries (especially where stairs are concerned), traction mats to prevent falls, and nightlights to improve visibility, can offer a level of security for both the pets and their owners. Additionally, ensuring easy access to the pet's necessities, including food and water bowls, litter boxes, and potty pads, is important to help maintain independence and reduce anxiety.

Just as safety concerns can increase with worsening CDS signs inside the home, risks of injury can also increase outdoors. Of particular concern is water safety when it comes to pools and backyard ponds. Bodies of water can often be overlooked by families as a safety risk, especially when a pet has spent years enjoying the water. As CDS progresses, even a familiar body of water can become a significant danger. A compromised pet who suddenly falls into a pool or pond, regardless of depth, may panic and become disoriented and exhausted, leading to a drowning event. While it may not be the first consideration during a clinic visit, veterinary professionals should be prepared to inquire about the pet's access to water and to discuss the importance of reliable barriers (pool gates, fences, etc.) and increased owner vigilance.

Within the same vein of concern is the importance of addressing the possibility of wandering outside of normal outdoor boundaries. Often, families feel confident that a pet will "always stay in the yard," or "never need a leash," but these beliefs are not accounting for CDS changes. Reinforcing the need for physical boundaries, updating identification information (collar tags and microchip registration), appropriate leashing, and monitoring CDS-afflicted pets when outside is an especially pressing topic for pets who are demonstrating wandering and disorientation symptoms.

Grooming and Hygiene

An often-frustrating aspect of CDS in both cats and dogs is house soiling. Defecating and urinating in inappropriate places in the home, incontinence while sleeping, and becoming less capable of maintaining normal self-grooming habits may all be signs of disease progression. Unfortunately, house soiling and incontinence are more than inconveniences; these behaviors changes can lead to secondary skin infections and scalding, create sanitation concerns in the home environment, and test the human–animal bond by worsening caretaker fatigue.

Families should be prepared to manage these signs of hygiene changes with supplies such as potty pads, low-walled litter boxes, waterproof bedding, waterless shampoo, and baby wipes. If urine and feces are trapped in the pet's haircoat, owners may need to consider sanitary grooming to shorten hair and remove debris—it is vital to keep perianal, prepuce, and vulva regions clean to reduce the risk of UTIs, dermatitis, and yeast infections. Additionally, keeping senior animals' nails and interdigital hair trimmed can also be important to their ability to continue to walk comfortably and with better traction. Because some pets will become increasingly sensitive to touch and manipulations of their limbs due to the compounding effects CDS and arthritis, grooming, bathing, and brushing may become increasingly challenging. If needed, sedative dosing with some of the anxiolytic options previously discussed may help to keep hygiene care manageable and safe.

Environmental Enrichment

In humans, a lifestyle of physical, social, and mental engagement has been proven to decrease the risk of cognitive decline in senior years, and the same applies to our pet population. For pets who are diagnosed with CDS, encouraging mental stimulation and regular, low-impact exercise can help to slow the progression and decrease the severity of clinical signs of CDS by releasing antianxiety endorphins, increasing learning, and maintaining memory.[22]

Environmental enrichment can be as simple as introducing new toys, rotating toys to maintain novelty, utilizing alternate feeding methods such as snuffle mats and graze feeding, and providing socialization times with conspecifics and family members.[7,24] Ensuring that time is reserved for these enrichment activities not only benefits the pet but can also be very important for maintaining the human–animal bond in the final stages of a pet's life. At a time when medications and hygiene may be large parts of the daily routine, finding moments of simple joy and creating new, happy memories with a senior best friend is sometimes the best medicine for both the human and the pet alike.

CAREGIVER SUPPORT AND END-OF-LIFE DISCUSSIONS

Because CDS tends to progress over weeks to months, veterinarians must consider the changes that will inevitably occur not only in their patient but also within the family unit. Unfortunately, caregiver burden and anticipatory grief will escalate exponentially with time and the severity of cognitive decline. While most pet guardians express complete dedication to their beloved pet, considering their role as caretakers to be an honor,[21] it is important to encourage families to share in the responsibilities of monitoring, hygiene needs, and medicating. When all responsibilities fall onto one person, it will inevitably lead to burnout, resentment within the family, guilt, and euthanasia considerations earlier in the disease process.

Because CDS can degrade so many aspects of our pets' lives, the negative impact of this health condition on the human–animal bond cannot be overlooked. Pet parents often become overwhelmed with the challenges that CDS brings as it advances or as it complicates comorbidities. Continued support from veterinary professionals is pivotal in reducing anxieties and confusion in caregivers.

According to the 2023 survey by Taylor and colleagues, when pet guardians were asked to name a health issue, their dog had been diagnosed with by a veterinarian. Only 4% of survey respondents named dementia.[21] However, up to 75% of dogs within this survey population met the required threshold scores using the DISHAA assessment, indicating a significant diagnosis gap.[21] Almost all the canines who had received a veterinary diagnosis were moderately or severely affected by the disease, supporting the perception that diagnosis mostly occurs in advanced presentations.[21] Taylor and colleagues also found that prescription rates for CCD-specific medications (including selegiline) were extremely low in dogs with all levels of CDS; only 7% of dogs with severe CDS scores had been prescribed medications to help alleviate clinical signs.[21]

While the low occurrence of diagnosis and medication prescribing in this study population may be due to various perceptions (symptom-overlap with other health concerns, uncertainty of drug effectiveness or drug interactions, or owner ignorance when considering relevant clinical signs), it is alarming to see how underestimated this disease and its possible treatments were within the study population. These findings reinforce the need for veterinarians to invest time and knowledge into CDS (diagnosis and management) as a lack of such leads to increased caregiver burden and reduced quality of life for the entire family. Veterinary support staff, veterinary social workers, and pet loss grief counselors are also valuable resources for families who may require additional time, advice, and support through the progression of CDS, especially when considering end-of-life decisions.

CDS is not typically a disease that is financially costly to treat or manage when compared to health conditions like cancer or diabetes; however, time constraints and emotional strength budgets may be stretched by the clinical signs. When any caregiver budgets are becoming exhausted, the consideration for humane euthanasia to prevent further decline of the pet, avoid further stress on the human–animal bond, and ensure a peaceful quality of death is justified.

SUMMARY

While CDS is not a disease that creates a sense of urgency in the veterinary community, it is a significant, devastating neurodegenerative disease that gradually degrades a pet's quality of life mentally, physically, and socially. Because the signs of CDS mimic so many other age-related health conditions, it is important to conduct a thorough general workup including a detailed patient history, physical exam, neurologic assessment, blood work, blood pressure, and possibly imaging including radiograph and ultrasound. Any comorbidities that are identified should be addressed to the best of the veterinarian's ability, as CDS may only exaggerate uncontrolled symptoms.

Use of researched CDS assessment tools can be extremely helpful in a clinical setting to diagnose and stage symptoms of neurodegeneration. The DISHAA, CADES, and CCDR are all excellent options, and while these are typically used in canine patients, can generally be applied to feline patients as well. Assessment tools should be evaluated with the help of a veterinary professional to ensure accuracy and help avoid owners misreading clinical behaviors as simply signs of a pet "getting old."

With the complexities of CDS in mind, treatment requires a tailored, multimodal approach that considers the neurobehavioral nature of the disease. Prescription medications like selegiline (Anipryl) and supplements rich in omega-3 fatty acids have been shown to aid as neuroprotectants, slowing the progression of neuronal death and inflammation. It is often necessary to consider anxiolytics, gabapentin, and benzodiazepines, which can be used alone or in combination to help decrease the frequency and severity of anxiety, sleep disturbances, and other related behavior changes.

The chronic and progressive nature of this syndrome can be a double-edged sword; while it means that the family typically has time to share with their pet, the gradual decline may also increase anticipatory grief and make decisions for the end of life very difficult. For these reasons, early and ongoing support from veterinary professionals is imperative as clinical signs of CDS advance.

Veterinary medicine has always advanced with the goal of prolonging the lives of animals. But, as the pet population continues to exceed lifespan expectations, our profession has a responsibility to increase research into diseases and health concerns of senior and geriatric animals. By improving our understanding of the pathophysiology of CDS, we may be able to improve early diagnostics, prevention measures, and treatment options. The veterinary community's increasing knowledge and confidence in managing this disease will in turn allow affected families to be better educated, supported, and empowered so that their last miles of their senior pets' lives can be walked with love and dignity.

CLINICS CARE POINTS

- Diagnosis of CDS is often one of rule-out. Evaluation should include physical and neurologic examinations, blood work, blood pressure, and imaging for possible health concerns or comorbidities. Use assessment tools like DISHAA, CADES, or CCDR early on if CDS is suspected.
- Because client conversations about CDS may be lengthy and require extra time in a clinic setting, consider training nursing staff on how to use CDS assessment tools and answer general client questions.
- If suspected, begin treatment for CDS as early as possible for best results. Selegiline is the only FDA-approved medication for the treatment of CDS in small animals; use of medications to help slow neuronal loss of CDS is most effective when started early.
- A multimodal approach to CDS management is recommended for best outcomes—often, this includes prescription medications to reduce sleep disturbances and anxiety, nutraceuticals to improve cognitive health, nutrition high in omega-3 fatty acids, and environmental enrichment.
- Home environment safety considerations for pets with CDS should be discussed to avoid potential emergency situations such as falls, drowning events, and wandering from the home.
- Caregiver support is an important, often neglected, aspect of navigating CDS, considering the chronic nature of the disease. Encourage family members to share responsibilities, offer access to support for anticipatory grief counseling, and do not shy away from discussions about when end-of-life decisions may be appropriate to consider.

DISCLOSURES

The author has nothing to disclose.

REFERENCES

1. Alzheimer's Association. Stages of Alzheimer's. Alzheimer's Disease and Dementia, Available at: https://www.alz.org/alzheimers-dementia/stages, 2025, (Accessed 25 August 2025).
2. Managing cognitive dysfunction and behavioral anxiety. AAHA, Available at: https://www.aaha.org/resources/2023-aaha-senior-care-guidelines-for-dogs-and-cats/managing-cognitive-dysfunction-and-behavioral-anxiety/, 2024, (Accessed 25 August 2025).
3. Luca C, Casini L, Cecchi F, et al. The canine cognitive dysfunction syndrome: epidemiology, pathophysiology and diagnosis. Dog Behavior 2023;9(2).
4. MacQuiddy B, Moreno JA, Kusick B, et al. Assessment of risk factors in dogs with presumptive advanced canine cognitive dysfunction. Front Vet Sci 2022;9:958488.

5. Landsberg GM, Denenberg S, Araujo JA. Cognitive dysfunction in cats: a syndrome we used to dismiss as 'old age'. J Feline Med Surg 2010;12(11):837–48.
6. Kim SH, Hao J. Recent advances in diagnostic and therapeutic strategies for canine cognitive dysfunction. Am J Vet Res 2025;86(8):1–8. Advance online publication.
7. Woodruff D. Essay 8: cognitive dysfunction and related sleep disturbances. In Gardner M, McVety D, editors. Treatment and care of the geriatric veterinary patient. Hoboken (NJ): Wiley Blackwell; 2017. p. 57–76.
8. Cummings BJ, Head E, Afagh AJ, et al. Beta-amyloid accumulation correlates with cognitive dysfunction in the aged canine. Neurobiol Learn Mem 1996; 66(1):11–23.
9. Di Benedetto G, Burgaletto C, Bellanca CM, et al. Role of microglia and astrocytes in Alzheimer's Disease: from neuroinflammation to Ca^{2+} homeostasis dysregulation. Cells 2022;11(17):2728.
10. Mohandas E, Rajmohan V, Raghunath B. Neurobiology of Alzheimer's disease. Indian J Psychiatry 2009;51(1):55–61.
11. Habiba U, Ozawa M, Chambers JK, et al. Neuronal deposition of Amyloid-β oligomers and hyperphosphorylated Tau is closely connected with cognitive dysfunction in aged dogs. Journal of Alzheimer's disease reports 2021;5(1): 749–60.
12. Abey A, Davies D, Goldsbury C, et al. Distribution of tau hyperphosphorylation in canine dementia resembles early Alzheimer's disease and other tauopathies. Brain Pathol 2021;31(1):144–62.
13. Hines AD, McGrath S, Latham AS, et al. Activated gliosis, accumulation of amyloid β, and hyperphosphorylation of tau in aging canines with and without cognitive decline. Front Aging Neurosci 2023;15:1128521.
14. Landsberg GM, Nichol J, Araujo JA. Cognitive dysfunction syndrome: a disease of canine and feline brain aging. Vet Clin Small Anim Pract 2012;42(4):749–vii.
15. Dewey CW, Davies ES, Xie H, et al. Canine cognitive dysfunction: pathophysiology, diagnosis, and treatment. Vet Clin Small Anim Pract 2019;49(3):477–99.
16. Ehrenzweig J, Hunter RP. Canine cognitive decline and Alzheimer disease: clinical insights to solve a shared one-health problem. J Am Vet Med Assoc 2023; 261(11):1597–604.
17. Haake J, Meller S, Meyerhoff N, et al. Comparing standard screening questionnaires of canine behavior for assessment of cognitive dysfunction. Front Vet Sci 2024;11:1374511.
18. Madari A, Farbakova J, Katina S, et al. Assessment of severity and progression of canine cognitive dysfunction syndrome using the CAnine DEmentia Scale (CADES). Appl Anim Behav Sci 2015;171:138–45.
19. Salvin HE, McGreevy PD, Sachdev PS, et al. The canine cognitive dysfunction rating scale (CCDR): a data-driven and ecologically relevant assessment tool. Vet J (London, England: 1997) 2011;188(3):331–6.
20. Campbell S, Trettien A, Kozan B. A noncomparative open-label study evaluating the effect of selegiline hydrochloride in a clinical setting. Vet Therapeut: research in applied veterinary medicine 2001;2(1):24–39.
21. Taylor TL, Smith BP, Hazel SJ. Guardians' perceptions of caring for a dog with canine cognitive dysfunction. Vet Rec 2024;194(2):e3266.
22. Mohamadi MH, Bavafa A, Salehi S, et al. Cognitive effect of levetiracetam in patients with Alzheimer's disease or mild cognitive impairment: a systematic review. Curr Ther Res Clin Exp 2025;103:100798.

23. Blanchard T, Eppe J, Mugnier A, et al. Enhancing cognitive functions in aged dogs and cats: a systematic review of enriched diets and nutraceuticals. GeroScience 2025;47(3):2925–47.
24. Taylor T, Fernandez E, Handley K, et al. Non-pharmacological interventions for the treatment of canine cognitive dysfunction: a scoping review. Appl Anim Behav Sci 2023;269:106097. https://doi.org/10.1016/j.applanim.2023.106097.

Managing Comorbidity

Coordinating Care for Complex Geriatric Cases

Tyler Carmack, DVM, CVA, CHPV, CVFT, CTPEP, CPEV, CVPP

KEYWORDS

- Multimorbidity • Comorbidity • Polypharmacy • Quality of life (QoL)
- Functional status • Veterinary hospice • Palliative care

KEY POINTS

- Multimorbidity is common in senior pets, often complicating diagnosis and requiring holistic, patient-centered care.
- Disease processes frequently interact (eg, hyperthyroidism masking kidney disease), making contextualized monitoring essential.
- Polypharmacy is often necessary but must be balanced against risks of adverse interactions and caregiver burden.
- Functional assessments and quality of life tools are critical in guiding care decisions beyond disease control.
- Coordinated, interdisciplinary veterinary care, combined with empathetic communication and education, supports both patient comfort and caregiver resilience.

INTRODUCTION

As companion animals live longer, veterinary professionals are increasingly called upon to manage geriatric patients with multiple coexisting chronic conditions—referred to as comorbidities or, in more complex cases, multimorbidity. The American Geriatrics Society defines comorbidity as the presence of one or more additional diseases alongside a primary or "index" condition.[1] For instance, it is very common for a senior dog diagnosed with lymphoma to also have mild osteoarthritis. Multimorbidity, by contrast, refers to multiple concurrent chronic conditions without a single dominant disease, as in an older cat simultaneously managing diabetes, hyperthyroidism, and kidney disease.[1] These presentations are not only common but often define the clinical landscape of senior veterinary practice.

Recent studies estimate that multimorbidity affects 22.6% to 65.8% of senior dogs, with similarly high prevalence in older cats.[2] In an Australian study, 52% of dogs and cats of all ages showed intercurrent conditions at the time of vaccination.[3] Risk factors

Hospice and Palliative Care, Caring Pathways, 4740 Baxter Road #105, Virginia Beach, VA 23462, USA
E-mail address: dr.tyler@caringpathways.com

Vet Clin Small Anim 56 (2026) 419–430
https://doi.org/10.1016/j.cvsm.2025.09.029 vetsmall.theclinics.com

Abbreviations	
CGA	Comprehensive Geriatric Assessment
CMI	clinical metrology instrument
NSAIDs	nonsteroidal anti-inflammatory drugs
QoL	quality of life

include advancing age, neuter status, and breed predispositions.[4] These findings underscore that complex disease management is often the rule rather than the exception in geriatric veterinary patients.

Effective management of multimorbid pets requires a contextualized, patient-centered approach that integrates medical, ethical, and emotional considerations. Holistic geriatric care prioritizes quality of life (QoL), accounts for age-related changes in physiology and pharmacology, and recognizes the potential for both treatment burden and caregiver fatigue.[5,6] Clear communication with pet owners is essential, as treatment decisions must reflect the animal's well-being and the caregiver's capacity.[7] Modern guidelines for senior pet care emphasize evidence-based medicine, client education, and palliative strategies to optimize comfort and extend a meaningful life.[8]

Veterinary teams must also navigate the ethical dimensions of geriatric care. Advanced interventions can improve clinical outcomes but may inadvertently prolong suffering.[9,10] Strategies such as proactive client education, setting humane endpoints, and incorporating clinical metrology instruments (CMIs) are recommended to guide decision-making. By balancing sophisticated medical care with compassionate, context-driven management, veterinarians can best serve the needs of complex geriatric patients and their caregivers. Success hinges on integrating evidence-based medicine with palliative principles, ethical deliberation, and empathetic client communication.

UNDERSTANDING CO-MORBIDITIES IN GERIATRIC ANIMALS

Common Co-morbid Conditions

Senior dogs and cats frequently develop age-related diseases, with distinctive patterns in each species. In dogs, common disorders include osteoarthritis, periodontal disease, otitis externa, and obesity, all of which can substantially affect comfort and mobility.[4] Age-related trends also shift clinical priorities: preventive medicine visits are predominant in younger dogs, whereas active management of heart disease, kidney disease, and Cushing's disease is more prevalent causes for hospital visits in older dogs.[11] Cats commonly develop cardiovascular disease, chronic kidney disease, and malignant neoplasia in their senior years.[12] Breed-specific analyses reveal that dental calculus, tooth extractions, and dog bites remain frequent concerns across canine populations.[13]

Cognitive dysfunction, sensory decline, and chronic pain are frequent, but underrecognized contributors to multimorbidity. Dogs aged 8 years or older show high rates of one or more sensory (visual, auditory, and olfactory) impairments, which are strongly associated with age-related cognitive deterioration[14,15] This mirrors human findings in which sensory impairments are independently predictive of cognitive decline and dementia.[16] This relationship is likely bidirectional; sensory impairments can both contribute to and be affected by cognitive decline, as seen in human Alzheimer's disease.[17] Training and enrichment activities may offer cognitive protection, highlighting the importance of the veterinary team prescribing early behavioral and environmental interventions.[15]

Pathophysiologic Interactions of Comorbidities

Pharmacologic concerns of comorbidities

Managing comorbid conditions in geriatric companion animals frequently involves utilizing polypharmacy, which inherently increases the risk of drug–drug and drug–disease interactions. Veterinarians must carefully assess potential drug–drug and drug–disease interactions, considering how medications may interact with existing therapies or exacerbate underlying conditions. Incorporating both pharmacologic and non-pharmacologic modalities in pain management strategies, as advocated in the *AAHA/AAFP Pain Management Guidelines for Dogs and Cats,* is crucial.[18] This holistic approach not only addresses pain effectively but also minimizes the risk of adverse drug reactions in older pets, ensuring comprehensive care tailored to their specific health needs.

Drug–drug interactions. Clinically significant impacts may occur when commonly prescribed medications interact. Additionally, the use of multiple concurrent medications raises the possibility of adverse events, such as serotonin syndrome, when serotonergic agents are combined. Careful selection, dosing, and monitoring of drugs—along with routine reassessment of the medication list—are essential to minimize these risks and optimize therapeutic outcomes in senior patients.[6,18]

Drug–disease interactions. In geriatric companion animal patients, managing drug–disease interactions requires a nuanced approach due to the prevalence of subclinical organ dysfunction, as well as overt diseases that can substantially impact drug pharmacology. As highlighted by KuKanich in 2012, these conditions may alter drug metabolism and clearance, influencing treatment efficacy and safety. Older patients often have age-related physiologic changes, such as altered hepatic metabolism or reduced renal clearance, that can exacerbate risks. For example, the use of long-term furosemide therapy in patients with cardiac disease may lead to dehydration and further strain on kidney function, necessitating careful monitoring and dose adjustments.[19,20]

Functional Versus Disease-Based Assessment

In geriatric companion animal care, there is a noticeable shift from a purely disease-based approach to a more holistic functional assessment centered on managing QoL. Traditionally, veterinary care often prioritized curing ailments, but as pets age, the emphasis increasingly leans toward optimizing their daily functioning and overall well-being. This paradigmatic change underscores the importance of validated CMIs in veterinary practice. The use of validated and non-validated QoL assessment tools has been shown to increase the frequency of care plan discussions with the veterinary team.[21] As the focus continues to shift toward enhancing the lives of geriatric companion animals, the integration of validated QoL assessments, chronic pain scales, sleep questionnaires, and cognitive dysfunction screening assessments stands pivotal in guiding effective management strategies that prioritize comfort, functionality, response to treatment, and overall QoL.

DIAGNOSTIC AND MONITORING STRATEGIES

Managing comorbidities in geriatric companion animals requires a systematic, multidimensional approach guided by the Comprehensive Geriatric Assessment (CGA) strategy widely used in human medicine. In veterinary practice, a CGA involves evaluating medical conditions, functional status, nutrition, cognitive and behavioral health, and the pet's home environment to develop a holistic, individualized care plan for the patient and their caregivers. History-taking in complex geriatric cases should go beyond current clinical signs, capturing longitudinal information such as progression of chronic diseases, treatment responses, and subtle changes in daily activity or cognition reported by caregivers. Owners often provide crucial insights into appetite trends, mobility patterns, and behavioral shifts that may signal that medication adjustments, education, and investigation are warranted (**Fig. 1**).

Baseline and serial monitoring form the foundation for managing multiple chronic conditions, enabling clinicians to detect clinically significant trends rather than isolated

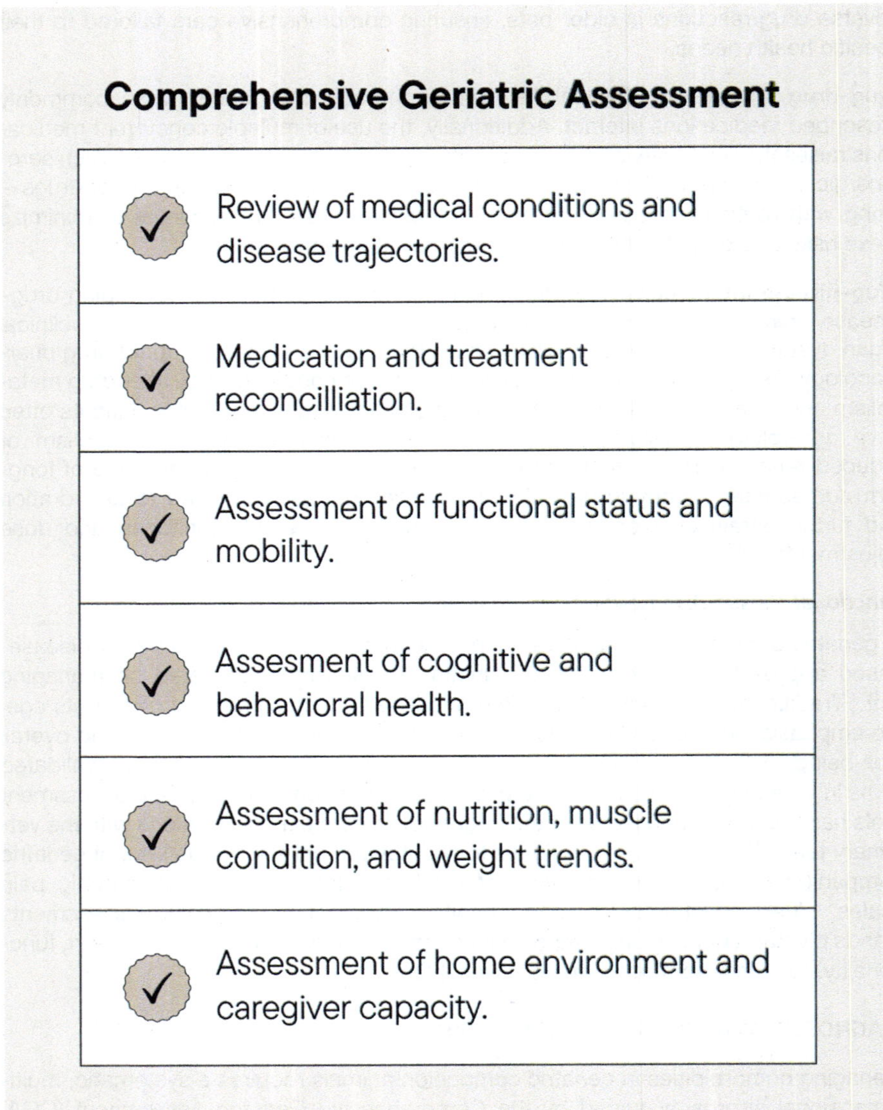

Fig. 1. A modified veterinary equivalent of the Comprehensive Geriatric Assessment (CGA) used in human medicine provides a useful structure for managing multimorbidities in geriatric veterinary patients.

abnormalities. Routine laboratory work, including complete blood count, serum chemistry, urinalysis, and endocrine screening, helps identify emerging complications such as renal insufficiency, electrolyte disturbances, or medication-induced adverse effects. Imaging modalities like thoracic radiographs, abdominal ultrasound, or targeted orthopedic radiographs provide structural context and can guide interventions when symptoms overlap between comorbidities. Importantly, client-reported outcomes, including mobility and pain scores, appetite and activity trackers, and QoL questionnaires, offer a real-time perspective on the pet's daily function and comfort that may not be evident during periodic clinic visits. Interpreting changes in laboratory or imaging results requires careful contextualization, for example, a mild creatinine elevation may be less concerning in a stable stage 2 chronic kidney disease patient than in one experiencing concurrent dehydration from gastrointestinal disease. Integrating multiple data streams, objective diagnostics, and subjective owner observations allow veterinarians to better distinguish between disease progression, treatment effects, and natural variability, guiding timely and appropriate adjustments to the care plan. It is also important to consider and plan for a threshold when diagnostic results may not have a substantial actionable impact on the patient's care plan. For example, many end-stage osteoarthritis patients would be immobile if pain medications were reduced or removed. In this scenario, even if bloodwork provided evidence of compromised hepatic or renal function, discussing the risks and benefits of continuing a nonsteroidal medication without further bloodwork monitoring may be most appropriate to maintain the pet's comfort and caregiver's compliance.

Risk stratification and prognostication are crucial for aligning medical interventions with both patient welfare and family expectations. Estimating life expectancy in geriatric patients with comorbidities is inherently difficult. Education about the possible interplay between primary disease trajectories, potential complications, anticipated clinical symptoms, and the pet's baseline resilience is important information for the pet's family. Early, transparent discussions with caregivers about anticipated disease course(s) and likely endpoints foster shared decision-making and minimize crisis-driven choices. Goals of care should be reassessed whenever there is a substantial change in clinical status, such as a new diagnosis, acute decompensation, or a notable decline in function. This high-touch approach allows the care plan to evolve, transitioning from curative or disease-stabilizing strategies toward palliative, comfort-focused interventions when appropriate. By integrating human gerontology principles like the CGA, ongoing monitoring, and proactive education, veterinarians can manage complex comorbidities in geriatric companion animals while optimizing both lifespan and healthspan.

DEVELOPING INTEGRATED TREATMENT PLANS

Principles of Polypharmacy Management

Managing multiple comorbidities in geriatric companion animals often necessitates the use of polypharmacy, which can increase the risk of drug interactions, adverse effects, and treatment complexity. A core principle is to routinely evaluate every medication for necessity, efficacy, and compatibility with the patient's overall health status. Veterinary professionals should perform regular medication reconciliations, particularly when new prescriptions are introduced, to identify potential contraindications such as nonsteroidal anti-inflammatory drugs (NSAIDs) combined with corticosteroids or overlapping nephrotoxic agents in patients with kidney compromise. As long-term risks of medications become less of a concern, it is also important to consider that short-term risks, such as gastrointestinal upset, may have a more substantial impact on QoL for the pet and the caregiver than they would in a younger animal and can influence the timing of euthanasia. Anticipating and preparing the families for potential complications can help mitigate the severity of these risks.

Communication with pet owners is crucial to ensure accurate dosing, compliance, and monitoring for side effects. In the context of advanced geriatric hospice care, deprescribing strategies take on special significance. As disease progresses and QoL priorities shift, decreasing the medication burden, whether by reducing the number of medications, the doses of medications, or utilizing more convenient formulations, may improve comfort, simplify caregiving, and minimize the risk of drug interactions. Tapering or discontinuing nonessential drugs, such as long-term preventive therapies or supplements that no longer contribute meaningfully to the animal's well-being, should be approached thoughtfully and collaboratively with the owner, aligning decisions with the goals of care and the pet's remaining life expectancy.

Pain and Symptom Management

Effective management of chronic pain and clinical symptoms is central to supporting geriatric animals with multiple health challenges. Multimodal pain control, using complementary pharmacologic and non-pharmacologic strategies, can address the diverse mechanisms of pain seen in degenerative joint disease, neuropathies, and cancer-related discomfort[18] For example, in osteoarthritis cases, combining NSAIDs, gabapentin/pregabalin, amantadine, acetaminophen, and other adjunctive therapies such as acupuncture, prescribed exercise, pulsed electromagnetic pulse therapy, and/or photobiomodulation may enhance comfort while limiting reliance on any single drug. Holistic comfort and QoL management extend beyond pain to other common comorbid manifestations like nausea, inappetence, weakness, and incontinence. Appetite stimulants, antiemetics, and careful use of gastrointestinal protectants can improve nutritional intake and QoL. Incontinence, whether due to age-related sphincter weakness, decreased mobility, or endocrine disease, can often be mitigated with medications, absorbent bedding, or elevated hygiene practices to reduce owner stress and maintain the pet's independence and dignity. Veterinary teams must remain vigilant to the cumulative effect of seemingly minor symptoms. For example, uncontrolled nausea, chronic diarrhea, and/or sleep disruption can have a profound cumulative impact on welfare. Regular reassessment ensures that interventions remain proportionate to the pet's changing needs, the family's caregiving capacity, and do not inadvertently contribute to suffering.

Nutrition, Mobility, and Environmental Modifications

Optimizing nutrition and environmental support plays an essential role in managing comorbidities in older pets. Diet formulation should reflect both the animal's underlying health conditions and the practical realities of feeding at home. For example, a senior dog with concurrent chronic kidney disease, cognitive dysfunction, dental disease, and osteoarthritis may require a renal-supportive diet enriched with omega-3 fatty acids and antioxidants while also needing to be soft, palatable, and energy-dense to prevent muscle loss.[22–25] Veterinary nutritionists can help balance multiple dietary goals, sometimes using home-cooked or hybrid feeding strategies. Mobility support is equally critical, as declining strength, coordination, and joint function compound the challenges of multimorbidity in geriatric pets. Tools such as harnesses, slings, ramps, traction devices, and non-slip flooring reduce the risk of injury and enable continued engagement in daily activities. In-home environmental modifications, such as restricting access to stairs, elevating food and water bowls, or providing orthopedically supportive bedding, can dramatically enhance comfort and independence.[25] Integrating environmental enrichment, even in modified or simplified forms, supports cognitive health and emotional well-being, helping pets maintain a sense of routine and engagement despite physical limitations. Combined with the recommended nutritional support, these interventions work synergistically to slow cognitive decline.[26,27]

Individualizing Care Plans

The successful management of geriatric animals with multimorbidities ultimately depends on individualized, owner-centered care planning. Veterinarians must consider the caregiver's capabilities, preferences, and emotional readiness when designing treatment plans, recognizing that the most medically comprehensive approach is not always the most sustainable or compassionate. Cultural perspectives, lifestyle constraints, and financial realities all shape the range of feasible interventions. Open communication fosters trust and allows for collaborative decision-making, ensuring that owners feel supported rather than overwhelmed, exhausted, or judged. Care plans should remain dynamic, with goals reassessed regularly to reflect the animal's condition, response to treatment, and the family's evolving priorities.

At some point, the medical focus should transition from disease modification to comfort-oriented palliative care, emphasizing symptom control and daily enjoyment over extending total lifespan.[28] Documenting and frequently reassessing QoL scales and other relevant clinical measurement instruments facilitates timely adjustments and prevents unnecessary suffering. By tailoring interventions to the unique intersection of medical needs, caregiver burden, and human-animal bond considerations, veterinarians can honor both the patient's autonomy and dignity as well as the caregiver's values, even in the face of complex and progressive illness.

COORDINATING THE VETERINARY TEAM

Interdisciplinary Collaboration

Effective care for geriatric pets with multiple disease processes relies on the collaboration of an interdisciplinary veterinary team, ensuring that each patient benefits from the diverse expertise of multiple providers and pet professionals. The general practitioner typically serves as the central provider, overseeing routine health assessments, monitoring chronic conditions, and issuing referrals to specialists as needed. Internal medicine specialists may be engaged for complex diseases such as renal insufficiency or endocrine disorders, while oncologists, cardiologists, and neurologists contribute to the diagnosis and management of advanced conditions that commonly arise in older pets. Rehabilitation practices are often integral in maintaining mobility, muscle mass, and overall function, while veterinary hospice and palliative care teams guide comfort-focused interventions and end-of-life planning. Coordinating these services requires clear case management to prevent fragmented care, with an emphasis on continuity as the pet transitions between primary, specialty, and supportive care settings. Proactive scheduling of follow-up visits, clear communication between and among care teams, and consensus regarding care priorities ensure that interventions are complementary rather than duplicative or conflicting, ultimately supporting the pet's QoL. It's also important to consider the overall demand on the patient and caregiver. Utilization of telemedicine and house-call services, when appropriate, can offer flexibility for the caregiver while encouraging communication and reassessment.

Client Communication and Education

Geriatric pet care can quickly become overwhelming for owners, particularly when multiple conditions and specialists are involved, making client communication a central tenet of effective care coordination. Veterinary professionals must balance the complexity and nuances of medical recommendations while maintaining clarity and empathy, and help pet owners make informed decisions without inducing confusion or guilt. Shared decision-making models are particularly valuable, involving owners as partners in planning while respecting their emotional, financial, and logistical capacities.[29] Conversations should address prognosis honestly, educate about potential complications relevant to the specific comorbidities present, outline stepwise care plans, and incorporate QoL assessments to guide both intervention and observation periods. Studies have shown that using participatory QoL assessment tools can significantly increase the frequency of discussions during veterinary consultations.[21] Other CMIs are likely to have a similar effect. Client experiences of caregiver burden, anticipatory grief, and QoL are distinct, but interconnected, and influence both decision-making and emotional functioning.[30] Anticipatory grief, owners' emotional distress before the actual loss of their pet, often arises as pets develop more and more clinical symptoms of multimorbidities.[30] Proactive education helps the veterinary team frame discussions with sensitivity and allows owners to consider their medical options, as well as end-of-life plans, prior to the heightened emotions that can make decision-making difficult. By fostering open dialogue and aligning recommendations with the family's values and care goals, veterinary teams can create a supportive environment where owners feel empowered rather than overwhelmed, leading to more consistent compliance. Involvement of a veterinary social worker or referral to another mental health professional is recommended for caregivers experiencing substantial levels of caregiver burden, anticipatory grief, and perceived decreases in their own QoL.

Medical Records and Continuity of Care

Accurate, centralized medical records are the backbone of coordinated geriatric care, ensuring that all team members remain informed and aligned in their recommendations. Detailed documentation of presumptive and definitive diagnoses, diagnostic results, treatments (and outcomes), and quality-of-life discussions allows general practitioners, specialists, mobile veterinarians, and hospice providers to work from the same foundation of information. Clear and timely communications are essential when pets transition between their primary care veterinarian, specialists, and any home-based services. For example, when a pet receiving chemotherapy from an oncologist experiences a decline managed by an at-home hospice team, the prompt exchange of updated treatment notes and observations can inform future treatment decisions, minimize future adverse events, and avoid unnecessary or unwanted interventions. In human health care, multiprofessional communication improves service satisfaction, QoL, and reduces hospital readmissions for older patients during care transitions.[31] By prioritizing thorough documentation and structured communication, veterinary teams reduce the risk of missed information, reinforce client confidence in the collaborative process, and ensure that geriatric pets receive care that is both consistent and compassionate across every stage of life. It also allows the caregiver to speak openly and honestly about their evolving goals of care and be sure the entire care team understands.

ETHICAL CONSIDERATIONS AND END-OF-LIFE TRANSITIONS

Veterinary end-of-life care presents complex ethical challenges for health care providers, patients, and their families. Decisions during this period often involve balancing the pursuit of life-prolonging treatments against the patient's autonomy, comfort, dignity, and overall QoL. Ethical considerations guide the transition from curative to palliative care and support both patients and clinical teams through emotionally demanding choices.

Balancing Quality Versus Quantity of Life

One of the central ethical dilemmas in veterinary geriatric and end-of-life care is determining whether to prioritize extending life or enhancing its quality. Aggressive interventions may prolong survival but can cause suffering, reduce independence, or diminish the human–animal bond. Ethical frameworks encourage shared decision-making that incorporates client values, patient prognosis, and most likely outcome scenarios. Providers must assess whether continued interventions align with the caregiver's goals or represent a disproportionate burden. This balance requires sensitive communication and respect.

Indicators for Palliative Versus Curative Approach

Recognizing when to shift from a curative to a palliative approach is crucial. Indicators include declining functional status, repeated hospitalizations, poor response to treatments, or progression of one or more of the multimorbid conditions despite interventions. Ethical practice involves acknowledging the limits of medical technology and engaging patients and families in honest conversations about realistic outcomes. A palliative focus does not signify abandonment; rather, it prioritizes comfort, symptom management, and emotional support, often improving the patient's remaining QoL.

Hospice Planning and Euthanasia Decision-Making

Hospice care embodies a palliative philosophy, offering interdisciplinary support for patients with a prognosis of 6 months or less. Planning for hospice care requires transparency and sensitivity to the cultural, spiritual, and personal beliefs of the individual. Discussions around euthanasia further complicate ethical decision-making. These conversations must respect patient autonomy, caregiver budgets (financial, emotional, physical, and support) while considering professional codes of ethics and the moral perspectives of the veterinary team.

Ethical end-of-life transitions demand a holistic approach that balances quality and length of life, carefully weighs palliative versus curative interventions, and addresses the profound emotional dimensions of hospice and euthanasia considerations.

SUMMARY

The care of geriatric companion animals is inherently complex due to overlapping chronic diseases, sensory and cognitive decline, and heightened risks of drug interactions. Recognizing common comorbidities and their interactions, while adopting individualized and multimodal management approaches, is essential for improving both longevity and QoL in aging companion animals.

This article has highlighted the importance of comprehensive assessment, early identification of concurrent conditions, and individualized care planning. Successful outcomes rely on balancing disease-specific treatments with overall QoL, carefully considering how interventions for one condition may affect others. Central to this process is an understanding that our care goals must extend beyond simply extending life; we must also focus on preserving QoL.

Adaptability is a cornerstone of effective geriatric care. Clinical plans must evolve as patients age, new conditions or symptoms develop, established conditions progress, and caregivers' circumstances change. Collaboration—both within the veterinary health care team and with pet owners—is equally vital. Open communication, shared decision-making, and coordination among primary care providers, specialists, and caregivers ensure that treatment strategies remain patient-centered and tailored to each individual's needs. This approach fosters trust, supports compliance, and ultimately leads to better outcomes for the pet.

Looking to the future, geriatric veterinary medicine is poised to benefit from advances in diagnostics, aging sciences, and telemedicine capabilities, as well as a growing emphasis on hospice and palliative care. Emerging research in biomarkers, CMIs, and disease interventions will further refine our ability to monitor and support aging pets with multiple health challenges. By embracing an adaptable, collaborative, and patient-focused approach, veterinarians can meet the unique needs of senior animals and their families, ensuring that the later stages of life are managed with compassion, dignity, and clinical excellence.

CLINICS CARE POINTS

General Principles of Comorbidity Management

- Multimorbidity is the rule—not the exception—in geriatric patients, affecting over half of older dogs and cats.
- Distinguish between comorbidity (one dominant condition) and multimorbidity (no dominant condition), as management priorities differ.
- Integrate functional assessment and caregiver capacity into decision-making alongside disease-specific treatments.
- Avoid over-reliance on laboratory data alone; longitudinal client observations are often the first indicator of decline.

Diagnostic and Monitoring Strategies

- Apply a modified CGA: evaluate medical status, mobility, cognitive function, nutrition, and caregiving environment.
- Prioritize high-yield, low-burden diagnostics in frail patients to limit stress and maximize actionable findings.
- Use serial monitoring to identify trends rather than relying on single data points—especially important in chronic kidney disease (CKD), diabetes, and cognitive decline.
- Incorporate client-reported quality-of-life and mobility scores at every recheck; these are often more sensitive than physical examination alone and prompt discussion.

Pharmacology and Polypharmacy

- Conduct regular medication reconciliation to minimize polypharmacy risks—especially NSAID–corticosteroid overlaps or nephrotoxic stacking.
- Watch for drug–disease interactions in patients with subclinical organ dysfunction; adjust dosing based on renal and hepatic changes with age.
- Deprescribe medications or supplements that no longer offer benefit in end-stage care, particularly when goals shift to comfort.
- Assess the cumulative burden of care and risk of short-term side effects for any medications added.

Pain, Mobility, and Caregiver Communication

- Use validated CMIs such as pain scores to track pain and function across visits.
- Chronic pain can exacerbate cognitive decline and other conditions; treat even mild osteoarthritis proactively to preserve cognitive function and mobility.
- Enlist caregiver input when evaluating appetite, behavior, and daily routine—many signs of decompensation occur at home, not in the clinic.
- Normalize and address anticipatory grief early in disease discussions; this reduces caregiver guilt and improves care plan adherence.

DECLARATION OF AI AND AI-ASSISTED TECHNOLOGIES IN THE WRITING PROCESS

During the preparation of this work the author(s) used [Name tool/Service] in order to [Reason]. After using this tool/service, the author(s) reviewed and edited the content as needed and take(s) full responsibility for the content of the publication.

DISCLOSURE

No competing interests exist.

REFERENCES

1. Boyd CM, Ritchie CS, Tipton EF, et al. From bedside to bench: summary from the American Geriatrics Society/National Institute on aging research conference on comorbidity and multiple morbidity in older adults. Aging Clin Exp Res 2008; 20(3):181–8.
2. O'Neill DG, Church DB, McGreevy PD, et al. Prevalence of disorders recorded in cats attending primary-care veterinary practices in England. Vet J 2014;202(2): 286–91.
3. Banyard M. Prevalence of intercurrent disease in dogs and cats presented for vaccination at a veterinary practice. Aust Vet J 1998;76(9):600–1.
4. O'Neill DG, James H, Brodbelt DC, et al. Prevalence of commonly diagnosed disorders in UK dogs under primary veterinary care: results and applications. BMC Vet Res 2021;17(1):69.
5. Gardner M, McVety D, editors. Treatment and care of the geriatric veterinary patient. 1st edition. Wiley; 2017. https://doi.org/10.1002/9781119187240.
6. KuKanich B. Geriatric veterinary pharmacology. Vet Clin North Am Small Anim Pract 2012;42(4):631–42.
7. Grieve J. Contextualised care a welcome recalibration. Vet Rec 2024;195(8): 340–1.
8. Dhaliwal R, Boynton E, Carrera-Justiz S, et al. AAHA senior care guidelines for dogs and cats. J Am Anim Hosp Assoc 2023;59(1):1–21.
9. Quain A, Ward MP, Mullan S. Ethical challenges posed by advanced veterinary care in companion animal veterinary practice. Animals 2021;11(11):3010.
10. Rollin BE. Ethical issues in geriatric feline medicine. J Feline Med Surg 2007;9(4): 326–34.
11. Kim E, Choe C, Yoo JG, et al. Major medical causes by breed and life stage for dogs presented at veterinary clinics in the Republic of Korea: a survey of electronic medical records. PeerJ 2018;6:e5161. https://doi.org/10.7717/peerj.5161.
12. Gates M, Hinds H, Dale A. Preliminary description of aging cats and dogs presented to a New Zealand first-opinion veterinary clinic at end-of-life. N Z Vet J 2017;65(6):313–7.
13. Forsyth KK, McCoy BM, Schmid SM, et al. Lifetime prevalence of owner-reported medical conditions in the 25 most common dog breeds in the dog aging project pack. Front Vet Sci 2023;10:1140417. https://doi.org/10.3389/fvets.2023.1140417.
14. Hopper RG, Bromberg RB, Salzman MM, et al. Dual sensory impairments in companion dogs: prevalence and relationship to cognitive impairment. In: Santacà M, editor. PLoS One 2024;19(10):e0310299. https://doi.org/10.1371/journal.pone.0310299.
15. Szabó D, Miklósi Á, Kubinyi E. Owner-reported sensory impairments affect behavioural signs associated with cognitive decline in dogs. Behav Process 2018;157:354–60.

16. Maharani A, Dawes P, Nazroo J, et al. Associations between self-reported sensory impairment and risk of cognitive decline and impairment in the health and retirement study cohort. In: Anderson N, editor. J Gerontol Ser B 2020;75(6):1230–42.
17. Zhang NK, Zhang SK, Zhang LI, et al. Sensory processing deficits and related cortical pathological changes in Alzheimer's disease. Front Aging Neurosci 2023;15:1213379. https://doi.org/10.3389/fnagi.2023.1213379.
18. Epstein ME, Rodanm I, Griffenhagen G, et al. AAHA/AAFP pain management guidelines for dogs and cats. J Feline Med Surg 2015;17(3):251–72.
19. Ware WA, Bonagura JD, Scansen BA. Drugs for the treatment of heart failure. In: Ware WA, Bonagura JD, editors. Cardiovascular disease in companion animals. 2nd edition. Boca Raton: CRC Press; 2021. p. 317–36. https://doi.org/10.1201/9780429186639-24.
20. Pardo M, Spencer E, Odunayo A, et al. 2024 AAHA fluid therapy guidelines for dogs and cats. J Am Anim Hosp Assoc 2024;60(4):131–63.
21. Yeates JW, Mullan S, Stone M, et al. Promoting discussions and decisions about dogs' quality-of-life. J Small Anim Pract 2011;52(9):459–63.
22. Stockman J. Nutrition and aging in dogs and cats. Adv Exp Med Biol 2024;-(1446):203–15.
23. Bartges JW. Chronic kidney disease in dogs and cats. Vet Clin North Am Small Anim Pract 2012;42(4):669–92.
24. Blanchard T, Eppe J, Mugnier A, et al. Enhancing cognitive functions in aged dogs and cats: a systematic review of enriched diets and nutraceuticals. GeroScience 2025;47(3):2925–47.
25. Frye C, Carr BJ, Lenfest M, et al. Canine geriatric rehabilitation: considerations and strategies for assessment, functional scoring, and follow up. Front Vet Sci 2022;9:842458. https://doi.org/10.3389/fvets.2022.842458.
26. Zicker SC. Cognitive and behavioral assessment in dogs and pet food market applications. Prog Neuropsychopharmacol Biol Psychiatry 2005;29(3):455–9.
27. Araujo JA, Studzinski CM, Head E, et al. Assessment of nutritional interventions for modification of age-associated cognitive decline using a canine model of human aging. AGE 2005;27(1):27–37.
28. Bishop G, Cooney K, Cox S, et al. AAHA/IAAHPC end-Of-life care guidelines. J Am Anim Hosp Assoc 2016;52(6):341–56.
29. Cornell KK, Kopcha M. Client-veterinarian communication: skills for client centered dialogue and shared decision making. Vet Clin North Am Small Anim Pract 2007;37(1):37–47.
30. Spitznagel MB, Anderson JR, Marchitelli B, et al. Owner quality of life, caregiver burden and anticipatory grief: how they differ, why it matters. Vet Rec 2021;188(9):e74. https://doi.org/10.1002/vetr.74.
31. Allen J, Ottmann G, Roberts G. Multi-professional communication for older people in transitional care: a review of the literature. Int J Older People Nurs 2013;8(4):253–69.

Client Education

Empowering Pet Owners Through the Geriatric Journey

Eric D. Garcia

KEYWORDS

- Senior pet care education • Geriatric pet health communication strategies
- Pet owner engagement in senior pet care • Senior pet wellness communication
- Veterinary palliative care education • End-of-life pet care communication
- Veterinary communication strategies

KEY POINTS

- Digital media offers unprecedented opportunities for educating pet owners about the unique needs of senior pets, from preventive care to end-of-life decision-making.
- A cohesive client education plan blends digital and nondigital tools to reach owners across generational and technological divides.
- Consistent, empathetic communication fosters trust, compliance, and improved quality of life for geriatric patients.
- Data-driven strategies and personalized messaging increase owner engagement and adherence to care plans.
- Veterinary teams play a critical role as the trusted, go-to source for accurate and actionable geriatric care information.

INTRODUCTION AND BACKGROUND

When we talk about client education in veterinary medicine, it is often framed around preventive care, puppy and kitten guidance, and *sometimes*, chronic disease management. However, there is one stage of life that demands a uniquely tailored, consistent, and empathetic educational approach—the geriatric stage.

Geriatric pets are not just "older adults" in the veterinary sense. They are often deeply woven into the emotional fabric of their families, and the decisions their owners make in these years are shaped as much by love, grief, and guilt as they are by clinical data. I have seen this repeatedly in my work with practices across North America and beyond: owners of senior pets are eager for guidance but are often navigating

Tapir, Animal Health Digital Strategist, 615 Channelside Drive, Suite 207, Tampa, FL 33602, USA
E-mail address: eric@tapir.vet

Vet Clin Small Anim 56 (2026) 431–443
https://doi.org/10.1016/j.cvsm.2025.09.025 **vetsmall.theclinics.com**
0195-5616/26/

unfamiliar territory. So, where are they to turn? Dr Google. Yet, you, the veterinary practice, can and should be who they turn to first. Pet owners need practical, digestible, and compassionate information—delivered in ways they can easily access and trust.

The Evolving Landscape of Client Education

When I first began working with veterinary practices, most client education only took place in the examination room or through a printed handout. Today, the conversation extends far beyond the clinic walls. The rise of digital tools—Web sites, email reminder campaigns, social media, apps, and telemedicine—has dramatically expanded how and when we can connect with pet owners.

- Access: Information is now available on-demand, 24/7.
- Reach: A single educational post can reach hundreds of clients easily.
- Format diversity: Video, infographics, interactive quizzes, and mobile apps give us new ways to present information that fits different learning styles.

The challenge, of course, is that our clients are also exposed to *misinformation* at unprecedented levels. Pet owners can Google "best diet for senior dogs" and be met with thousands of results—many of them inaccurate, biased, or even harmful. This is where veterinary teams have the opportunity, and I would argue the responsibility to become the go-to trusted source of truth for senior pet care.

Why Geriatric Care Requires a Different Communication Approach

Educating owners of senior pets is different from educating the owner of a young, healthy animal.

- Complexity of care: Senior pets often have multiple health concerns, from arthritis to chronic kidney disease, which require layered education.
- Emotional stakes: Owners may be facing the reality of a limited lifespan, making every conversation more emotionally charged.
- Proactive versus reactive: Without early and regular education, many owners wait until a crisis to seek help—missing opportunities for prevention or early intervention.

A Blend of Digital and Nondigital.

While this article leans heavily on digital strategies, the reality is that no single channel works for every client. The most effective education plan blends both worlds:

- Digital tools for efficiency, consistency, and reach.
- Nondigital interactions for personal connection and nuanced conversations.

The goal is not just to *inform* owners but to *empower* them—helping them understand what is happening, anticipate changes, and feel supported every step of the way. Done well, this approach strengthens the client–veterinarian bond, improves compliance, and, most importantly, enhances the quality of life for senior pets.

Core Educational Goals for the Geriatric Journey

In my experience, one of the most common mistakes practices make is delivering geriatric education reactively—waiting for a crisis before giving the client the information they need. By then, the window for prevention or early intervention is often closed, and the owner is making decisions under stress.

A proactive, structured education plan starts with clear goals. These goals should serve as guideposts for every digital post, email, handout, or in-person conversation.

1. Preventive Care in the Senior Years

   Owners often assume preventive care matters less as pets age, but the opposite is true. Education should reinforce:
   - Biannual wellness examinations to detect changes early.
   - Vaccination and parasite prevention tailored to lifestyle and health status.
   - Nutritional adjustments to support weight management, joint health, and organ function.
2. Early Disease Detection

   Many age-related conditions—like chronic kidney disease or arthritis—start subtly. Clients should understand:
   - What screening tests are recommended and why.
   - The value of trending laboratory work over time.
   - Observable early signs of common senior conditions.

   This is where visual education shines. Short videos showing early mobility changes or appetite shifts help owners identify subtle symptoms they might otherwise dismiss. Showing pet owners bloodwork results from the previous year to show them you are trending and finding what is *"normal"* for their pet, while expressing that their pet is unique.
3. Symptom Recognition and Tracking

   Educating owners to spot and record changes can help you intervene earlier. Key topics include
   - Pain indicators (changes in posture, reluctance to jump).
   - Cognitive changes (disorientation, altered sleep patterns).
   - Appetite and weight fluctuations.

   Digital tools like pet health tracking apps can be integrated into your education plan, allowing owners to share real-time updates with your team.
4. Palliative and Hospice Care Awareness

   For many owners, these concepts are unfamiliar or emotionally loaded. Education here should
   - Normalize palliative care as a way to improve comfort and quality of life.
   - Outline what hospice care involves, including home modifications, pain management, and ongoing monitoring.

   This discussion often benefits from recorded content or written guides that clients can revisit when ready.
5. End-of-Life Decision-Making Support

   Clear, compassionate guidance helps reduce guilt and uncertainty. Owners should have
   - Tools for quality-of-life assessment (scoring charts, symptom trackers).
   - Information on euthanasia options, aftercare, and memorializing their pet.
   - Access to grief support resources.
6. Financial Planning for Long-Term or End-of-Life Care

   Education should include realistic cost expectations and available options:
   - Pet insurance coverage for senior care.
   - Wellness plans or financing options.
   - How early planning can prevent difficult financial decisions later.

Key takeaway

Educational goals for the geriatric journey must address both the clinical and the emotional needs of the client. When owners know what to expect and when to act, they are more likely to follow through—leading to better outcomes for the pet.

DIGITAL CLIENT EDUCATION STRATEGIES

In today's veterinary landscape, digital tools are not just an optional add-on to client communication; they are central to how we educate, engage, and support pet owners. When done well, digital strategies allow you to meet clients where they already spend their time, reinforce messages between visits, and make it easier for them to take action.

In working with practices across the country, I have seen the most successful ones use multiple digital touchpoints that align with the client's journey, from early senior care through end-of-life. The magic happens when these tools work together, rather than in isolation.

Practice Web site

Your Web site should function as the hub for all digital education. Everything else—emails, social media posts, even in-clinic materials—should point back to it.

Best practices for a senior pet care hub:

- Dedicated Senior Pet Page: Centralize resources on one page, including wellness checklists, mobility guides, and links to quality-of-life tools.
- Downloadable Resources: Provide printable symptom trackers, home safety checklists, and nutrition guides.
- Search Optimization: Use terms pet owners actually search for—eg, "signs of arthritis in dogs" or "cat cognitive decline"—so your content is discoverable.
- Video Integration[2]: Short educational videos embedded on the page can increase retention.

Email Campaigns and Automated Reminders

Email is one of the most underutilized tools in veterinary communication—especially for long-term education.

How to use it for geriatric care:

- Lifecycle Campaigns: Triggered when a pet reaches a certain age, these can deliver educational content in digestible chunks over weeks or months.
- Lab Work Reminders: Automated emails explaining the *why* behind biannual bloodwork.
- Postvisit Follow-Ups: Summaries of instructions with links to videos and resources.

Social Media

Many owners *start* their pet health research on social platforms,[3] whether that is a good thing or not. The advantage is that you can control the narrative with accurate, empathetic, and visually engaging content.

What works best for geriatric education:

- Facebook: Longer posts with images for storytelling, like senior pet spotlights or case studies.
- Instagram/TikTok: Bite-sized videos with tips, mobility exercises, or "myth vs. fact" education.
- Live Q&A Sessions: Real-time interaction to answer questions and build trust.

Content themes:

- "Day in the Life" videos showing adaptations for a senior pet.
- "Did You Know?" facts about aging pets.
- Testimonials from other pet owners who followed through on recommended care.

Telemedicine and Virtual Consults

While telemedicine gained momentum during the pandemic,[4] it is particularly well suited for senior pet care:

- Progress Check-Ins: Quick video calls to assess mobility, comfort, or cognitive changes.
- Medication Reviews: Ensuring correct administration without the stress of a clinic visit.
- Caregiver Education: Involving multiple family members in the discussion without requiring everyone to be physically present.

When integrated with your digital education plan, telemedicine becomes a powerful reinforcement tool—allowing you to review symptom logs, answer questions, and provide ongoing guidance between in-person exams.

It is important to note that telemedicine requires training to ensure clinical effectiveness and compliance with regulations.[5] State, provincial, and international laws vary widely regarding what can and cannot be done through virtual care. Veterinary teams should always check with their local veterinary governing bodies to understand and follow applicable guidelines before implementing telemedicine services.

Video Education

Video is an engaging format for senior pet education:

- Short Form (1–3 min): Ideal for showing how to give medications, assist mobility, or recognize early signs of pain.
- Longer Videos (and even webinars for pet owners!) (15–20 min): Deep dives into topics like cognitive dysfunction, arthritis, or nutrition.
- Personalization: Simple smartphone videos recorded by the veterinarian addressing the pet by name can have a major emotional impact.

Apps and Digital Tracking Tools

Many owners want to be proactive but need help staying organized. Apps can:

- Track pain scores or mobility changes.
- Remind owners about medication schedules.
- Log appetite, water intake, and behavior changes.

Some platforms allow direct sharing with your clinic, giving your team real-time insight and allowing earlier intervention.

Key takeaway
Digital tools extend your reach, reinforce your message, and make education accessible 24/7. The best results happen when these tools work together, creating a consistent experience for the client and reducing the information gaps that can compromise senior pet care.

LEVERAGING REMINDERS IN THE PRACTICE INFORMATION MANAGEMENT SYSTEM

Reminders are one of the most underutilized tools in many practices, yet they are one of the most powerful ways to drive compliance, especially for senior pet care. When reminders are strategically set up and thoughtfully worded, they can become a cornerstone of your geriatric client education strategy.

Why Reminders Matter for Geriatric Care

Senior pets often require more frequent check-ins, diagnostics, and follow-up care than younger patients. Reminders ensure that:

- Preventive care and screenings happen on time.
- Chronic conditions are monitored consistently.
- Owners do not forget follow-ups after a change in treatment or medication.

For older pets, these reminders can be the difference between catching a developing condition early and managing a crisis later.

Make Reminders Specific and Action-Oriented

Generic reminders like *"Fido is due for a check-up"* can easily be ignored or misunderstood. Instead, make them clear and connected to the pet's needs:

- *"Bella is due for her senior wellness screening, including arthritis evaluation and bloodwork."*
- *"Max is due for his cognitive health check—let's review any changes you've noticed."*

The more specific the reminder, the more relevant it feels to the owner, and the more likely they are to act on it.

Ensure Reminders Are Unique Across the System

In some practices, multiple team members set up reminders in different ways, leading to duplicates, conflicting timelines, or inconsistent messaging. This can confuse clients and undermine trust.

- Audit your reminder types regularly to eliminate duplicates.
- Standardize naming conventions and intervals in the PIMS.
- Train all team members on how and when to set reminders, ensuring a unified approach.

Integrating Reminders with Education

Reminders should not just be prompts; they should also educate. Include links to relevant resources or invite clients to call with questions. For example:

- *"Charlie is due for his mobility recheck. Click here to watch a quick video on what to expect during the visit."*
- *"Molly's next kidney function test is due—here's why regular monitoring is so important."*

This turns a reminder into both a nudge and an educational moment.

Key takeaway
Well-crafted, unique reminders within your practice management system and communication platform are a powerful driver of compliance and client engagement. They keep geriatric patients on track with their care plans and provide ongoing opportunities to educate owners in a timely, relevant way.

NONDIGITAL EDUCATION METHODS

While digital platforms have transformed client communication, not all pet owners will rely exclusively on them. An effective geriatric education strategy should ensure that every client, regardless of age, technological comfort, or access, has multiple pathways to receive and absorb important information. Nondigital methods remain critical for building personal connections, reinforcing digital messages, and ensuring that vital education reaches every household.

In-Clinic Materials

Printed resources are still a mainstay of client education and can be powerful when well designed and easy to understand.

- Handouts and Booklets: Focus on a single topic per piece, using clear language and visuals.
- Exam Room Posters: Highlight common senior health concerns or care tips in an approachable format.
- Discharge Instructions: Summarize postvisit recommendations, with space for personalized notes from the veterinary team.

Printed materials work best when they complement, rather than replace, digital resources.[6] For example, a handout can reference a web link or QR code for further information.

One-on-One Conversations

The examination room conversation remains the most trusted form of veterinary communication.

- Speak in plain language, avoiding unnecessary jargon.
- Confirm understanding by asking clients to explain recommendations back in their own words.
- Use visual aids—such as anatomic models or diagrams—to illustrate complex topics.

The tone of these discussions is as important as the content; empathy and patience encourage clients to engage, ask questions, and absorb the information.

In-Person Events

Group education sessions can strengthen client relationships and provide a supportive environment for owners of senior pets.

- Topics might include pain management strategies, mobility exercises, or nutrition for aging pets.
- Events can be paired with senior pet wellness days, allowing owners to receive education and services in the same visit.

These sessions also encourage peer-to-peer sharing, which can reinforce key messages.

Phone Calls and Follow-Ups

A simple follow-up call after a senior pet's visit can:

- Reinforce recommendations.
- Answer questions that arise after the appointment.
- Demonstrate ongoing support and care.

These calls are particularly valuable after emotionally charged discussions, such as those involving palliative or end-of-life care.

Support Groups

Facilitated support groups, within the practice or in partnership with community organizations, provide owners with emotional support and a place to share strategies for caring for senior pets.

- Can be focused on general geriatric care, or on specific conditions like cognitive decline or mobility issues.
- Helps normalize challenges and create a sense of community.

Key takeaway

Nondigital methods are essential for reaching clients who prefer face-to-face, print-based, or verbal communication. They also deepen personal connection, making digital follow-up more effective by building trust and rapport first.

INTEGRATING DIGITAL AND NONDIGITAL FOR A COHESIVE EDUCATION PLAN

Just as veterinarians take a multimodal approach to medicine—using tools like NSAIDs, pain relievers, laser therapy, and physical therapy together for arthritis—the most effective geriatric care communication strategies are also multimodal. Digital and nondigital education methods should not be treated as separate tracks. When they are aligned, each reinforces the other, creating a consistent and accessible experience for the client while reducing redundancy for the veterinary team.

Why Integration Matters

People absorb information differently based on their personal preferences, access to technology, and emotional state.[7] Providing multiple, coordinated channels ensures:

- The same core message reaches the client in more than one way.
- Clients can choose the format that works best for them without missing essential information.
- The veterinary team can deliver education more efficiently, using templates and repeatable processes.

Creating Consistency Across Channels

- Unified Messaging: The language, tone, and recommendations should be consistent whether a client reads a printed handout, a web site article, or hears it in an exam room conversation.
- Shared Resource Library: Develop a master library of educational materials that can be adapted for print, email, and social media to ensure accuracy and branding remain consistent.
- Cross-Referencing: Printed materials should point to online resources for further detail, while digital platforms can promote in-clinic events or printed guides.

Using One Channel to Drive Engagement in Another

- Mention your online resources during appointments and provide the direct link or QR code in take-home materials.
- Use email to remind clients about upcoming in-person workshops or support groups.
- Share photos or recaps of in-clinic events on social media to encourage future attendance.

Reducing Staff Workload Through Integration

When digital and nondigital tools are developed together, veterinary teams can

- Avoid duplicating work by repurposing the same content across multiple formats.
- Automate delivery of digital follow-ups to extend the value of in-person conversations.
- Rely on a consistent set of visuals, talking points, and templates to save time.

Key takeaway
Integration ensures that client education is cohesive, consistent, and accessible—no matter how the client prefers to engage. By designing your geriatric education strategy to flow between in-person and digital touchpoints, you create a stronger connection with the client, improve retention of information, and support better patient outcomes.

MEASURING IMPACT OF EDUCATION EFFORTS

Client education is only effective if it translates into improved compliance, better decision-making, and enhanced patient outcomes. Measuring results not only validates the investment of time and resources but also highlights where adjustments are needed to maximize impact.

Why Measurement Matters

Without tracking results, education remains a good intention rather than a proven strategy. Data-driven evaluation

- Shows whether clients are engaging with the content.
- Identifies gaps in understanding or compliance.
- Helps prioritize which methods and messages are most effective.

Key Metrics to Monitor

1. Compliance Metrics
   - Preventive Care Uptake: Biannual exam attendance, vaccination rates, and senior screening compliance.
   - Follow-Through on Recommendations: Lab rechecks, imaging follow-ups, and medication adherence.
   - Palliative and Hospice Participation: Enrollment rates in supportive care programs.
2. Digital Engagement Metrics
   - Web site Analytics: Page views, time spent on senior care resources, and download counts for tools like pain scales or checklists.
   - Email Campaign Performance: Open rates, click-through rates, and content engagement trends.
   - Social Media Insights: Post reach, shares, comments, and engagement on senior care topics.
3. Client Satisfaction and Feedback
   - Postappointment surveys to assess whether clients felt informed and supported.
   - Feedback forms linked in digital follow-ups.
   - In-person check-ins where staff ask, "Was the information we gave you helpful?" and record responses.
4. Patient Outcome Indicators
   - Earlier detection of conditions due to the owner reporting of subtle symptoms.
   - Reduced emergency visits for preventable conditions.

- Improved quality-of-life scores over time for patients in palliative care.

Building a Feedback Loop

Data should be reviewed regularly—monthly or quarterly—to inform adjustments in your approach. For example,

- If email open rates are low, test new subject lines or adjust sending times.
- If preventive care compliance is high but quality-of-life tools are underused, revisit how those tools are introduced to clients.
- If Web site traffic is high but average time on page is low, simplify content or add more visual elements.

Key takeaway

Measuring impact ensures that your geriatric client education program is not just active, but effective. When metrics show progress, you can scale what's working; when they show gaps, you have a clear direction for improvement.

OVERCOMING CHALLENGES AND PITFALLS

Even the most thoughtfully designed geriatric education program will face obstacles. Anticipating these challenges and building strategies to address them is essential for sustaining momentum and ensuring that client education remains effective and efficient.

1. Digital Fatigue

   Many people receive constant notifications, emails, and social media prompts. Overloading them with messages, no matter how valuable, can lead to disengagement. In fact, 40% of US consumers unsubscribe from brand emails or text messages weekly, and over half will do so if they receive 4 or more messages from the same company within 30 days.[8]

   Solution:
   - Focus on quality over quantity.
   - Space out educational messages so they feel intentional rather than overwhelming.
   - Personalize communications based on the pet's needs and the client's past engagement.
2. Information Overload

   Geriatric care involves multiple layers—nutrition, mobility, disease management, palliative care, which can overwhelm clients if delivered all at once.

   Solution:
   - Prioritize the most urgent or immediately relevant information.
   - Use phased education, releasing new topics over time.
   - Provide recap tools, such as checklists or resource hubs, so clients can revisit information when ready.
3. Inconsistent Messaging

   If information differs depending on who in the clinic delivers it—or between digital and nondigital formats, clients can become confused or lose trust.

   Solution:
   - Create standardized talking points and educational templates.
   - Keep a shared library of approved resources for the whole team to use.
   - Align messaging during team meetings to ensure consistency.
4. Keeping Content Current

   Medical guidelines, technology, and best practices evolve quickly. Outdated resources can diminish credibility.

Solution:

- Schedule regular reviews of all educational content—digital and print—at least twice a year.
- Assign a team member or small committee to maintain and update resources.
- Remove outdated materials from circulation promptly.

5. Inclusivity and Accessibility

Not all clients have equal access to digital platforms, and some may have visual, hearing, or literacy limitations. Literacy-related disparities in technology access and use are widespread, with lower-literate individuals being less likely to own smartphones and use digital services.[9]

Solution:

- Offer information in multiple formats.
- Ensure digital resources are mobile-friendly and accessible (eg, alt text for images, captions on videos).
- Translate materials when possible to serve a broader client base.

6. Team Bandwidth

One of the #1 things I'm aware of that I often hear is that education initiatives will stall if they create too much additional work for the team.

Solution:

- Automate where possible, such as scheduling recurring email campaigns.
- Repurpose the same content across multiple channels.
- Use preapproved templates so team members do not need to start from scratch.

Key Takeaway

Challenges are inevitable, but with planning and structure, they become manageable. The practices that succeed in geriatric client education treat obstacles as opportunities to refine their approach and strengthen their connection with clients.

CASE STUDIES AND REAL-WORLD APPLICATIONS

The principles of geriatric client education become most powerful when applied consistently and adapted to fit a practice's unique culture, client base, and resources. While the specific details will vary from one clinic to another, the following scenarios illustrate how digital and nondigital strategies can be blended for meaningful impact.

Scenario 1: Improving Preventive Care Compliance in Senior Pets

A multidoctor practice recognized that senior wellness screenings were often delayed or declined by owners who did not fully understand their value. They implemented a multichannel education campaign:

- Digital: Automated emails explaining the importance of biannual bloodwork, linking to a webpage with FAQs and a short educational video.
- Nondigital: Printed brochures in the lobby and brief conversations during each exam to reinforce the message. Within 1 year, compliance improved significantly, and owners began initiating conversations about scheduling screenings.

Scenario 2: Supporting Owners Through Cognitive Decline

Owners often miss early signs of cognitive dysfunction, leading to delayed intervention. A clinic created a phased education plan:

- Step 1: Awareness content on social media, highlighting subtle behavioral changes to watch for.

- Step 2: A downloadable symptom checklist on the website for owners to track changes.
- Step 3: Follow-up phone calls to review completed checklists and discuss treatment options.

This approach gave owners tangible tools while keeping the conversation going over time.

Scenario 3: Integrating End-of-Life Education Early

Rather than waiting until a crisis point, a practice integrated gentle end-of-life discussions into routine senior visits:

- During Appointments: Quality-of-life scoring introduced as a standard conversation, normalized as part of proactive care.
- Digital Support: A web portal with educational articles, video explanations, and grief resources.
- Follow-Up: Personalized phone calls after quality-of-life discussions to answer questions and offer emotional support. This early integration reduced client anxiety when difficult decisions arose later.

Scenario 4: Streamlining Education for Busy Clients

Some owners struggle to absorb information during a visit due to time constraints. To address this:

- At the Appointment: Key recommendations summarized verbally, supported by a short printed checklist.
- After the Appointment: Automated email sent the same day with links to videos, handouts, and instructions. This method ensured owners had accurate, accessible information without extending appointment times.

Key Takeaway

Effective geriatric education does not require a complete overhaul of a practice's workflow. By combining consistent messaging, multiple delivery formats, and ongoing reinforcement, veterinary teams can significantly improve client understanding, compliance, and confidence, ultimately enhancing the quality of life for senior pets.

SUMMARY

Empowering pet owners through the geriatric journey is not a single conversation, it is an ongoing, evolving relationship. Senior pets have unique medical, emotional, and lifestyle needs, and their owners often require extra guidance, reassurance, and support to navigate these years with confidence.

Digital tools have expanded the possibilities for client education, allowing veterinary teams to deliver timely, relevant, and personalized information well beyond the walls of the clinic. At the same time, nondigital methods remain vital for personal connection, trust building, and ensuring accessibility. The real strength lies in integrating both approaches into a cohesive, consistent plan that meets owners where they are—emotionally, technologically, and culturally.

As veterinary professionals, we hold the privilege and responsibility of being the trusted source for accurate, compassionate information. In fact, over 90% of animal owners trust and appreciate veterinary teams.[10] When we combine our medical expertise with strategic communication, we do more than educate—we empower.

This empowerment not only improves compliance and clinical outcomes but also deepens the bond between client, patient, and practice.

The geriatric journey can be challenging, but it can also be filled with meaningful moments, improved quality of life, and a sense of partnership between veterinary teams and pet owners. By committing to intentional, measured, and empathetic client education, we ensure that senior pets and their families are supported every step of the way.

CLINICS CARE POINTS

- Personalize client education at the point of care by linking information to each pet's condition and the owner's emotional readiness, avoiding one-size-fits-all messaging.
- Use digital tools to reinforce in-person discussions, not replace them. Follow up with brief, actionable summaries and links to reliable resources.
- Audit reminder systems and educational materials regularly to ensure they are accurate, unique, and aligned with current geriatric protocols and telemedicine regulations.
- Be mindful of client overload by spacing out communications and using plain language to promote understanding and long-term engagement.

DISCLOSURE

None.

REFERENCES

1. Avma, Available at: https://www.avma.org/resources-tools/pet-owners/petcare/senior-pets (Accessed 23 October 2025).
2. Speech, Available at: https://speach.me/blog/7-stats-that-prove-why-video-instructions-are-more-effective-than-written (Accessed 23 October 2025).
3. PubMed, Available at: https://pubmed.ncbi.nlm.nih.gov/34051032/ (Accessed 23 October 2025).
4. PubMed, Available at: https://pmc.ncbi.nlm.nih.gov/articles/PMC11128645/ (Accessed 23 October 2025).
5. AVMA, Available at: https://www.avma.org/resources-tools/animal-health-and-welfare/telehealth-telemedicine-veterinary-practice/veterinary-telehealth-basics (Accessed 23 October 2025).
6. PubMed, Available at: https://pmc.ncbi.nlm.nih.gov/articles/PMC8475791/ (Accessed 23 October 2025).
7. PubMed, Available at: https://pmc.ncbi.nlm.nih.gov/articles/PMC5573739/ (Accessed 23 October 2025).
8. Business wire, Available at: https://www.businesswire.com/news/home/20241007772448/en/40-of-U.S.-Consumers-Unsubscribe-From-Marketing-Emails-Weekly Strategies-for-Businesses-to-Re-Engage (Accessed 23 October 2025).
9. PubMed, Available at: https://pmc.ncbi.nlm.nih.gov/articles/PMC4417455/ (Accessed 23 October 2025).
10. Boehringer ingelheim, Available at: https://www.boehringer-ingelheim.com/animal-health/our-responsibility/new-survey-shows-over-90-pet-owners-trust-vets-overlook-their-challenges (Accessed 23 October 2025).

Goals of Care

Prioritizing What Truly Matters at Life's End

Rebecca K. Frank, DVM, CVHEP, CT (Certified in Thanatology: Death, Dying, Loss, and Bereavement)[a,*], Rachel Welch, DVM[b]

KEYWORDS

• Goals of care • Tough conversations • Hospice • Palliative care

KEY POINTS

- There is a wide range of approaches to end of life care of pets.
- In order to establish goals in end of life care, rapport and trust must be established with care.
- There are several categories of goals, and some are more important to pet owners than others.
- Establishing goals in end of life care can strengthen bonds with pets and smooth the entire end of life care phase.

GOALS: WHY HAVE THEM IN END OF LIFE CARE?

Paralleling human medicine, veterinary care for pets has evolved to help loved ones as they age, prolonging life and bringing change to the end of life experience. While dignity is a major contributor to human end of life decisions, there are many dimensions in end of life decision-making for pets, including

- Physical needs
- Psychological needs
- Social/human–animal bond
- Cultural needs
- Spiritual needs

When we address these needs, we can help tame anxiety and fear surrounding the dying process, giving families the comfort of a plan, which may translate to peace of mind.[1]

Advance Medical Directives (AMD) were proposed in the west by the Euthanasia Society of America in 1967 to bring a more holistic approach to end of life care and

[a] Lap of Love, IAAHPC, PO Box 4063, Reading, PA 19606, USA; [b] Lap of Love, 17804 N. US Highway 41, Lutz, FL 33549, USA
* Corresponding author.
E-mail address: drbecky@lapoflove.com

Vet Clin Small Anim 56 (2026) 445–454
https://doi.org/10.1016/j.cvsm.2025.10.001 vetsmall.theclinics.com

Abbreviations	
ACP	advanced care planning
AMD	advance medical directives
REMAP	reframe, expect emotion, map out patient goals
SMART	specific, measurable, achievable, relevant, and time-bound
SVICG	serious veterinary illness conversation guide

to respect individuals' wishes for how they would like to be treated at the end of their lives. Advanced Care Planning (ACP) came about in the 1990s in human medicine, taking the AMD and broadening it. Please note that while the AMD is a legal document, the ACP is not, though the latter is more likely what we are to model our own end of life care plans for our patients, as it encompasses values and life goals that may be more important to clients than whether or not to pursue invasive medical care for their pet.[2]

As a member of the community, a veterinarian and their team often serve as a helper through all phases of a pet's life, including their death. As such, we are an important part of the ritualization of the end of a pet's life, and often have direct control as to when and how a pet dies, specifically through euthanasia. While euthanasia may not be chosen for a pet for any number of reasons, we still play the important part of guiding a family through the dying process. Young clients and families may be unfamiliar with the process, especially in cultures where death is often difficult and taboo to discuss or experience. However, by guiding families through what the dying process looks like, and by making goals for the care of their beloved pet, we can satisfy the ritual of saying goodbye, as well as upholding the human-animal bond.

While it may not be practicable in all situations, taking the time to go over goals and the dying journey helps support the family, creating a space for them to honor their pet, while also fulfilling our role in the community. The effect has mostly been studied in human medicine, and the overall pattern is that open discussions and preparedness for death can lower the chance of complicated grief in postdeath bereavement, and may also help mitigate anticipatory grief.[3] Having these discussions ahead of time may also prepare families and increase efficiency if time-sensitive or emergency situations arise at end of life.[4] For this reason, if a family is open to communication, setting goals and plans for end of life care is a positive where applicable. In fact the goal of this article is to give the reader the tools and knowledge to feel confident in guiding families through some of the hardest days.

APPROACHING THE DISCUSSION

As many of us know, death is not a popular topic of discussion in day to day life. Most people in western society avoid the topic altogether, which can make the job of approaching a family to discuss the dying process, more challenging for some of us than surgery. The serious illness of a beloved pet shakes the foundations of most peoples' daily lives, and how they see the world. Thus it is imperative that we tread carefully and adopt a collaborative approach with caregivers.

In this endeavor, communication is the key. If we are to guide a family through the dying process, whether it involves euthanasia or not, we need to be very clear in our communication about a pet's prognosis and their current status in regards to that prognosis and disease progression. While we may easily see what a pet needs, keep in mind a pet parent's world has been altered with the diagnosis and prognosis, and they will need time to rebuild their world view, this time with the reality that their pet may not be with them for much longer. Giving them time to digest this information, as well as time to develop questions will go far in continuing rapport and trust.

Cultural considerations should also be at the forefront of our minds. For example, in western individualistic cultures, which emphasize the value of an individual's choices and liberty, families may see accepting death as giving up, or taking their pet's autonomy away, especially if a pet is still eating despite poor quality of life. There is a certain Lazarus effect in these cultures, that if they love enough, or spend enough, that a pet can *beat* the dying process. In more collectivist cultures, which emphasize the value of a family unit, or the cohesiveness of society as a whole, you may have multiple family members caring for the pet, and they may have different views on what is best for them. Some cultures consider even speaking about end of life care to be taboo and may refuse to enter into conversation about it.

Often religion is tied to culture as well, though there is much variation. To that end, we may see 1 Christian family as willing to euthanize a pet. They see their role in that culture and religion as caring for the pet and having the authority to prevent suffering by partnering with a veterinarian to euthanize their pet, and give them a good death. Another Christian family may question if they have the authority to do so, equating allowing a pet to be euthanized with playing God. Some Buddhist families see allowing an animal to continue to feel pain and suffering to reflect poorly on their soul, while other Buddhist families see even death as an important learning experience for their pet, and do not want to interfere with their pet in the dying process, which they see as important to experience. There is no black and white view for the link between religion and euthanasia preparedness.

EXAMPLE STORY PART 1

Charlie is an 11-year-old male neutered black lab. He has come in with his owner, Brenna, who is a 24-year-old woman. Her older parents are with her, and they often dog-sit Charlie when she has to work.

Charlie has come in for his yearly vaccines, but on examination you notice that he is pale, and his belly is a bit tender. All your other findings are normal. Brenna consents to bloodwork and radiographs at your suggestion. Unfortunately, the bloodwork shows he is anemic, and the radiographs show that he has what is likely a splenic mass, with some free blood in the abdomen. At this point the family is stressed and worried; Charlie was just coming in to get vaccines and now you may have found cancer? Brenna seems very worried and confides that her childhood dog died horribly, and she doesn't want that to happen to Charlie. Meanwhile, her parents declare that they *Don't want to just kill him. He looks fine!*

What is the best way to approach this conversation?

In order to even think about approaching this conversation and making goals, we need to establish a connection. There is a lot of great information out there about approaching these conversations, from body language to opening words. Having a road map for these conversations is almost essential, because you only get one chance to get this right.

In general, making sure that you are at eye level or below the family, as well as having nothing in between you, like a table, will help keep the conversation and connection open. Families sometimes surprise us with what they know, and jumping right into a spiel about a disease is not usually the right move. We want the client to be able to ask questions and communicate with us. Once we've assessed what they might know about a diagnosis, or prognosis, we can share our information, checking with them along the way to make sure they understand. In the clinic, this can be time consuming, so it is ok to take breaks in the conversation as needed. A family may need time to digest a lot of the medical heavy information you've given them.[5]

Once you've shared your information and concerns, pass the conversation back to them to start establishing goals for care of the patient. A lot of goals come from the fears a family may have, whether it is a pet dying alone, or the monetary cost of chemo versus palliative care, or even the time it will take to care for the patient. This is where categories of goals will be very helpful to assess, and even write down.

CATEGORIES OF GOALS

Developing goals of care at a pet's end of life helps to ensure everyone is on the same page, that the veterinary team is able to adequately support the pet and their family through this process, and that we can address the family's individual wishes. Palliative goals often differ from those earlier in a pet's life, and may require a shift in mindset and priorities, focusing more on comfort and quality of life.[6] These goals will also be unique for each individual pet and their family and should be tailored as such. The goals of care conversation can take place at varying times in the end of life journey. In our example case, an unexpected finding on a routine examination initiated the conversation. They can also happen when treatment efficacy for a serious or chronic illness begins to wane, or when a pet's quality of life begins to decline.[7,8]

Types of goals and the conversations that elucidate them can take many forms. At present, these conversations often happen without prompts or guidelines, and given their highly emotional nature, can be stressful for both the veterinary team and the families. By providing structure, we can assess the situation, formulate a plan, and support the family more efficiently and successfully.

Goals can be broken down into different types and involve both the pet and their family. In human medicine, these goals often reflect the patient's personal wishes for themselves. Given the nature of veterinary medicine, these goals can be more complex as they take into account both the pet and their family, who are making decisions in their best interest and are instrumentally involved in their care. Goals include physical, psychological, social, and cultural or spiritual needs, though there is often overlap in these types of care.

Categories of goals

- Physical
  - Often more obvious and tend to be some of the first goals we think of
  - More easily seen and conceptualized by owners and veterinary team
  - Includes pain management, hygiene, environmental needs, and symptomatic care based on the underlying diseases and issues each pet is facing
  - Pain management is a key aspect of physical care
- Psychological
  - Sometimes less overt than physical care but equally important.
  - Many pets experience increased anxiety and stress at the end of their lives, caused by increased pain, limited mobility, cognitive decline, or simply changes in their routine
  - Addressing their physical needs can help alleviate some psychological distress
- Social
  - Often an important factor for families as their bond with their pet is paramount and can be negatively impacted at life's end
  - Human–animal bond can be strained by increased veterinary care, treatments provided at home, and physical pain or psychological issues
  - Changes at the end of a pet's life also affect their relationship with other pets or people in their home or environment

- Spiritual and cultural
  - Can inform a family's decision to pursue diagnostics and treatment,
  - Affect their decisions surrounding euthanasia
  - Influence the family's comfort level when discussing end of life

We can also consider the owners personal financial, emotional, physical, or time budgets. As the owner is often the primary caregiver for the pet and is instrumental in facilitating the care plan, it is essential to ensure that the goals and plans are achievable given each family's personal budgets.[9] By addressing each aspect of care, we can ensure all of the pet's and family's needs are considered and met.

TOOLS FOR GOAL SETTING

There are various tools already available to help the veterinary team guide families in developing goals of care. Veterinary end of life conversation guides and outlines have begun to emerge as we learn from the human hospice and palliative medicine field. Some have been borrowed and adapted from human medicine, tailoring them to pets and their families, including the Serious Veterinary Illness Conversation Guide, which was adapted from the Serious Illness Conversation Guide by Ariadne Labs.[7,8] Other helpful resources include the 2016 American Animal Hospital Association (AAHA)/Internation Association for Animal Hospice and Palliative Care (IAAHPC) End-of-Life Care Guidelines and the 2023 American Association of Feline Practitioners (AAFP)/IAAHPC Feline Hospice and Palliative Care Guidelines.[9,10]

The Serious Veterinary Illness Conversation Guide (SVICG), created by Katherine Goldberg, lays out a framework for goals of care conversations. The guide is broken down into 8 sections, beginning with *understanding* and *information preference*. These focus on acquiring an understanding of what the family already knows, initial questions they may have, and the amount and type of information they prefer to receive moving forward. After setting a foundation for the conversation, the next step *Prognosis* involves sharing information about their pet's prognosis and disease processes, taking into account what the family has shared in the first steps. With this mutual understanding in place, the guide moves on to goals, *fears/worries*, *function*, and *trade-offs*. Here, the focus is on determining the priorities each family has in these scenarios with respect to their pet's end of life. In these sections, the physical, psychological, social needs we discussed earlier will come into play. Finally, the guide ends with *Aid in dying*. This part clearly diverges from the human version as euthanasia is a treatment option for veterinary patients. This section in particular also takes into account the owners' spiritual and cultural goals in relation to death and euthanasia.[7]

Another example is the REMAP (Reframe, Expect emotion, Map out patient goals framework), which helps guide end of life conversations between oncologists and their patients. REMAP is a mnemonic that stands for Reframe, Expect emotion, Map out patient goals, Align with goals, and Propose a plan. Though made for human patients, this can easily be adjusted for our veterinary patients. In the original framework, the initial step often takes place when the oncology treatment is no longer working and the physician and patient need to reevaluate the goals of care. For the veterinary team, this may mean initialing a conversation after a terminal diagnosis or for a senior pet whose quality of life is in serious decline to *reframe* the conversation toward hospice or palliative care. As in the SVICG, this first step seeks to gain understanding of what a family already knows and gently steer the conversation toward palliative care. When discussing these sensitive topics, it is normal to *expect emotion*.

Acknowledging these emotions helps build rapport and trust with the family and allows the conversation to progress to the next step, *mapping out patient values*. Here we are focusing on the family's values and wishes for their pet. We can use open ended questions to assess physical, psychological, and social goals the family may have. Next, use this information to *align with values*, repeating back what you've learned and summarizing their goals. Finally, we can *propose a plan* given what we've learned to maximize the goals and values discussed.[11]

Readers can adapt resources themselves to make personalized frameworks or questionnaires used to guide their conversations, or handouts to provide to their clients to facilitate these conversations at a later time. For example, you can print a copy of the SVICG or make your own framework to keep in each examination room to pull out at senior visits or after a poor prognosis is made. Many resources created and available for people at their end of life, like the REMAP framework, can be easily tailored to our patients and their families. The following questionnaire was adapted by a veterinarian from a human advanced directive.

VETERINARY ADVANCED DIRECTIVE EXAMPLE (DESIGNED BY DR. FRANK)

Medical Care

If your pet is seriously ill, or nearing the end of life, how much medical treatment would feel right to you?

Would you feel better getting a full diagnosis? Would you prefer your pet to not undergo all diagnostics or treatments if they might be invasive, even if they might help?

What worries you most about future health care needs your pet may have?

The financial burden? The Emotional Burden? The time and physical strength to take care of them?

What does a *good death* mean to you?

For example, would your loved one like to be surrounded by family, or would they prefer just those closest to them? Would they like to avoid pain? Would they and you prefer having certain songs playing or to be in their favorite bed?

Are there any spiritual beliefs that affect the kind of care you would like for your pet?

By having an idea of what you would like for your pet, it may help bring a sense of calm and organization when the time comes. This can be done at any time in a pet's life.

With these goals and tools in mind, we can continue the conversation with some active listening, repeating back to the family what you've heard to in turn help them feel heard.

EXAMPLE STORY PART 2

You decide to sit on the chair next to the family, and open with *Would it be alright if we talk about what these things mean for Charlie?* Keeping the patient in care and focus is always a good idea. Once you get the go ahead, you ask what they know about splenic tumors.

Surprisingly, the daughter knows a bit. Their last dog had one, and it was very traumatic for her to watch the dog die at home. It seemed to happen so fast. You agree that yes it can happen fast, going over fast and slow bleeds. You also go over options for referral to oncology/surgery, as well as hospice care. You ask if they understand the information so far. Then you ask the family what they are most worried about.

The daughter does not want to go through something so traumatic again and has limited time to care for Charlie while traveling for work. The parents are worried about saying goodbye too early, as Charlie still looks good. They also worry about physically getting Charlie somewhere if

> he cannot get up. They are not interested in putting Charlie through surgery and absolutely don't want him to suffer.
>
> Essentially, their goals for Charlie are to keep him comfortable, and to help him pass before he has a major bleed. The daughter does not want it to be an emergency, and you reiterate that it would be best to help him say goodbye on a good day. They have physical and emotional budgets, which are very important to them. You have given them a lot of information today and know that they are not ready to euthanize yet, but you can try to keep him comfortable and happy in the meantime.
>
> "I can tell you love Charlie a whole lot, and I wish we had more time to chat. I want to give you some time to digest everything. For now our plan is to add a couple of medications to keep Charlie comfortable. To keep with our goals of making sure Charlie doesn't suffer, and to keep him from being unable to move at home, we will want to schedule to help him pass on a good day in this time frame. I have some information and papers here you can look at when you're ready, and if you have any questions, please just give us a call. We're here for you and Charlie. We'll give you a call in a few days to check up on you and Charlie as well."

In our example story, the veterinarian used the Serious Veterinary Illness Conversation Guide as a framework, helping guide the unexpected conversation. She began by discerning the family's current understanding of the disease and situation, then moved on to discuss more about the disease and prognosis. This led into the family's goals, fears, and worries for their pet and themselves. They discussed tradeoffs and finished by coming up with a plan for the time being, which was informed by the prior conversation. As these conversations can be long and very emotional, they may need to be broken up over time. Providing the family with an advanced directive handout allows for them to digest the information and further consider their preferences and goals, both individually and as a family. Finally, the veterinarian scheduled a follow-up (visit or phone call), allowing for the continued care of the pet, to address any questions or concerns that may arise, and to ensure follow-up is not forgotten.

In some cases, it is not possible to have the goals of care conversation at the time of diagnosis or in one sitting. There may not be enough time, or perhaps the family reacts in anger or simply isn't ready to have a conversation to establish goals. Having written information on common diseases allows families to take home verified information to help them understand disease trajectory. Along with this information, especially in the case of terminal diseases, you can provide an advance pet directive or questionnaire to help put their goals into writing.[5] Providing a gentle questionnaire or handout after a senior pet visit can allow the family to start considering their wishes and goals ahead of time, even if a terminal diagnosis is not made. A follow-up visit, whether in person or virtually, is especially important in these cases, and should be scheduled to continue the conversation, cooperatively develop goals of care, and address any questions that may arise.

Not all goal setting is the same, however. We want to make sure the goals we set with families are realistic, while still addressing what a family and pet want and need. The following section helps us do just that.

HOW TO CREATE GOALS WITH SPECIFIC, MEASURABLE, ACHIEVABLE, RELEVANT, AND TIME-BOUND MEASURES

SMART is an acronym, standing for Specific, Measurable, Achievable, Relevant, and Time-bound. It is used in many functions in life today, but its success related to end of life care may not be entirely intuitive, so let's go through these parameters together.

SPECIFIC: Many families come to us with very wide conceptions of saying goodbye. How many simply tell us *I just don't want him to suffer, doc*, or *I just don't want him to be in pain*? Meanwhile, they have a very hard time defining suffering, or a very individual idea of it. For some people, pain means a pet is vocalizing, when we know that pain happens often long before a pet ever vocalizes it. For this measure, we need to interpret and narrow down what they are looking for while using gentle curiosity to get them to be more specific. *When you say suffering, are you referring to pain? Let's talk about what pain and discomfort looks like in cats with kidney failure so we can watch for that...* Nausea is a large concern for kidney failure cats, so let's say her appetite is going to be a specific parameter we will be watching, as it correlates to how much she may be feeling.

MEASURABLE: This can take many forms. As doctors we often think of CBCs and Chem 15's, but even something like only eating 1 meal a day, down from 2, is measurable. Following our kitty with kidney failure example, only using the litter box once a day instead of 3 times, or only eating a few tablespoons of food, versus her usual one-fourth cup, is a measurement of how she is doing as her disease progresses. We may think of introducing an antinausea med if her weight reaches a specific number, or she is only eating a certain amount of food a day that isn't life sustaining (ie, eating less than one-eighth of a cup a day).

ACHIEVABLE: Achievability in end of life care may not seem as intuitive as the other parameters. However, we need to help families gain a realistic view of how they would like the last days of their pet's life to be. A lot of families, including our own, would love their pet to live forever, or die quietly in their sleep, but most of the times, that's not achievable. What is achievable is a peaceful passing at home or at a clinic. Going through a bucket list of things with their pet is achievable. For our running example of a kitty with kidney failure, we may set an achievable goal of spending 15 minutes each day brushing her on her heated bed, or giving her a week with new meds and sub-q fluids before reassessing how she's doing. These parameters are within our reach.

RELEVANT: This parameter is so intuitive, it almost goes without saying. Think of this as a check on how a goal is forming so far. These goals are focused around the human-animal bond, containing physical, social, psychological, financial, and emotional lenses. In this way, we can dismiss input from outside sources, like *My mother doesn't want my kitty to die on her birthday*. Not only is this not necessarily achievable (though specific and measurable), it is not centered around the caregiver and the bond they have with their kitty. We need to keep the bond at the center of our goal-setting.

TIME-BOUND: While we wish we had a crystal ball to predict the exact time a patient will have a seizure, their spleen will rupture, or their heart will give out, we simply don't. Time-bound goals help us move forward into the unknown, while also allowing us to reassess and change our goals from time to time as a patient's condition changes either for better or worse. This could be anything from setting an end-point of hospice care, now warranting euthanasia, or reassessment of how a patient is responding to current care and treatment so that we can set another time bound goal for recheck. In the case of our kitty with kidney failure, we may set a time-bound red flag, that if she doesn't eat despite medication for 24 hours, it's time for euthanasia. Or in the latter case, let's recheck her bloodwork in 2 weeks with medication and subcutaneous fluid treatments.[12]

Over time, setting goals like this will become second nature, and be a real help to families in regards to end of life care. Some examples of goals pertaining to different diseases may look like this:

Examples of goals pertaining to different diseases

1. Hemangiosarcoma: It sounds like you are very concerned with Max dying suddenly. Our goal is to make sure Max and you don't experience the suffering or trauma of a fast bleed, so we are going to set a day for euthanasia in 1 week so you have time to spend with him, while also giving him peace on a good day.
2. Osteoarthritis: We now know that Buddy's panting and paw licking has been self-soothing since he's in pain. We are going to try this medication to see if that behavior reduces by at least 75%, and I would like to see you in 2 weeks to see if this is working for him. Make sure to record the time he is or isn't doing this behavior.
3. Cardiac Failure: Princess's heart is moving into a later stage of heart failure. Based on what you've told me, we want to say goodbye at home and not at an emergency center. To do this, we are going to do resting respiratory rate measurements twice a day, and when they reach between 30 and 40 breaths per minute, we are going to schedule euthanasia for her.

REASSESSMENT OF GOALS

Once the initial conversation has taken place and goals of care have been determined, it is essential to follow up and reassess these goals over time. The timeline for each patient will vary based on the goals and diseases, but should be discussed and documented. While many pets will require follow-up care for laboratory work or rechecks, visits focused solely on quality of life and goals of care can be important as well. Families may also have further questions or concerns after taking time to digest the information and monitor the pet at home. They may have taken time to discuss with other family members or assess their pet in a new light, which may lead to adjustments of the goals of care.

This is a great time to implement technician visits to follow up and evaluate a pet's progress.[6,13] The veterinary technician can be a critical link between the veterinary team and the family. Technicians can follow up after an initial visit, evaluate vital signs and evidence of disease progression during rechecks, and teach the family signs of various diseases so they are better prepared to monitor their pets at home. If a team member is able to visit the pet in their home, this can deepen the veterinary-patient–client relationship while involving the family and assessing the pet in their environment. A skilled palliative care technician can alleviate the veterinarian's work load while providing a supportive resource for the family as they navigate this difficult time.[12]

While the initial work leading up to and including the goals of care conversation is the main focus, frequent check-ins are incredibly helpful and meaningful to families in this difficult and emotional time. This could involve in-office or in-home rechecks with the pet, a telemedicine visit with someone from the veterinary team, or even an email sent by a trained technician. Follow through will help ensure the family feels supported and the pet's comfort and wellbeing are considered throughout the end of life journey.

CLINICS CARE POINTS

- Use active listening to help owners feel heard and to reach an agreement on goals.
- Be direct but compassionate in speech to meet owners where they are in the process.
- If the conversation derails, bring it back to focus on the pet.
- If an owner isn't ready to have this conversation, give them the go ahead to approach you when they are, and periodically check in.

DISCLOSURE

Authors are associate veterinarians at Lap of Love and have made no profit in the writing of this article.

REFERENCES

1. Corr CA, Corr DM, Doka KJ. Death and dying, life and living. 8th edition. Boston: Cengage; 2018.
2. Servaty-Seib HL, Chapple HS. Handbook of thanatology: the essential body of knowledge for the study of death, dying, and bereavement. 3rd edition. Association for Death Education and Counseling; 2021.
3. Schulz R, Boerner K, Klinger J, et al. Preparedness for death and adjustment to bereavement among caregivers of recently placed nursing home residents. J Palliat Med 2015;18(2):127–33.
4. Shearer T. Nonpharmacologic methods to improve the euthanasia experience. Vet Clin Small Anim Pract 2020;50(3):627–38.
5. Robertson S. The tender conversation. Available at: https://lap-of-love.helpjuice.com/grief-additional-resources/the-tender-conversation?from_search=194166607. Accessed May 16, 2025.
6. da Costa JM, Guerra Barroso T, Correia Prata J. Research priorities in veterinary palliative care. Vet J 2024;306. https://doi.org/10.1016/j.tvjl.2024.106184.
7. Goldberg KJ. Goals of care. Vet Clin Small Anim Pract 2019;49(3):399–415.
8. Ariadne labs: a joint Center for health systems innovation (www.ariadnelabs.org) between Brigham and women's Hospital and the Harvard T.H. Chan School of public health, in collaboration with Dana-Farber cancer Institute. Serious illness conversation guide. 2023. Available at: https://www.ariadnelabs.org/wp-content/uploads/2023/05/Serious-Illness-Conversation-Guide.2023-05-18.pdf. Accessed April 1, 2025.
9. Eigner DR, Breitreiter K, Carmack T, et al. AAFP/IAAHPC feline hospice and palliative care guidelines. J Feline Med Surg 2023;25(9).
10. Bishop G, Cooney K, Cox S, et al. AAHA/IAAHPC end-of-life care guidelines. J Am Anim Hosp Assoc 2016;52(6):341–56.
11. Childers JW, Back AL, Tulsky JA, et al. REMAP: a framework for goals of care conversations. J Oncol Pract 2017;13(10):e844–50.
12. Boogaard K. How to write SMART goals. Available at: https://www.atlassian.com/blog/productivity/how-to-write-smart-goals.12/26/2023. Accessed May 16, 2025.
13. Carter K. The role of the veterinary technician in end-of-life care. Vet Clin Small Anim Pract 2020;50(3):639–45.

Veterinary Hospice—Enhancing Quality Without Prolonging Suffering

Tyler Carmack, DVM, CVA, CHPV, CVFT, CTPEP, CPEV, CVPP

KEYWORDS

- Veterinary hospice • Palliative care • Quality of life • Symptom management
- End-of-life decision-making • Palliated death • Euthanasia planning

KEY POINTS

- Veterinary hospice is a philosophy of care that prioritizes comfort, dignity, and quality of life (QoL) when curative treatment is no longer beneficial or desired.
- Early, proactive communication, including prognosis discussions, quality-of-life assessments, common QoL challenges, and *what if* scenarios, supports thoughtful decision-making and reduces crisis-driven choices.
- Effective hospice care integrates multimodal analgesia, symptom management, environmental adaptations, and caregiver empowerment to maximize patient comfort.
- Euthanasia planning, including discussion of anticipatory grief, benchmarks for QoL thresholds, home versus hospital procedures, and memorialization options, is central to end-of-life care.
- Hospice care strengthens the human–animal bond by supporting families emotionally, providing anticipatory grief resources and ensuring that pets experience a peaceful, dignified final stage of life.

INTRODUCTION

Defining Veterinary Hospice in Small Animal Medicine

Veterinary hospice is a philosophy and model of care that focuses on maximizing comfort, maintaining dignity, and supporting the human–animal bond during a pet's final life stage. It is appropriate for animals with a life-limiting diagnosis, geriatric medical concerns, or progressive disease(s) when curative treatment is no longer beneficial or desired. Hospice care shifts the care goal from prolonging life expectancy to enhancing its quality and offering tailored medical, emotional, and practical caregiving and planning support to both the patient and their family. While many of the principles and strategies for providing care mirror human hospice, there are also some key differences. While medical aid in dying is increasingly recognized as an endpoint in

Caring Pathways, 4740 Baxter Road #105, Virginia Beach, VA 23462, USA
E-mail address: dr.tyler@caringpathways.com

Vet Clin Small Anim 56 (2026) 455–473
https://doi.org/10.1016/j.cvsm.2025.10.004 vetsmall.theclinics.com

Abbreviations	
COAST	canine osteoarthritis staging tool
EMKs	emergency medication kits
IRIS	International Renal Interest Society
LOAD	Liverpool Osteoarthritis in Dogs
QoL	quality of life

human hospice, with approximately 20% of Americans living in jurisdictions where it is legal, the veterinary model has long incorporated euthanasia as a compassionate tool to prevent and end suffering.[1,2] The growing pet insurance industry may further shape how families access and use hospice services for their animals but does not have strictly defined hospice benefit periods or limitations of care, the way human hospice does. For example, a person qualifies for hospice care if they have a 6-month or less life expectancy, and they are typically not eligible for curative treatments at the same time they are receiving hospice services (defined as concurrent care).[3]

Hospice versus palliative care

Although closely related, hospice and palliative care are not identical. Palliative care may be provided alongside curative or life-prolonging treatments at any disease stage, aiming to relieve symptoms and improve comfort. Hospice, by contrast, is reserved for the last phase of life—when prognosis is limited and the focus is exclusively on comfort rather than extending lifespan or curing a disease. In hospice, all interventions are weighed against the patient's remaining quality of life (QoL) and the risk of prolonging suffering.

Hospice versus euthanasia-only services

Euthanasia-only services provide a compassionate and humane death without a preceding period of supportive care by that same provider. Typically clients are receiving these services by their general practice veterinarian. Hospice incorporates euthanasia as one possible outcome, but it is framed as part of a larger care process. Through proactive ongoing symptom management, client education, end-of-life planning, and quality-of-life monitoring, hospice helps families recognize how and when euthanasia decisions are most appropriate for their pet. This in-depth approach can give owners time to prepare emotionally, address practical matters, and say goodbye in a manner that most aligns with their values.

Ethical positioning

The ethical foundation of veterinary hospice is the deliberate balance between maximizing QoL and avoiding unnecessary suffering. This requires open and frank communication, shared decision-making responsibilities, and proactive, frequent reassessment.[4] The field is guided by bioethical principles, including respect for autonomy, nonmaleficence, beneficence, and justice.[4] The veterinarian serves as both the medical guide and advocate for the patient, ensuring that compassionate care, not the prolongation of life or provision of futile care, remains the central priority.

Growing Client Demand for Veterinary End-of-Life Options

Pet owners are increasingly seeking individualized, compassionate approaches to end-of-life care for their animals, and this is reflected in the growing utilization of hospice and palliative care services.[5] As pets live longer due to advances in nutrition, preventive medicine, and chronic disease management, more families face decisions about terminal illness and age-related decline.[2] Many owners are now exploring options beyond continued aggressive treatment or immediate euthanasia, instead preferring a path that prioritizes comfort, dignity, and their family goals and values. Clients often seek veterinarians who can offer practical guidance, symptom management, and emotional support throughout the final stage of their pet's life. Using hospice services can support and strengthen the human–animal bond by allowing families to share meaningful, comfortable time together while ensuring their pet's final days are comfortable and content.

Providing Veterinary Hospice Services

Role of the primary care veterinarian

The general practitioner is uniquely positioned to guide families through their pet's life stage transitions, including the final one into hospice care. General practitioners often have long-term relationships with clients, detailed knowledge of the patient's medical history, and the trust necessary for sensitive conversations.[6] In this role, the veterinarian must provide clear information about prognosis, outline all care options (including hospice), and help families align treatment choices with their values and the animal's welfare. By initiating timely discussions and facilitating gradual shifts in care goals, primary care veterinarians help ensure that end-of-life decisions are made thoughtfully, without unnecessary suffering, and are not crisis-driven choices.

Veterinary hospice naturally aligns with structured geriatric care programs, serving as the final phase of a continuum that begins with wellness care and extends through chronic disease management and geriatric care. Integrating hospice into geriatric protocols allows for earlier conversations about QoL, advance care planning, and helps set realistic expectations.[6] This integration ensures that the transition to end-of-life care is seamless, with the same veterinary team maintaining oversight from early aging changes to the final goodbye. It also allows for proactive preparation, such as mobility support, pain management adjustments, and environmental modifications, before crises occur.

Role of the veterinary specialist

Unlike human medicine—where hospice enrollment historically requires discontinuation of curative treatment—veterinary hospice allows for concurrent care, enabling pets to receive palliative interventions alongside disease-directed therapies.[5,7] This flexibility can ease the emotional transition for owners, maintain hope, and address both comfort and longevity goals without forcing an abrupt shift in treatment philosophy. Veterinary specialists, therefore, can play a pivotal role in hospice and palliative care by providing advanced diagnostics (when desired), targeted treatment recommendations, and disease-specific prognostic guidance.[8] Their expertise helps refine the care plan, ensuring that symptom management strategies are evidence-based and tailored to the underlying condition. Specialist teams—including veterinary technicians, rehabilitation therapists, and client liaisons—can offer ongoing caregiver support, educate owners in home care techniques, and coordinate with the interdisciplinary hospice team to maintain continuity of care and work to minimize owner confusion and caregiving burden. This collaboration ensures that even complex medical cases receive compassionate, high-quality end-of-life care that focuses on both patient comfort and family goals.

Role of the hospice veterinarian

While many veterinarians find themselves in the position of providing hospice care, especially in general practice, as noted previously, it is important to note that there are dedicated practices limited to hospice and palliative care services. Using these services can be beneficial for the patient, caregivers, and the busy veterinary team. Hospice case management is typically very time-intensive and presents unique challenges that may not fit within the guidelines and standards of other cases within the practice. Dedicated hospice and palliative care veterinarians serve as holistic medical coordinators in the end-of-life care team, working in partnership with the primary care veterinarian, relevant specialists, and the pet's family to guide the hospice process from start to finish. Their advanced training in pain management, symptom control, communication, and caregiver support allows them to address both the medical and emotional aspects of care with exceptional depth.[9] Appointments are often far longer than standard veterinary visits, providing time for thorough assessments, detailed education, exploration of goals, and collaborative decision-making. Many hospice veterinarians operate in-home service models, which can reduce patient fear, anxiety, and stress, allow for real-time environmental assessments, and give families a more intimate, supportive setting in which to say goodbye.[10,11] Many dedicated hospice services also provide teleadvice services and virtual second-opinion consultations, offering detailed QoL discussions that can support families while easing the workload of busy primary care teams. Hospice veterinarians leading a comprehensive, team-based approach ensure care plans are individualized, regularly reassessed, and centered on maximizing comfort and QoL in a familiar environment.

DISCUSSION

Philosophic and Ethical Framework

Core hospice principles

The core philosophies of hospice care, whether in people or animals, center on prioritizing comfort, dignity, and QoL when curing is no longer the goal. Both human and veterinary hospices embrace a patient-centered and family-centered approach that addresses physical, emotional, and, when relevant, spiritual needs, recognizing the interconnectedness of well-being across all parties involved. In veterinary medicine, these values are underpinned by established animal welfare principles, such as the *Five Freedoms* and the *Five Domains Model*, which emphasize freedom from pain, distress, and discomfort while promoting the opportunity to experience positive states.[12,13]

QoL evaluation has become crucial in veterinary care, particularly for terminally ill pets, balancing life prolongation with welfare.[13] Veterinarians play a significant role in guiding clients' decision-making regarding seriously ill companion animals and therefore should receive training in ethical approaches to euthanasia decisions, client communication skills, and implement standardized protocols including QoL assessment tools.[14,15]

Ethical concerns

Veterinarians consistently face ethical conflicts and moral distress in modern small animal practice, particularly when balancing patient welfare against client emotional needs and financial constraints.[16,17] End-of-life care, in particular, can present complex ethical challenges for veterinary providers, patients, and families. Key issues include balancing patient and caregiver autonomy with beneficence (acting in the patient's best interest), nonmaleficence (avoiding harm), weighing quality versus quantity of life, and justice in providing fair and compassionate care; all while addressing a variety of cultural and religious perspectives.[18,19]

End-of-life care presents particular challenges, with veterinarians needing to weigh euthanasia decisions while maximizing patient comfort and supporting clients emotionally.[6] The majority of veterinarians report experiencing moderate to severe distress due to obstacles in providing appropriate care, with many feeling unprepared to handle these conflicts.[16] Veterinary hospice also requires an added layer of advocacy for the patient, ensuring that interventions align with their welfare rather than solely the emotional needs of the caregiver. Trends with modern advanced human medicine can translate into a similar *treat until the end* culture with our veterinary patients, which can lead to provider stress regarding providing futile care. A comfort-first hospice approach represents a compromise between the binary outcomes typically presented to owners: advanced care or euthanasia. Recent studies have highlighted the prevalence and impact of futile care in both veterinary and human medicine. In small animal veterinary practice, up to 99.2% of surveyed veterinarians reported encountering futile care during their careers, with 42.4% experiencing it frequently, highlighting its role as a significant source of ethical conflict and moral distress.[16,20] Similarly, in human critical care, 19.6% of patients were perceived to receive futile or probably futile treatment, accounting for 6.7% of intensive care unit (ICU) days and substantial costs.[21] Being able to shift these conversations with caregivers to focus on comfort and QoL can help relieve the moral stress of an owner not being ready for euthanasia but the reality that advanced and aggressive care is no longer likely to be successful. Across species, hospice care seeks not to hasten or postpone death but to ensure the final stage of life is lived as fully and comfortably as possible, in a manner consistent with ethical obligations, professional guidelines, and animal welfare standards.

Ethical dilemmas can arise in decisions regarding euthanasia for a variety of psychosocial reasons, and when experienced regularly, these can contribute to moral stress of the veterinary team.[22] Financial concerns, caregiver burden, and QoL considerations play significant roles in euthanasia decisions and may represent frequent sources of ethical dilemmas.[23]

Guidelines and professional standards

Practice guidelines provide an evidence-based framework that helps veterinarians deliver consistent, high-quality hospice and palliative care.[6] By following established recommendations, such as those listed later, practitioners can ensure appropriate pain and symptom management, client communication, and decision-making processes. These guidelines also support continuity of care, reduce variability between providers, and reinforce the profession's commitment to patient welfare and compassionate end-of-life support.

Relevant practice guidelines, toolkits, and position statements

- Hospice and Palliative Care
  - 2025 (International Association for Animal Hospice and Palliative Care [IAAHPC]) Hospice and Palliative Care Guidelines
  - 2023 (Feline Veterinary Medical Association [AAFP])/IAAHPC Feline Hospice and Palliative Care Guidelines
  - 2021 AAFP End of Life Toolkit
  - 2016 IAAHPC/American Animal Hospital Association (AAHA) End-of-Life Care Guidelines
  - 2013 IAAHPC Hospice and Palliative Care Guidelines
- Chronic Pain
  - 2024 FVMA Chronic Pain Educational Toolkit
  - 2024 ISFM and AAFP consensus guidelines on the long-term use of non-steroidal antiinflammatories (NSAIDs) in cats
  - 2022 World Small Animal Veterinary Association (WSAVA) guidelines for the recognition, assessment, and treatment of pain
  - 2022 AAHA Pain Management Guidelines & Toolkit for Dogs and Cats
- Euthanasia & Aftercare
  - American Veterinary Medical Association (AVMA) Guidelines for the Euthanasia of Animals: 2020 Edition

Patient Selection and Timing of Hospice Enrollment

Identifying candidates

Determining when a small animal patient is an appropriate candidate for hospice care requires careful consideration of medical prognosis, overall QoL, and the caregiver's goals and values.[24] Introducing the idea of hospice care to pet families also needs to be broached with sensitivity and thoughtfulness. Ideally, the expected progression from *adult* to *senior* to *geriatric* status, and then entrance into hospice care, would be introduced early in the pet's life, revisited and expanded upon at each subsequent visit, and benchmarks would be set for each of those transitions before deterioration of the pet's clinical status. This proactive approach can be aided with educational materials, clinical metrology instruments, and practice protocols to ensure all pet families receive detailed and individualized guidance throughout these transitions.

Prognosis-based criteria often serve as the starting point for entering hospice care. These criteria include a life expectancy of approximately 6 months or less, as determined by disease stage, progression, and response to therapy.[25,26] Since veterinary medicine allows for concurrent care, a definitive prognosis or discontinuation of curative treatment is not required, as it often is in adult human medicine. Common examples of diseases qualifying for hospice care include advanced neoplasia, end-stage organ failure (such as congestive heart failure or chronic kidney disease), progressive neurologic disorders, or severe degenerative joint disease when surgical or curative options are no longer viable. In these cases, the primary treatment goal shifts from prolonging survival to maximizing comfort and dignity.

Nonprognosis-based criteria are equally important in identifying hospice candidates, particularly when survival time is difficult to predict. Declining QoL despite optimal medical management, manifested by persistent pain, sarcopenia, inappetence or anorexia, respiratory distress, incontinence, or inability to ambulate, can indicate that the animal's remaining time should focus on comfort rather than cure. Client factors also play a critical role: owners may choose hospice if ongoing curative treatment conflicts with their values, resources, or the perceived well-being of the pet. In some situations, a pet may meet hospice criteria because the family wishes to avoid repeated hospitalizations, intensive interventions, or the emotional toll of aggressive care.

Ultimately, identifying hospice candidates requires a combination of clinical assessment, honest discussion with the owner, and alignment of care goals. Early recognition allows for a timely transition into comfort-focused management, giving both the patient and family the opportunity for a more peaceful, prepared, and supported end-of-life journey.[27]

Prognostication tools

In human medicine, prognostication tools such as the Palliative Performance Scale, Karnofsky Performance Status, and disease-specific staging systems are widely used to estimate life expectancy and guide transitions into hospice care.[28–30] These tools help physicians objectively track functional decline, identify when patients meet eligibility criteria (such as a prognosis of $\leq$6 months), and support consistent, evidence-based decision-making across care teams.

While veterinary medicine does not yet have standard, global prognostication tools, several disease-specific staging tools do exist and can be used in this manner. For canine osteoarthritis, the Canine OsteoArthritis Staging Tool (COAST) incorporates owner and veterinarian assessments to evaluate both preclinical and established cases, potentially improving pain control and management.[31] The International Renal Interest Society (IRIS) guidelines for chronic kidney disease staging help guide targeted treatment, including dietary modifications and management of associated conditions like hypertension and anemia.[32] In these cases, symmetric dimethylarginine has been shown to serve as a sensitive biomarker for early diagnosis and staging in both dogs and cats.[33] The 2016 AAHA Oncology Guidelines recommend a patient-specific approach involving diagnosis, staging, and appropriate therapeutic interventions, emphasizing the importance of considering various treatment modalities based on tumor type, grade, and stage.[34] Other disease-specific screening tools, such as DISHAA and CADES scales for cognitive dysfunction, chronic pain scales, QoL questionnaires, and the University of Tennessee's End-of-Life Values and Goals Worksheets, can all be useful in determining when patients should be transitioned into a hospice care program.

Assessing and Monitoring Hospice Patients

When managing animal hospice and palliative cases, providing high-quality care should include a 5-step care plan for efficiency and consistency.[26,35] A structured plan provides veterinarians and families with a clear, compassionate roadmap for guiding pets through the final stages of life. *Step 1:* Evaluation of the pet owner's needs, beliefs, and goals ensures that the care approach aligns with the family's values and expectations, fostering trust and shared decision-making. *Step 2:* Education about the disease process (es) empowers owners to understand the progression of illness, anticipate changes, consider alternative interventions, and recognize early signs of declining QoL. *Step 3:* Development of a personalized plan tailors medical, emotional, and environmental strategies to both the patient's condition and the caregiver's abilities, creating a realistic, sustainable approach. The care plan should be delivered both verbally and in written materials for the caregiver to reference when needed. *Step 4:* Application of hospice or palliative care techniques focuses on symptom relief, comfort measures, and practical interventions that can be carried out at home, most often by the family as primary caregivers, but can also involve the veterinary team, groomers, pet sitters, and other support persons. *Step 5:* Emotional support during the care process and after the death of the pet acknowledges the profound impact of the impending loss, offering grief resources and continued connection to help families navigate bereavement. This support can begin with the veterinary team, but should also utilize mental health professionals when appropriate. This systematic approach not only improves patient comfort but also supports the human–animal bond and eases the caregiver's journey through end-of-life care (**Fig. 1**).

Assessing quality of life

The increasing importance of QoL assessments in veterinary medicine mirrors trends in human health care.[36] These tools are particularly relevant for terminally ill and geriatric pets, when veterinary providers are balancing efforts to maximize lifespan with animal welfare.[13] The World Health Organization defines QoL as *an individual's perception of their position in life in the context of the culture and value systems in which they live and in relation to their goals, expectations, standards, and concerns*.[37] Based on this definition, patient-reported outcomes are the gold standard in monitoring QoL. In veterinary medicine, much like in pediatric medicine, providers have to make QoL assessments based on observer (pet owner)-reported outcomes. Veterinarians play a significant role in interpreting observer-reported outcomes and guiding clients' decision-making regarding seriously ill companion animals.[14] It's recommended to implement standardized protocols, including QoL assessment tools for these evaluations and sensitive discussions.[14,15] The use of any QoL assessment tool increases the frequency of owner-veterinarian consultations and can help families feel more a part of their pet's care.[38,39] (**Tables 1** and **2**).

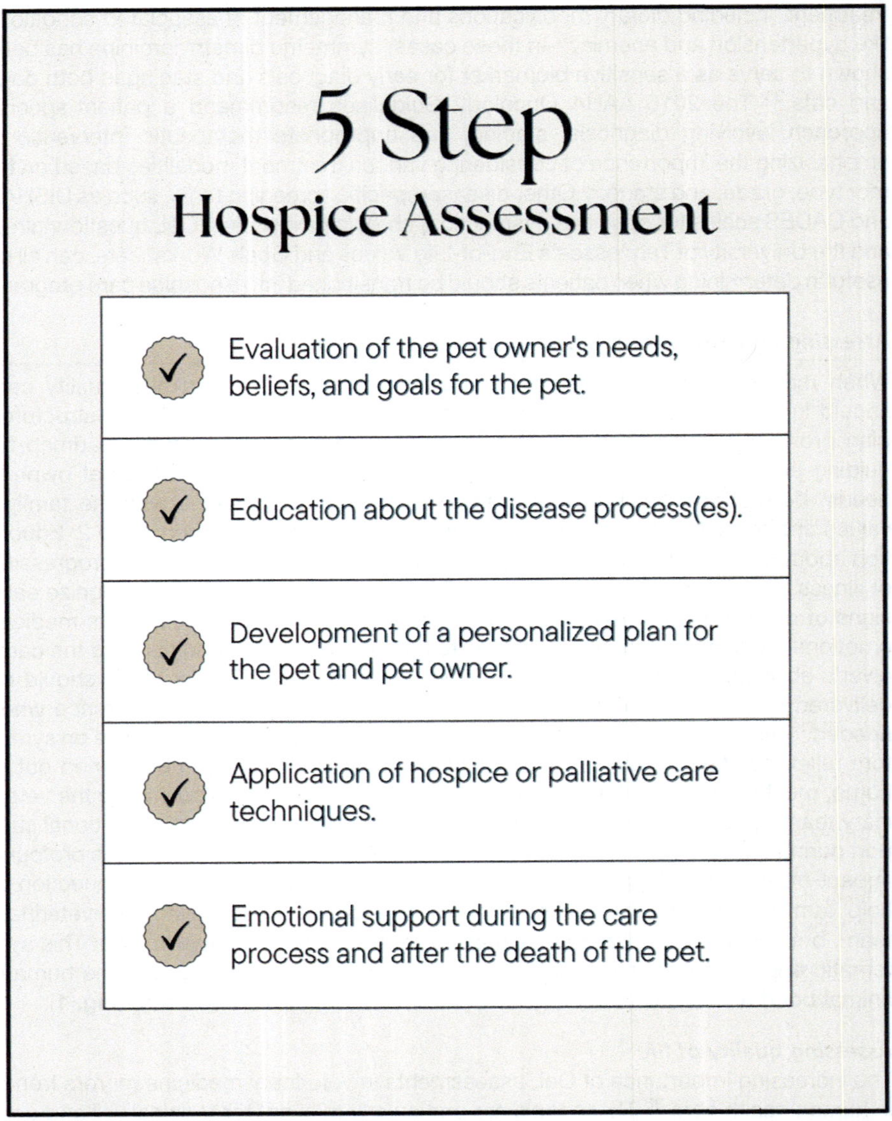

Fig. 1. The Step Hospice Assessment provides a systematic approach to ensure consistency of care. (Tamara S. Shearer, Pet Hospice and Palliative Care Protocols, Veterinary Clinics of North America: Small Animal Practice, 41 (3), 2011, 507-518, https://doi.org/10.1016/j.cvsm.2011.03.002.)

The ultimate goal of a QOL assessment is to prioritize holistic well-being as the primary consideration in making health care decisions.[40] In this respect, a QOL survey has the potential to influence therapy decisions and assess treatment response, particularly when the goal is palliative.[41] Other benefits of a QOL questionnaire include raising awareness among pet owners and clinical staff of factors that influence well-being in individual animals, monitoring changes in the pet's QOL over time, improving treatment compliance, increasing the client's sense of involvement in the dog's treatment plan, and improving the practice's relationship with its clients.[42,43] To illustrate,

Table 1
Overview of quality-of-life tools available for dogs

Category	Represents Tool Example	Key Focus Areas
Generic QoL	HHHHHMM, Lap of Love, OSU *How Will I Know?*, Midtown Moblie Veterinary Hospice Services, JOURNEYS, VetMetrica HR-QOL,[a] Yeates 2011,[a] Lavan 2013,[a] CHQLS-21/15[a] (healthy dogs)	Multidomain QoL assessment
Disease-Specific QoL	LOAD questionnaire[a](arthritis), COAST[a] (arthritis), FETCH Questionnaire[a] (cardiac), CDQoL-TSQ[a] (canine allergic dermatitis), CORQ[a] (cancer)	Condition-specific QoL assessment
Acute Pain Scales	GCMPS,[a] Melbourne Pain Scale,[a] CSU Acute Pain Scale	Objective acute pain assessment
Chronic Pain Scales	Canine Brief Pain Inventory,[a] HCPI,[a] Visual Analog Scale,[a] CSU Chronic Pain Scale, BEAP Pain Scale, client specific outcome measures	Objective chronic pain assessment

Abbreviations: BEAP, breathing, eyes, ambulation, activity, appetite, activity, attitude, posture, palpation; CDQoL-TSQ, canine dermatitis QoL and treatment satisfaction questionnaire; COAST, canine osteoarthritis staging tool; CORQ, canine owner-reported QoL questionnaire; CSU, Colorado State University; FETCH, functional evaluation of cardiac health; GCMPS, Glasgow composite measure pain scale; HCPI, Helsinki chronic pain index; HHHHHMM, hurt, hunger, hydration, hygiene, happiness, mobility, more good days than bad days; OSU, Ohio State University.
[a] Indicates validation study.

81% of dog owners undergoing cancer treatment reported that completing a QOL survey made them feel more involved in their pet's treatment.[38]

Client education for monitoring

Veterinary client education is central to successful hospice care, as families serve as the primary caregivers and observers of their pet's day-to-day condition.[2] Owners should

Table 2
Overview of quality-of-life tools available for cats

Category	Tool Example	Key Focus Areas
Generic QoL	CHEW Questionnaire,[a] VetMetrica HRQOL,[a] CatQoL,[a] HHHHHMM, OSU *How Will I Know?* Vetmetrica HRQOL,[a] Lap of Love, Midtown Mobile Veterinary Hospice Services, JOURNEYS QoL	Multidomain QoL assessment
Disease-Specific QoL	Hyperthyroid HRQoL[a] (hyperthyroidism), DIAQoL-pet[a] (diabetes), CATCH Questionnaire[a] (cardiac), Feline Musculoskeletal Pain Index,[a] Noli 2016[a] (skin disease)	Condition-specific QoL assessment
Acute Pain Scales	FGS,[a] UNESP-Botucatu Multidimensional Composite Pain Scale,[a] GFCMPS,[a] CSU Acute Pain Scale	Objective acute pain assessment
Chronic Pain Scales	CSU Chronic Pain Scale, BEAP Pain Scale, Client Specific Outcome Measures[a]	Objective chronic pain assessment

Abbreviations: BEAP, breathing, eyes, ambulation, activity, appetite, activity, attitude, posture, palpation; CATCH, cats' assessment tool for cardiac health; CHEW, cat health and wellbeing; CSU, Colorado State University; FGS, feline grimace scale; GFCMPS, Glasgow feline composite measure pain scale; HHHHHMM, hurt, hunger, hydration, hygiene, happiness, mobility, more good days than bad days; OSU, Ohio State University.
[a] Indicates validation study.

be equipped with client-specific outcome measures that reflect both medical priorities and the pet's unique lifestyle, such as maintaining appetite, enjoying favorite activities, or the ability to rest comfortably. Veterinarians can provide pain scales, disease-specific staging tools (such as American College of Veterinary Interal Medicine's heart failure stages, IRIS kidney staging, or the COAST and Liverpool Osteoarthritis in Dogs (LOAD) tools for osteoarthritis), and QoL tools to standardize observations and guide decision-making.[13,26] Encouraging daily journals or the use of photo and video diaries helps families track subtle changes over time, reducing the likelihood that functional decline goes unnoticed or is dismissed lightly. Education should also emphasize red flag signs of distress—such as persistent anorexia, uncontrolled pain, dyspnea, collapse, or sudden behavior changes—that require immediate communication with the veterinary team. By engaging clients as active participants with structured tools and clear guidance, veterinarians empower families to monitor effectively, make timely adjustments to care, and ensure that comfort remains the central focus.[6]

Longitudinal assessment

Longitudinal assessment of clinical symptoms and overall QoL allow veterinarians and families to evaluate the pet's condition over time rather than relying on isolated observations. By tracking trend data, including appetite, mobility, pain scores, and quality-of-life assessments, caregivers can recognize gradual declines that may otherwise be overlooked.[42] These patterns provide an objective framework for discussions about prognosis and benchmarks to determine when current or future distress outweighs comfort, ensuring euthanasia decisions are made thoughtfully, with compassion, and based on evidence rather than during an acute decompensation episode with heightened emotions. For further discussion, see article *Guiding End-of-Life Decisions and Quality of Life Assessments* by Moen.

SYMPTOM MANAGEMENT AND COMFORT CARE

Pain Management in Hospice Care

Pain is one of the most common and distressing symptoms in veterinary hospice patients, and its management is central to preserving QoL. In hospice care, the goal shifts from minimizing long-term side effects to prioritizing comfort, even if that requires higher or more frequent dosing, alternative formulations, or novel approaches. A proactive, individualized plan not only improves patient welfare but also supports families in providing care at home. For a more comprehensive discussion of chronic pain strategies and the role of rehabilitation, see articles *Chronic Pain- Effective Relief Strategies for Geriatric Pets* by Petty and *Movement Is Medicine: How Rehabilitation Revitalizes Aging Pets* by Alvarez of this issue.

Practical considerations

When designing a home analgesia plan, veterinarians should

1. Educate owners on recognizing pain, including instruction in using the most appropriate CMIs, and monitoring for side effects.
2. Provide written instructions and demonstrate administration techniques. Special focus should be placed on administration techniques that will not stress the human–animal bond.
3. Schedule regular reassessments, with clear protocols for escalating therapy if needed.
4. Plan for acute pain flares and potential sudden decompensation.

One of the greatest challenges in hospice care is helping pet owners recognize the subtle signs of chronic pain, which can be easily overlooked as pets adapt and owners normalize gradual decline.[4,44] Families often become accustomed to reduced activity, reluctance to climb stairs, or changes in demeanor, interpreting them as *just old age* rather than indicators of discomfort. This phenomenon, where *bad becomes the new normal*, can delay timely interventions and inadvertently prolong suffering. Clear communication, use of validated and client-friendly pain scales, and comparison to earlier baselines can help illustrate the extent of decline. By reframing these subtle changes as treatable signs of chronic pain, veterinarians can empower owners to make more compassionate, informed decisions. A team-oriented approach, including the caregiving family, is vital for maximizing pain recognition and treatment.[2,44]

Ultimately, pain management in hospice care is both a medical and ethical imperative. A thoughtful, multimodal approach can transform the end-of-life experience from one of suffering to one dedicated to comfort. Veterinarians should educate clients about the aging process and provide comprehensive care plans that may include both pharmacologic and nonpharmacologic interventions.[26,45] This approach can enhance and potentially extend the lives of senior pets.[45]

Nonpain Symptom Control in Hospice Care

While pain control is central to hospice care, many small animal patients experience other symptoms that substantially impact comfort, function, and QoL. In hospice medicine, symptom management is proactive and tailored to the individual, minimizing distress without introducing burdensome interventions. Some of the most common categories warrant particular attention.

Dyspnea

Respiratory distress is one of the most concerning hospice symptoms for pets and families. Management focuses on comfort rather than diagnostics: oxygen therapy (clinic or home-based) can provide relief in the short-term; opioids reduce air hunger; and anxiolytics mitigate panic. Owners should be trained to anticipate and recognize crises and have an emergency plan in place.

Cachexia/anorexia

Loss of appetite and muscle wasting are common in advanced disease. Appetite stimulants, assisted feeding (hand feeding, syringe feeding, and short-term feeding tubes), and highly palatable, calorie-dense foods offered in small, stress-free meals can improve comfort. Emphasis should be on desire and enjoyment rather than strict nutrition. Feeding techniques should reinforce and not unnecessarily strain the human–animal bond.

Sarcopenia

Sarcopenia, the progressive loss of muscle mass and strength associated with aging, is increasingly recognized as a contributor to frailty and diminished QoL in companion animals.[46,47] In hospice care, addressing sarcopenia involves educating owners about early recognition, providing nutritional support with adequate protein and omega-3 fatty acids, and encouraging gentle exercise or passive range-of-motion to preserve function. In people (and likely animals), even modest interventions can help maintain mobility, reduce the risk of injury, and enhance overall comfort during the end-of-life stage.[48]

Nausea/vomiting

Nausea may result from disease, treatment, or metabolic imbalance. Antiemetics, prokinetics, and antacids can restore comfort and appetite. Owners should administer medications before meals and monitor for persistent nausea or vomiting as a sign of diminished QoL.

Constipation/diarrhea
Bowel changes cause discomfort and complicate care. Constipation may be managed with hydration, fiber, stool softeners, or enemas when necessary. Diarrhea can be a substantial stressor to caregivers and should be treated prophylactically if expected as an adverse event and decisively if it presents as an unexpected complication. Diarrhea often improves with bland diets, probiotics, herbal supplements, or medications. The goal is comfort while avoiding burdensome interventions.

Hygiene
Incontinence, decreased tolerance for grooming, drooling, or wound drainage can lead to irritation and odor, impacting comfort and stress levels. Bedding changes, absorbent pads, barrier creams, and gentle cleaning help prevent infection and preserve comfort.

Urinary and fecal incontinence
Incontinence is common in hospice patients due to neurologic decline, mobility loss, and chronic disease, and can cause discomfort, skin irritation, frustration/anxiety, and reduced QoL. Management focuses on maintaining hygiene. Diapers or belly bands, if tolerated, can be used to simplify hygiene care for pets. These measures improve comfort for the pet and ease caregiving for families. Families can also be taught to adjust feeding schedules and manually stimulate bowel movements when outside to help minimize indoor cleaning demands.

Sensory accommodations
For full discussion, see article *Sensory Decline: Real-World Tactics for Managing Vision & Hearing Loss* by Adelman and Tarantino.

Cognitive changes
For full discussion, see article *Addressing Cognitive Dysfunction: Education, Diagnosis, and Practical Care* by Lynch.

Sleep disturbances
Dogs and cats in hospice, especially those with cognitive dysfunction, chronic pain, or chronic illness, may experience fragmented sleep, sundowning syndrome, nighttime pacing, or restlessness. Management includes maintaining consistent daily routines, mental enrichment, providing comfortable and quiet sleeping areas, and using night lights to reduce disorientation. In most advanced cases, medications are needed to help regulate sleep patterns and improve overall restfulness. Treating underlying pain and other clinical symptoms is imperative to encouraging better sleep. The inability of both pets and caregivers to sleep throughout the night is frequently reported to the author be a driver of euthanasia decision-making.

Mobility
A thoughtfully adapted home environment is a powerful, low-intervention way to improve QoL for veterinary hospice patients. By optimizing comfort, safety, and accessibility, environmental modifications can minimize distress, reduce the risk of injury, and allow pets to continue engaging in modified daily activities for as long as possible. Declining mobility can cause frustration and anxiety in both patients and caregivers. In addition to pain management and comfort techniques, traction tools, slings, harnesses, ramps, nonslip flooring, adjustments to food/water dishes and litterboxes, and rearranging the home all improve safety, maintain independence, and reduce strain on caregivers. Training pets to accept and use these tools before discomfort and instability is optimal and should be recommended very early in wellness, senior, and geriatric care.

Nonpain symptom control is a core component of veterinary hospice care. By anticipating common problems and providing simple, owner-friendly interventions, veterinarians can dramatically improve the patient's comfort and the family's caregiving experience. In all cases, treatment choices should be individualized, with ongoing reassessment to ensure interventions remain aligned with the goals of hospice care.

Emergency Planning in Hospice Care

A central component of veterinary hospice care is preparing families for the possibility of crises. Many communities do not have reliable access to 24/7 emergency services, and some families strongly wish for their pets to remain at home, even through the dying process. Without a plan, sudden distress, such as respiratory compromise, seizures, or severe pain, can leave families feeling helpless and patients vulnerable to unnecessary suffering. Hospice planning, therefore, emphasizes proactive education, discussion of anticipated scenarios, and the provision of tools that empower owners to act compassionately when a veterinarian is not immediately available.[26] By equipping families with a clear, 24-hour plan of action, hospice care ensures pets are supported with dignity and comfort at every stage, regardless of timing or access to clinical resources.

Emergency medication kits

Emergency medication kits, also referred to as *comfort kits* or *crisis kits* are an important tool in veterinary hospice care, designed to prepare families for anticipated crises such as acute dyspnea, severe pain, or distressing agitation.[49] Human hospice studies show that Emergency Medication Kits (EMKs) are used in 50% to 66% of hospice cases and are perceived as valuable by both caregivers and health care providers.[50,51] These kits are tailored to the individual patient's most likely end-of-life emergencies and contain predispensed medications, such as injectable opioids, diuretics, antiepileptic medications, sedatives, or antianxiety agents, that owners can administer under veterinary guidance (**Table 3**). Their primary purpose is not to prolong life but to provide immediate comfort, stabilize the patient, and relieve suffering until further veterinary care can be accessed. In many cases, use of an emergency kit serves as a bridge to euthanasia, allowing families the time to gather loved ones, contact their veterinarian, and/or arrange for in-home euthanasia.

To ensure safe and compliant use, veterinarians should check state prescription monitoring program regulations, as many have specific caveats for hospice patients. If controlled substances are dispensed, drug enforcement administration (DEA)-compliant labeling must be used, and all medications should be provided in child-proof packaging. Families should receive a clear, signed consent form outlining the purpose and use of the kit, along with written instructions for safe storage and proper disposal of any unused medications. By offering families both a plan of action and the means to act swiftly, EMKs not only reduce panic during crises but also maintain patient dignity and provide reassurance that distress can be managed compassionately even outside of regular veterinary hours.

Client Communication and Decision-Making Support

Setting clear expectations at the beginning of hospice care is essential for ensuring compassionate, effective support for both pets and their families. Early, honest communication about prognosis allows veterinarians to guide owners through the anticipated course of illness, while integrating tools such as QoL scales to help track patient comfort over time.[52] Advance care planning, including discussions of potential *what if* scenarios, prepares families for difficult decisions and reduces the likelihood of

Table 3
Common emergency kit medications in veterinary hospice

Crisis	Medication Protocol	Route
Pain	Methadone 0.25 mg/kg + Acepromazine 0.015 mg/kg	SQ
	Hydromorphone 0.05–0.1 mg/kg + Acepromazine 0.015 mg/kg	SQ
Respiratory distress	Butorphanol 0.2 mg/kg + Acepromazine 0.015 mg/kg	SQ
	Furosemide 2 mg/kg	SQ
	Flow-by oxygen	
Hemoabdomen	Methadone 0.25 mg/kg + Acepromazine 0.015 mg/kg	SQ
	Pro-Coagulant Medications: • Aminocaproic Acid 50 mg/kg q8–12h (up to 100 mg/kg for active bleed) • Tranexamic Acid 15–20 mg/kg PO q6–12h • Yunnan Baiyo (emergency teapill + increased capsule dosing) • San Qi Formula	Oral
Epistaxis	Oxymetazoline hydrochloride (OTC)	Intranasal via atomizer
	Epinephrine 0.1 mL with 0.4 mL saline	Intranasal via atomizer
Seizures	Midazolam 0.2–0.4 mg/kg (≤1 mL per nostril)	Intranasal via atomizer

crisis-driven choices. Veterinary technicians also play a key role by providing hands-on nursing care, emotional support, and assistance during euthanasia, helping to uphold patient welfare and client trust.[53] Because these conversations are complex and emotionally charged, veterinary professionals benefit from training and practice in communication skills to foster shared understanding and outcomes that honor both the pet's dignity and the family's needs.[52]

Euthanasia planning

Thoughtful preparation for death is a cornerstone of veterinary hospice care, helping families make decisions that are guided by compassion rather than crisis. Establishing clear criteria for QoL thresholds, such as persistent pain, loss of mobility, or substantially declining QoL scores, provides owners with an objective framework to recognize when euthanasia is the most humane option.[54] Discussions should also include the logistics of home, veterinary clinic, urgent care, or emergency hospital euthanasia. Research shows that pet owners report more positive experiences at home (80%) compared with a hospital setting (43%).[55] Families are also more likely to report a positive experience when they have at least one day to prepare and when a pre-euthanasia consultation is offered to review the procedure, address questions, and explain the process.[55] By planning proactively, veterinary teams can help ensure euthanasia is experienced as a peaceful, dignified, and compassionate final act of care.

Palliated or hospice-supported death

In some cases, families may decline euthanasia for religious, spiritual, cultural, or deeply personal reasons, and veterinarians are then called to support death with the highest degree of palliation possible. A palliated or hospice-supported death involves close monitoring, frequent reassessment, and the use of medications to control pain, dyspnea, anxiety, and other distressing symptoms, ensuring that the pet's final days and hours are as comfortable and dignified as possible. This contrasts sharply with an unpalliated death, in which no symptom-directed medications or veterinary oversight are provided; the pet may experience unmanaged suffering, and families are left unsupported in a time of great distress. By offering hospice-guided palliation, veterinarians can honor the family's beliefs while upholding their professional responsibility to minimize suffering.[26]

Anticipatory grief and bereavement support

Supporting families through the emotional challenges of hospice care includes acknowledging anticipatory grief, the sadness and anxiety that occur before a pet's death, as well as the profound loss that follows. Veterinarians and their teams can help by normalizing these feelings, providing caregiver resources to reduce caregiver fatigue and burnout, and offering structured pet loss support, such as grief counseling referrals, support groups, or hotlines. Sharing written materials and connecting families with trusted organizations ensures that owners feel supported. Although pet owners do expect their veterinarian to discuss bereavement, it is not expected that their veterinarian take on the role of counselor, and therefore, utilizing the interdisciplinary team, including veterinary social workers or other mental health professionals, is recommended.[55]

SUMMARY OF CORE CONCEPTS

Veterinary hospice care represents a compassionate, patient-centered approach that emphasizes comfort, dignity, and QoL over curative intent. By integrating hospice into geriatric and chronic disease management, veterinarians can provide continuity of care that supports both the animal and the family through the final life stage. The use of validated quality-of-life tools, structured communication strategies, and proactive symptom management ensures decisions are thoughtful, individualized, and guided by the patient's welfare. Hospice also reframes end-of-life care as a process, not a single event, helping families prepare emotionally, practically, and ethically for death or euthanasia when it becomes the most compassionate option.

As the field continues to evolve, ongoing education, research, and collaboration across general practice, specialty care, and dedicated hospice services are vital. Veterinarians and their teams are uniquely positioned to advocate for the patient while supporting caregivers through anticipatory grief, decision-making, and bereavement. By embracing evidence-based strategies, interdisciplinary collaboration, and open, compassionate communication, veterinary hospice can transform the final chapter of a pet's life into one defined by comfort, connection, and peace rather than fear or suffering.

Call for Ongoing Education and Research in Veterinary Hospice

As interest in veterinary hospice grows, there is a pressing need for continued education and research to guide best practices in this evolving field.[5] Integrating hospice training into veterinary curricula has been shown to improve students' communication skills, confidence with euthanasia, and preparedness for end-of-life care across species.[56] At the same time, the use of clinical metrology instrument (CMI)s like QoL scales, pain scales, and frailty indices has advanced pain and quality-of-life assessment, yet further validation across diverse conditions and species is needed.

Collaborative efforts among academia, private practice, and industry will be critical for refining these tools, expanding the evidence base, and enhancing both patient comfort and caregiver support. Ongoing education for practitioners, coupled with rigorous research in pain management and QoL measurement, will ensure veterinary hospice continues to develop as a compassionate, evidence-driven discipline.

CLINICS CARE POINTS

Identifying and Transitioning to Hospice Care

- Use prognosis-based criteria ($\leq$6 months life expectancy, progressive untreatable disease) and non-prognosis criteria (declining quality of life [QoL] and caregiver goals) to identify hospice patients.
- Introduce hospice concepts early in senior and geriatric visits to normalize discussions and prevent crisis-driven choices.
- Employ QoL and pain scales to provide objective benchmarks.
- Avoid waiting for acute crises or allowing *bad to become normal* to delay timely intervention.

Symptom Management & Comfort Care

- Prioritize multimodal analgesia with clear goals for each drug; avoid indiscriminate polypharmacy.
- Consider integrative modalities to enhance comfort.
- Anticipate common nonpain symptoms before they create distress.
- Simple environmental modifications can dramatically reduce patient stress and caregiver burden.
- Avoid ignoring sarcopenia and subtle mobility decline until advanced stages, early support preserves function and dignity.

Communication and Decision-Making

- Establish expectations early with frank prognosis discussions and anticipated scenarios to support proactive decision-making.
- Leverage the veterinary team: technicians provide vital nursing care, caregiver education, and emotional support.
- Use structured tools (QoL scales, red-flag symptom lists, and client journals) to guide decisions and reduce ambiguity.
- Avoid delaying end of life conversations out of concern for being *too early*—owners value proactive and compassionate honesty.

Euthanasia and Emergency Planning

- Define clear, individualized criteria for *the right time* using QoL and functional benchmarks.
- Offer home euthanasia, or work with providers who do, whenever possible; as studies show higher owner satisfaction with the experience.
- Prepare families with emergency medication kits tailored to the most likely crises, allowing rapid crisis intervention and time to gather loved ones.
- Provide anticipatory grief resources, grief counseling referrals, and clear aftercare options during the planning process.
- Avoid leaving families without a 24-hour emergency plan; lack of preparedness increases suffering and caregiver distress.

DECLARATION OF AI AND AI-ASSISTED TECHNOLOGIES IN THE WRITING PROCESS

During the preparation of this work, the author used Elicit and Chat GPT in order to search, compile, and summarize relevant peer-reviewed research articles. After using this tool/service, the author reviewed and edited the content as needed and takes full responsibility for the content of the publication.

DISCLOSURE

No competing interests exist.

REFERENCES

1. VandeKieft G, Estep LA, Davis KA, et al. Medical aid in dying: developing communication strategies, staff support systems, and policy for hospices. J Pain Symptom Manag 2024;67(5):e577. https://doi.org/10.1016/j.jpainsymman.2024.02.380.
2. Johnson CL, Patterson-Kane E, Lamison A, et al. Elements of and factors important in veterinary hospice. J Am Vet Med Assoc 2011;238(2):148–50.
3. Harrison KL, Connor SR. First medicare demonstration of concurrent provision of curative and hospice services for end-of-life care. Am J Publ Health 2016;106(8): 1405–8.
4. Downing R. Pain management for veterinary palliative care and hospice patients. Vet Clin North Am Small Anim Pract 2011;41(3):531–50.
5. Goldberg KJ. Veterinary hospice and palliative care: a comprehensive review of the literature. Vet Rec 2016;178(15):369–74.
6. Bishop G, Cooney K, Cox S, et al. 2016 AAHA/ AAHPC end-of-life care guidelines. J Am Anim Hosp Assoc 2016;52(6):341–56.
7. Ernecoff NC, Anhang Price R. Concurrent care as the next frontier in end-of-life care. JAMA Health Forum 2023;4(8):e232603. https://doi.org/10.1001/jamahealthforum.2023.2603.
8. Shanan A, Pierce J, Shearer T, editors. Hospice and palliative care for companion animals: principles and practice. 1st edition. Wiley; 2017. https://doi.org/10.1002/9781119036722.
9. Shanan A, Pierce J, Shearer TS, editors. Hospice and palliative care for companion animals: principles and practice. Second edition. John Wiley & Sons, Inc; 2023. https://doi.org/10.1002/9781119808817.
10. Springer S, Axiak Flammer S, Dürnberger C. "Veterinary medicine is not finished when I have diagnosed an incurable disease, that's when it starts for me." A qualitative interview study with small animal veterinarians on hospice and palliative care. Front Vet Sci 2024;11:1440404. https://doi.org/10.3389/fvets.2024.1440404.
11. Kerrigan L. In-home hospice provision — a viable option for veterinary palliative care? Vet Nurse 2014;5(3):146–51.
12. Green T, Mellor D. Extending ideas about animal welfare assessment to include 'quality of life' and related concepts. N Z Vet J 2011;59(6):263–71.
13. Villalobos AE. Quality-of-life assessment techniques for veterinarians. Vet Clin North Am Small Anim Pract 2011;41(3):519–29.
14. Christiansen SB, Kristensen AT, Lassen J, et al. Veterinarians' role in clients' decision-making regarding seriously ill companion animal patients. Acta Vet Scand 2015;58(1):30.
15. Knesl O, Hart BL, Fine AH, et al. Veterinarians and humane endings: when is it the right time to euthanize a companion animal? Front Vet Sci 2017;4. https://doi.org/10.3389/fvets.2017.00045.
16. Moses L, Malowney MJ, Wesley Boyd J. Ethical conflict and moral distress in veterinary practice: a survey of North American veterinarians. J Vet Intern Med 2018; 32(6):2115–22.
17. Springer S, Sandøe P, Bøker Lund T, et al. "Patients' interests first, but , "–Austrian aeterinarians' Attitudes mo coral Challenges mn sodern amall pnimal Practice. Animals 2019;9(5):241.

18. Eigner DR, Breitreiter K, Carmack T, et al. 2023 AAFP/IAAHPC feline hospice and palliative care guidelines. J Feline Med Surg 2023;25(9):1098612X231201683. https://doi.org/10.1177/1098612X231201683.
19. Keshav K, Mane M, Kolaventi SS, et al. Assessing ethical challenges in end-of-life decision-making through a case study approach. Semin Med Writ Educ 2024; 3:499.
20. Peterson NW, Boyd JW, Moses L. Medical futility is commonly encountered in small animal clinical practice. J Am Vet Med Assoc 2022;260(12):1475–81.
21. Huynh TN, Kleerup EC, Wiley JF, et al. The frequency and cost of treatment perceived to be futile in critical care. JAMA Intern Med 2013;173(20):1887.
22. Kipperman B, Morris P, Rollin B. Ethical dilemmas encountered by small animal veterinarians: characterisation, responses, consequences and beliefs regarding euthanasia. Vet Rec 2018;182(19):548.
23. Spitznagel MB, Marchitelli B, Gardner M, et al. Euthanasia from the veterinary client's perspective. Vet Clin North Am Small Anim Pract 2020;50(3):591–605.
24. Kerrigan L. Veterinary palliative and hospice care - making the transition from 'cure' to 'care.'. Vet Nurse 2013;4(6):316–21.
25. Fox E, Landrum-McNiff K, Zhong Z, et al. Evaluation of prognostic criteria for determining hospice eligibility in patients with advanced lung, heart, or liver disease. JAMA 1999;282(17):1638.
26. Shearer TS. Pet hospice and palliative care protocols. Vet Clin North Am Small Anim Pract 2011;41(3):507–18.
27. Duggleby W, Berry P. Transitions and shifting goals of care for palliative patients and their families. Clin J Oncol Nurs 2005;9(4):425–8.
28. Cohen K. End-of-life prognostication in acute hospital palliative patients: is the palliative performance scale useful? Harefuah 2022. https://doi.org/10.26226/morressier.5c76c8bce2ea5a723761266f.
29. Baik D, Russell D, Jordan L, et al. Using the palliative performance scale to estimate survival for patients at the end of life: a systematic review of the literature. J Palliat Med 2018;21(11):1651–61.
30. Head B, Ritchie CS, Smoot TM. Prognostication in hospice care: can the palliative performance scale help? J Palliat Med 2005;8(3):492–502.
31. Cachon T, Frykman O, Innes JF, et al. Face validity of a proposed tool for staging canine osteoarthritis: Canine OsteoArthritis staging tool (COAST). Vet J 2018; 235:1–8.
32. Bartges JW. Chronic kidney disease in dogs and cats. Vet Clin North Am Small Anim Pract 2012;42(4):669–92.
33. Relford R, Robertson J, Clements C. Symmetric dimethylarginine. Vet Clin North Am Small Anim Pract 2016;46(6):941–60.
34. Biller B, Berg J, Garrett L, et al. 2016 AAHA oncology guidelines for dogs and cats. J Am Anim Hosp Assoc 2016;52(4):181–204.
35. Shearer T. Where have we been, where are we going. Vet Clin North Am Small Anim Pract 2019;49(3):325–38.
36. Pantaleon L. Why measuring outcomes is important in health care. J Vet Intern Med 2019;33(2):356–62.
37. WHOQOL: measuring quality of life. 2025. Available at: https://www.who.int/toolkits/whoqol. Accessed August 17, 2025.
38. Lynch S, Savary-Bataille K, Leeuw B, et al. Development of a questionnaire assessing health-related quality-of-life in dogs and cats with cancer. Vet Comp Oncol 2011;9(3):172–82.

39. Main D. Promoting quality of life discussions between the veterinary profession and the pet-owning public. Anim Welf 2007;16(S1):159–63.
40. McMillan FD. Quality of life in animals. J Am Vet Med Assoc 2000;216(12): 1904–10.
41. Freeman LM, Rush JE, Farabaugh AE, et al. Development and evaluation of a questionnaire for assessing health-related quality of life in dogs with cardiac disease. J Am Vet Med Assoc 2005;226(11):1864–8.
42. Yeates J, Main D. Assessment of companion animal quality of life in veterinary practice and research. J Small Anim Pract 2009;50(6):274–81.
43. Mullan S, Main D. Preliminary evaluation of a quality-of-life screening programme for pet dogs. J Small Anim Pract 2007;48(6):314–22.
44. Epstein ME, Rodanm I, Griffenhagen G, et al. AAHA/AAFP pain management guidelines for dogs and cats. J Feline Med Surg 2015;17(3):251–72.
45. Dhaliwal R, Boynton E, Carrera-Justiz S, et al. AAHA senior care guidelines for dogs and cats. J Am Anim Hosp Assoc 2023;59(1):1–21.
46. Saker KE. Nutritional concerns for cancer, cachexia, frailty, and sarcopenia in canine and feline pets. Vet Clin North Am Small Anim Pract 2021;51(3):729–44.
47. Freeman LM. Cachexia and sarcopenia: emerging syndromes of importance in dogs and cats. J Vet Intern Med 2012;26(1):3–17.
48. Calvani R, Miccheli A, Landi F, et al. Current nutritional recommendations and novel dietary strategies to manage sarcopenia. J Frailty Aging 2013;2(1):38–53.
49. Hendrix L. Animal hospice and palliative medicine for the house call veterinarian. Elsevier; 2023.
50. Bailey FA, Williams BR, Goode PS, et al. Impact of a hospice emergency kit for veterans and their caregivers: a prospective cohort study. J Palliat Med 2014; 17(8):931–8.
51. Leigh AE, Burgio KL, Williams BR, et al. Hospice emergency kit for veterans: a pilot study. J Palliat Med 2013;16(4):356–61.
52. Lummis M, Marchitelli B, Shearer T. Communication. Vet Clin North Am Small Anim Pract 2020;50(3):607–16.
53. Carter K. The role of the veterinary technician in end-of-life care. Vet Clin North Am Small Anim Pract 2020;50(3):639–45.
54. Matte AR, Khosa DK, Coe JB, et al. Exploring pet owners' experiences and self-reported satisfaction and grief following companion animal euthanasia. Vet Rec 2020;187(12):e122.
55. Cooney KA, Kogan LR, Brooks SL, et al. Pet owners' expectations for pet end-of-life support and after-death body care: exploration and practical applications. Top Companion Anim Med 2021;43:100503. https://doi.org/10.1016/j.tcam.2020.100503.
56. Corrigan VK, Cooney K, Foster R. Compassionate end-of-life care: development, implementation, and evaluation of a comprehensive euthanasia course in veterinary education from 2019–2024. Hum-Anim Interact 2025;20:0025. Published online May.

Guiding End-of-Life Decisions and Quality of Life Assessments

Kimberly Moen, DVM, CPEV

KEYWORDS

- QOL • QOD • Guiding end-of-life decisions

KEY POINTS

- End-of-life decisions should prioritize the pet's quality of life, considering physical, emotional, and social well-being.
- The 5 freedoms serve as a framework for assessing and addressing animal welfare during end-of-life care.
- Compassionate communication and family support are essential when guiding families through difficult euthanasia decisions.
- Recognizing the family's emotional, financial, and physical capacity time helps tailor end-of-life care and decision-making.
- Respect for diverse beliefs and values ensures a humane, individualized approach to euthanasia and quality of death.

INTRODUCTION/HISTORY/DEFINITIONS

We are detailing Guiding End-of-Life Decisions and Quality of Life Assessments for patients with critical, terminal, declining quality of life (QOL), and behavioral conditions. Because it is vital to handle these situations with kindness, finesse, compassion, and in a manner that allows for continued connection between the family and you, after the pet is no longer with us. So, we must consider the complete family dynamic.

- The patient's QOL
- The family's QOL
- The importance of a quality of death (QOD)
- These all play an important role for the patient and for the healing of the family's emotions.

QOL is always important when considering animal welfare. There are 5 basic freedoms each animal deserves.[1] These are under consideration when we choose a

Lap of Love Veterinary Hospice & In-Home Euthanasia, 17804 N. US HWY 41 Lutz, FL 33549, USA
E-mail address: drkimberly@lapoflove.com

Vet Clin Small Anim 56 (2026) 475–489
https://doi.org/10.1016/j.cvsm.2025.11.002 vetsmall.theclinics.com

Abbreviations	
QOD	quality of death
QOL	quality of life

treatment, pursue surgery, add additional treatments, continue treatment, and also during end-of-life decisions. When we notice that, despite our best efforts in practicing quality medicine, the patient has a dwindling QOL. It's time to consider what is in the best interest of the patient and its family.

- Do we continue to treat?
- Do we continue to test?
  - If the answer is yes, what is the goal behind the decision?
  - Is the patient's best interest in mind?
    - Is the family considered in the decision?
    - If the answer is no, please know that supporting the families through end-of-life decisions requires compassion and finesse for a QOD for the patient and a quality experience for its family.

The five freedoms and their applications to end-of-life discussions: encompassing physical, emotional, and social components.

1. Freedom from Hunger and Thirst: Ensuring easy access to clean water and a healthy diet, and for our end-of-life patients, this means:

Adequate opportunity to eat and drink, with clean dishes, so that they don't become food-averse. Some end-of-life patients will have increased thirst and/or hunger. For some advanced end-of-life patients, their natural response is to stop eating nutrients.

Not all end-of-life patients stop eating before it is their time! This depends on the disease process and personality of the pet. So, it certainly isn't the gold standard for deciding when to have a QOL discussion or when to base the ever-so-important decision of euthanasia on.

2. Freedom from Discomfort:

Means providing safe shelter from the environment and a comfortable place to rest. Our end-of-life patients need extra considerations to be comfortable, for example:

- Orthopedic beds
- Having a safe space away from hyperactive pets and children
- Mats to prevent slipping and sliding
- Safety from pools and stairs

3. Freedom from Pain, Injury, or Disease:

Providing protection, prevention, diagnosis, and appropriate treatment, where the disease is being cured or managed to improve QOL. In some cases, less treatment or a change in treatment is preferred when side effects are making the patient miserable. If the treatment is necessary to prevent suffering, but the patient isn't tolerating it, and there isn't a good alternative or if the family can't afford the treatment, it's time to consider having a QOL discussion with the family.

4. Freedom to Express Normal Behavior:

Maintaining adequate and clean space, environmental enrichment, and social interaction appropriate to the species. And for our end-of-life patients: This means maintaining connection to the family and other pets in the home. So, they may still enjoy their human–animal bond and the interactions with other pets in the home despite their end-of-life ailments.

They may now be afraid of the other pets in the home since they can be knocked over, may not get to the food fast enough, be picked on, pushed down, or stepped on. If so, please advise that they be kept separate from other pets, but still get normal interactions with safe family members.

However, if the patient is avoiding or snapping at its owner or

If the patient is becoming progressively clingy with the owner, it's time for a QOL discussion.

5. Freedom from Fear and Distress:

Ensuring safe conditions and kind treatment. Our end-of-life patients may need additional anxiety medications, and if they aren't helping, it's time for a QOL discussion.

BACKGROUND

1. The intricacies of QOL for the pet:

It must be kept calm, clean, comfortable, cared for, and enjoy life. The enjoying life part is dependent on age, condition, and positive social interaction.[2] For example, an old orthopedic Labrador may not be able to chase after the ball, but it still loves playing with the ball and with its owners.

The desire is and has always been to do what is best for the patient. It's in the Veterinarian's Oath. Can we extend life, with quality maintained, and the human–animal bond intact? We can, and when we focus on the patient and on the patient's family's well-being, maintaining the human–animal bond, we do it well. So then, it is just left to how we choose the "right time" to lead these delicate discussions?

2. The Intricacies of QOL for the family:
   - They are calm (concerning taking care of the patient) and content to help the patient. Client education and compassionate support can go a long way with regards to this; they often don't know when it is time to let go until the animal is suffering (they need our gentle guidance with determining this, too. Sometimes they are too close to see it). The families love their pets and don't like to see them suffer. In that same Veterinarian's oath is prevention and relief of suffering. Which means we can help them say goodbye while the pet is struggling, to prevent suffering from ever occurring at all. It's not always best to try every option and wait for suffering to ensue.
   - They can physically do what we ask of them comfortably and safely for them and the patient. Can they medicate, rotate, clean, and assist the pet, 3 to 6 times a day, treatment on top of the multilayered hospice medications? Is their pet amenable to treatment without hiding from or fighting its owner?
   - They comfortably have the financial resources to care for the pet, at a level that sustains QOL for the patient.
   - They have enough time to take care of the patient, at the level that maintains its QOL; and if not, they supplement the time they can help with other good caretakers, whether family members, friends, pet sitters, vet assistants, or vet techs.

The purpose of taking the family into consideration is that ultimately, they are responsible for the care of their furry loved one; it's their family member, and they will be providing the care day and night. Sometimes care for an end-of-life patient can be overwhelming, and caregivers (in this case, the families we serve) can experience caregiver fatigue, especially if there are other difficult circumstances in their lives.

Should a family suffer just because more can be done medically? Should they be left with guilt if they have not tried every last treatment or test, when the patient is still getting worse? If we insist on doing every treatment, without consideration for how the family is managing the care, their human–animal bond can be broken by caregiver fatigue,[3] and this is the last memory for the patient and the family. We can help them maintain their human–animal bond by taking the family into account.

The intricacies of the human–animal bond with regard to end-of-life patients are as follows.

We have the:

- "I can do all the things" client
- "I can do all the things with additional client education," client
- "I can do some things with additional client education and support" client
- "I cannot do anything," client

Paired with the:

- "I love you no matter what," pet
- "I'm willing to let you treat me, because I know you have my best interest in mind," pet
- "I Don't Like being treated, but I will tolerate it" pet
- "I am going to hide or fight you if you try to treat me" pet

How to balance the considerations for the patient and those of its family, when considering end-of-life decisions:

Some clients want to do everything, and they have the emotional, physical, financial, and time resources to do so. This is the ideal situation, since we have the immense desire and ability to support them in that decision. We love to save animals and have taken an oath to do so; and if the pet maintains QOL, as defined earlier, this is what is best for all involved.

Some clients have experienced a traumatic ending with one of their pets, suffering in its last moments. Because of this, they may choose to lean more toward preventing suffering with this pet. When QOL is declining or the patient is facing highly probable final moments in an Emergency Room, we can help support the family with clean consciences.

PRESERVING THE HUMAN–ANIMAL BOND, WHEN THE PET PARENT/OWNER IS ALL IN, TRYING EVERY TREATMENT

Is their pet still enjoying its life, or is it getting snippy, withdrawn, not wanting to be touched, expressing stress? Do we continue to treat, or is it time to switch to comfort care and start the euthanasia conversations gently? This places the focus on the patient, with the goal of preventing suffering.

Conversely, is the pet still experiencing enjoyment in life, but is urinating all over the house despite the owner's best efforts to treat and keep the patient calm? Are owners sleeping on the couch, not with their spouse, and having fights because the house can never be quite clean? Is the patient vocalizing at random hours in the night, making it difficult for the family to function at work or causing them to fight amongst themselves? Is the patient mostly sweet but has moments of trying to kill a family member or stranger, and they have tried behaviorists, medications, and trainers? Can we see the declining QOL for the patient and family and help guide them gently with end-of-life discussions?

- *If not, do we want to take these pets home?*
- *How will they do in the shelter?*

We have the opportunity to offer a QOD for the patients, before we may want to, for the sake of sanity and safety for the family, and to prevent suffering for the patients. Some families become so desperate that they are forced to relinquish their pet to animal control, likely only to have it killed. We could offer more comfort for both the pets and the families. Other families set them free, and the pets are lucky if they don't get hit by cars. Or they threaten to shoot the dog. These families loved their pet, but clearly, the human–animal bond was broken, and the family had reached their threshold.

DISCUSSION

Veterinarians have a desire to help animals heal, treat, save, and have the honor and responsibility to prevent and relieve suffering. With hospice, we are taking the pet's whole life and its family into consideration, a holistic approach.

PET CONSIDERATIONS

- Can points of care be achieved?
- Can we keep the animal's deserved freedoms intact while preserving the human–animal bond?
- If not, having a QOL discussion and giving gentle guidance is indicated.
- Is the pet suffering? If so, a loving recommendation of "it's time." If not, suggest ER to help, in-home euthanasia, or provide a comfort kit so the owner has a moment to align the knowledge they just received with the needs of their hearts.
- *Behavior/Personality of the pet:* Does it enjoy its life while being treated? Is it hating treatment and now hiding or biting the owner? If the animal is no longer enjoying life, despite still having life to live, it doesn't have all of its innate freedoms.

TYPICAL FAMILY CONSIDERATIONS

- Emotions: if the care burden is getting too much it's best to end on a good note, maintaining the loving human–animal bond.
- Finances: families can love their pet with their whole heart and still have other expenses in their lives, too.
- Physically: it's kind to guide them in a way that they don't feel pressure from us to risk hurting themselves, straining their back, risking falls, just to prove they love their pet.
- Time: most people need to work to provide for themselves. Some have jobs with long shifts. Not all have the budget or family to care for their pet when they cannot be there.

SPECIAL FAMILY CONSIDERATIONS

Intuition

- Only some people can sense when their pet is showing it's time or struggling.

Faith

- They may believe in an afterlife and either understand QOL and have faith that their pet will live on.
- They may feel guilty for "playing God."
- They may have faith and not believe in letting suffering occur.
- They may not believe in ending any life.
- They may believe all things are energy, or that life ceases to exist after death, in this case, these will be their final moments together.

Spiritual Considerations

- Is it wrong to take the life of an animal that feels like family, or is it okay if the animal is struggling?

There is a finesse to balancing these factors, choosing what is best for the pet while honoring the family's desires for *Quality of Death* after a wonderful life together.

It is important to remember that if the family is taking their time to seek our help, instead of dropping their pet off somewhere, letting it loose, or ending its life themselves, 99.9% of the time, they truly love their pet. Whether that means wanting what is best for it by keeping it calm and comfortable, or euthanasing, maybe even a moment too early for our comfort, the intention is love.

SOME POINTS OF CONSIDERATION

- "You'll know when it's time,"

This phrase frightens owners; it places the full weight of the decision on them.
We are the ones with medical degrees and knowledge of how the ending looks.
We can help families by teaming up with them and saying,

"We will decide together, when it's the pet's best time for a quality final moment."

Guiding them through the process supports their emotional healing.

- "When they stop eating, it's time."

Not all pets stop eating before it is their time. There have been Labrador Retrievers and Beagles in their final moments, unable to rise and minimally responsive, yet still willing to scarf down a treat, maybe even with a tail wag.

Families who believe this statement may wait until the pet is suffering or struggle with the decision when the pet is already declining.

- *"Watch for 'the look.'"*

Not all pets give "the look."

Only some pet parents are emotionally attuned enough to read subtle signs. This depends on the disease process and what truly measures QOL. Most families aren't attuned to every behavioral detail. Many cannot tell the difference between panting with anxiety versus excitement, or between increased respiratory effort and a normal breath. It seems kinder not to wait for a look that signals extreme distress or misery.

There must be other markers to determine QOL and the right time to say goodbye.

By the time the patients have a terminal diagnosis or a behavior that is out of control, despite our best efforts for treating them, they are dangerous, or they are in the gray scale; Where any time the pet isn't comfortable &/or enjoying life and the owner is at a place of peace with the decision, it may be an acceptable time to consider euthanasia, or at least have that delicate conversation. To provide for a QOD and pleasant last memories for the family.

If, on the other hand, the patient is terminal and still comfortable, calm, and connected, then a QOL discussion is more directed toward what we can do, to what point we can do it, and signs to watch for when things turn. And a gentle preparation of "it's time to prepare emotionally, make sure to do a bucket list, and enjoy every last moment together." Now we don't have a crystal ball, nor do the diseases all follow the medical book timelines, so knowing the closest perfect time isn't always possible. But if we and the family are both 100% sure, the pet is most certainly suffering.

The goal with QOL considerations is to extend life, when we can make it good (comfortable, calm, connected). Then, when we can no longer make it good, we kindly and gently guide the families toward peaceful passings. We are the patient's advocates, always, at times of health, at times of treating disease, and consistent with our oath at times of preventing and relieving suffering too.

Prolonging the suffering of any animal (or the family, because of the animal, in some cases) is never the goal. We extend comfort and calm, then prevent suffering from occurring at all. We help, but not to the point that helping becomes hurting,[4] to the patient, the family, or their bond. We help keep the families' memories of that beloved pet the best they can be, even to the end, for that will stay with them just like the loss of any family member. Let's help guide them to a beautiful goodbye at the right moment. A moment when it is kind and can be peaceful.

We also want to know how the family wants the final chapter to look. Is it a calm, peaceful, perfect place, and surrounded by loved ones, with delicious snacks? Is it just them and the pet? Is it providing all possible measures to get every single second possible? This can help guide us in determining the appropriate timing and what is possible before that time.

CASE STUDY/PRESENTATION

1. A handsome gray and white senior cat, an oncology patient. He had a limb previously amputated, which healed nicely, and is now scheduled for a partial mandibulectomy. To some people, this might look like we are butchering the cat or that the family is being selfish.

So, is this pushing the Quality-of-Life boundary, or is this in the best interest of the cat and family? It helps to know that this cat did really well with the amputation, is thriving at home, enjoys affection, interacts normally with the family and other pets, and seems comfortable and well-adjusted with 3 legs. The patient has a great appetite and enjoys spending time with the family doing all previously enjoyed activities.

Mom understands that this may only buy a little while longer, and this cat is the last thing she has to remind her of her recently deceased husband. She is happy and able to care for this patient from all aspects.

CONSIDERATIONS

- Keeping the patient comfortable and calm
- Gently preparing the owner for when it is time
- Providing grief resources

2. A handsome senior Doberman with degenerative myelopathy, arthritis, and cognitive decline, among other conditions.

The female owner was sleeping on the couch, apart from her loving husband, face-to-face with the patient. She would be awoken by the patient vocalizing, then searching for her, getting stuck in corners, and falling into his own urine.

This pet is still most lovely when lucid but needs constant attention, is on a pharmacy of medications, is attended to 24/7, is on the best diet, and the owner feels guilty about making the decision.

Is this pet truly comfortable? Anxiety-free?

Does the owner have a QOL? Her back hurts from lifting the patient. She is running low on energy due to being woken every couple of hours at night and being unable to leave the patient's side without the patient becoming anxious.

CONSIDERATIONS FOR GUIDANCE

- QOL for the pet and owner, discussion
- The owner needs to know that the euthanasia decision is in the best interest of the patient. Otherwise, she may feel more guilty if it is about her QOL, and she would keep going at what expense? Her job? Her mental health?

Her marriage?

SO, WHEN DO WE HAVE A QUALITY OF LIFE DISCUSSION WITH A FAMILY?

1. *Critical cases* are usually easier to identify. We ask: what life-saving measures can we take? If the outcome is grave, how do we support the client?
   - If the client is on board intellectually and emotionally (though still likely sad), they understand it is in the best interest of the patient. Guidance focuses on affirming the decision and guiding them through euthanasia. For example, "We are making the right decision for Fluffy."
   - If the client was caught off guard, had no idea this conversation was coming, or didn't expect to leave without their pet, guidance requires patience, clear explanations, and giving them a moment to process. The focus should be on the patient's comfort and their being at peace.
   - If the client is not ready, despite their pet being critical, gently but firmly advise them to seek care as soon as possible. Recommend at-home services and suggest they call or offer to call for them. Let them know what they can expect with a "natural" passing, not to scare, but so they can make an informed decision.
2. With *urgent patients with poor prognosis*, considerations include
   - Does the family need more time?
   - Can we keep the patient comfortable?
   - Is this financially feasible for the family?
   - Will they get a reasonable amount of time (reasonable is up to them) with their pet for that cost? For example, is $5,000 worth it for 6 months?

This depends on how financially stable the owner is and how emotionally attached they are to their pet. Is it still worth it for 2 weeks of extra time? What if the patient's condition worsens faster than expected? How will this family manage?

Guidance here is kind and honest communication:

- Here are the treatment options.
- Based on the disease, the prognosis is, which means ... if they follow the textbook, you may have X amount of time, it may be less or more.
- What are their thoughts and needs? This gives us direction for how best to support them.

3. With *terminal patients*, life is in its final chapter. There may be a good prognosis for longer life with treatable conditions and many medical options. However, when QOL is low for the patient, and neither it nor its family is enjoying good QOL, consider:
   - Teaming with the family to create a plan for comfort and calm measures.
   - Ensuring maintenance of the human–animal bond.
   - Creating an expectation of what the final stages will look like.
   - Determine how much the family can comfortably invest in this process, with all of their limitations.

Knowing what is feasible allows both for the patient's QOL and provides a wonderful opportunity to guide the owner toward a peaceful passing. Any time during this period, the family chooses euthanasia is acceptable. It serves to relieve the patient's struggle, prevents suffering, and preserves the family's final memories.

It is crucial to remain free from judgment, even if their choice differs from what you might do for your own pet. Ultimately, this process is about supporting the family. When we offer compassionate support, families are more likely to return to the clinic and are spared a traumatic experience in their pet's final moments.

This is a perfect opportunity to discuss both a QOL and QOD discussion.

Some helpful topics and resources to include for these owners:

A. Discuss if the patient's decline:
   - Is imminent, meaning the pet could worsen at any moment. This requires a more urgent decision if a peaceful QOD is desired.
   - May fluctuate, where the patient appears fine one moment and unwell the next, repeatedly. In these cases, mindful consideration of timing is needed because the patient will be fine one moment and unwell the next, and repeat until the bad moment persists or worsens
   - Will be gradual, with no immediate rush, purely QOL monitoring and thoughtful bucket list planning.
   - Is combined (fluctuating and gradual), focus your discussion based on the most severe or advanced disease process.
B. Discuss whether the patient's good moments are becoming fewer or shorter progressively, and note changes in symptoms, habits, behaviors, and social interactions.
C. Provide QOL documents to help families track their pet's condition. Tools like the following QOL scales:
   - Lap of Love[5] (**Table 1**)
   - Dr. Alice Villalobos' HHHHHMM[6] (**Table 2**)
   - The Ohio State University VMC[7]
   - MMVHS[8] =can assist owners in understanding their pet's condition, in ways owners may not intuitively recognize.
D. Suggest creating a bucket list. This helps families capture special memories and reduce regrets. The list can include favorite foods (saving risky treats for just before euthanasia), activities, outings, special gifts, visits with friends, photos, videos, and anything their heart desires.[3] Modify the list based on how the patient will feel during these activities.
E. Determine the family's vision for the final moments. Where will it take place? In the clinic, at a park, or at home? (If needed, home service veterinarians can help if the clinic staff cannot step away.) Who will be present? The primary owner, immediate family, extended family, friends, neighbors, or coworkers? Hint: Ask this as an open-ended question. Will there be snacks, music, pictures, poems, singing, prayers, or complete silence? Do the other family pets need closure?

Regarding other pets: Some young or playful pets may be too rough or careless around the patient. However, many pets appreciate closure. Depending on the pet's personality, it may want to observe the patient from a distance, sniff, or even cuddle before saying goodbye. This helps reduce anxiety and searching behavior for the remaining pets. If it can be done safely, having multiple pets present in the clinic room provides comfort and company for the way home.

Considerations regarding children: Parents generally know their children's emotional capacity best. The calmer and more centered the parents are, the easier the experience will be for the children. Children should be allowed to say goodbye if possible. If present, they need gentle guidance throughout the process. They should be reassured that their pet is comfortable, so their imaginations don't fill in scary or inaccurate details.

Table 1
Lap of Love QOL scale

Lap of Love
Pet Quality-of-Life Scale

When evaluating the quality of life of your pet, personalized patient and family information is important when reaching an educated, informed, and supported choice that fits not only your pet's medical condition, but also your wishes and expectations. In short, quality of life applies not only to the pet, it also applies to you!

SCORE EACH SUBSECTION ON A SCALE OF 0-2:

0 = agree with statement (describes my pet)
1 = some changes seen
2 = disagree with statement (does not describe my pet)

SOCIAL FUNCTIONS

_____ Desire to be with the family has not changed

_____ Interacts normally with family or other pets (i.e., no increased aggression or other changes)

HEALTH

_____ No changes in breathing or panting patterns

_____ No outward signs of pain (excessive panting, pacing, and whining are most commonly seen)

_____ No pacing around the house

_____ My pet's overall condition has not changed recently

MENTAL HEALTH

_____ Enjoys normal play activities

_____ Still dislikes the same thing (i.e., still hates the mailman = 0, or doesn't bark at the mailman anymore = 2)

_____ No outward signs of stress or anxiety

_____ Does not seem confused or apathetic

_____ Nighttime activity is normal, no changes seen

NATURAL FUNCTIONS

_____ Appetite has stayed the same

_____ Drinking has stayed the same

_____ Normal urination habits

_____ Normal bowel movement habits

_____ Ability to ambulate (walk around) has stayed the same

RESULTS

_____ Total score added from each section

0-8: Quality of life is most likely adequate. No medical intervention required yet, but guidance from your veterinarian may help you identify signs to look for in the future.

9–16: Quality of life is questionable and medical intervention is suggested. Your pet would certainly benefit from veterinary oversight and guidance to evaluate the disease process he/she is experiencing.

17-32: Quality of life is a definite concern. Changes will likely become more progressive and more severe in the near future. Veterinary guidance will help you better understand the end stages of your pet's disease process in order to make a more informed decision of whether to continue hospice care or elect peaceful euthanasia.

Scan the code or visit **Info.LapofLove.com/QOLscale** to access interactive versions of these tools.

Lap of Love
Veterinary Hospice & In-Home Euthanasia

Our dedicated Support Center is available 7:00 am - 11:00 pm ET, every day, including weekends and holidays.
Contact us at **(855) 933-5683** or **LapofLove.com**

(continued on next page)

Table 1
(*continued*)

Lap of Love
Pet Family Concerns

SCORE EACH ITEM ON A SCALE OF 0-2:

0 = I am not concerned at this time
1 = There is some concern
2 = I am concerned about this

I AM CONCERNED ABOUT THE FOLLOWING THINGS:

_____ Pet suffering	_____ Desire to perform nursing care for your pet
_____ Pet dying alone	_____ Ability to perform nursing care for your pet
_____ Not knowing the right time to euthanize	_____ Coping with loss
_____ Concern for other household animals	_____ Concern for other members of the family (i.e., children)

RESULTS

_____ Total score

0-4: Your concerns are minimal at this time. You may understand what lies ahead from the passing of a previous pet, or you may not want to face the inevitable loss of your pet. As difficult as it is to consider these things, now is the time to evaluate your concerns and limitations.

5–9: Your concerns are mounting. Prepare for the changes ahead by educating yourself on your pet's condition. Consult your veterinarian and ask if they can recommend reputable online sources of information.

10-16: Your concerns about the changes in your pet are valid. Remember to value your quality of life as a caregiver, too. Now is the time to build a support system around you. Veterinary guidance will help you prepare for the medical changes in your pet while counselors and other health professionals can help you with anticipatory grief.

DISCUSS THE QUESTIONS BELOW, AND THE ENTIRE QUALITY-OF-LIFE SCALE, WITH YOUR VETERINARIAN

Below are some open-ended questions that help gauge your family's time, emotional, and (when appropriate) financial budgets:

1. Have you ever been through the loss of a pet before? If so, what was your experience (good or bad, and why)?
2. What do you hope the life expectancy of your pet will be? What do you think it will be?
3. What is the ideal situation you wish for your pet's end-of-life experience? (at home, pass away in her sleep, etc.)

Suggestions on using this quality-of-life scale:

1. Complete the scale at different times of the day, note circadian fluctuations in well-being. (We find most pets tend to do better during the day and worse at night.)
2. Request multiple members of the family complete the scale; compare observations.
3. Take periodic photos of your pet to help you remember their physical appearance.

Resources:

1. AAHA/AAFP Pain Management Guidelines for Dogs and Cats, www.aahanet.org/Library/PainMgmt.aspx

Lap of Love
Veterinary Hospice & In-Home Euthanasia

Our dedicated Support Center is available 7:00 am - 11:00 pm ET, every day, including weekends and holidays. Contact us at **(855) 933-5683** or **LapofLove.com**

From Lap of Love. QOL scale. Published February 2013. Accessed August 30, 2025. https://www.lapoflove.com/how-will-i-know-it-is-time/lap-of-love-quality-of-life-scale.pdf.

Table 2
Dr Alice Villalobos' HHHHHMM

Quality of Life Scale (The HHHHHMM Scale)

Pet Caregivers Can Use This Quality of Life Scale to Determine the Success of Pawspice Care. Score Patients Using a Scale of: 0–10 (10 Being Ideal).

Score	Criterion
0–10	*HURT*: Adequate pain control and breathing ability are of top concern. Trouble breathing outweighs all concerns. Is the pet's pain well-managed? Can the pet breathe properly? Is oxygen supplementation necessary?
0–10	*HUNGER*: Is the pet eating enough? Does hand-feeding help? Does the pet need a feeding tube?
0–10	*HYDRATION*: Is the pet dehydrated? For patients not drinking enough water, use subcutaneous fluids daily or twice daily to supplement fluid intake
0–10	*HYGIENE*: The pet should be brushed and cleaned, particularly after eliminations. Avoid pressure sores with soft bedding and keep all wounds clean
0–10	*HAPPINESS*: Does the pet express joy and interest? Is the pet responsive to family, toys, etc.? Is the pet depressed, lonely, anxious, bored, or afraid? Can the pet's bed be moved to be close to family activities?
0–10	*MOBILITY*: Can the pet get up without assistance? Does the pet need human or mechanical help (e.g., a cart)? Does the pet feel like going for a walk? Is the pet having seizures or stumbling? (Some caregivers feel euthanasia is preferable to amputation, but an animal with limited mobility yet still alert, happy, and responsive can have a good quality of life as long as caregivers are committed to helping their pet.)
0–10	*MORE GOOD DAYS THAN BAD*: When bad days outnumber good days, quality of life might be too compromised. When a healthy human–animal bond is no longer possible, the caregiver must be made aware that the end is near. The decision for euthanasia needs to be made if the pet is suffering. If death comes peacefully and painlessly at home, that is okay
*TOTAL	*A total over 35 points represents an acceptable life quality to continue with pet hospice (Pawspice)

Original concept, *Oncology Outlook*, by Dr. Alice Villalobos, *Quality of Life Scale Helps Make Final Call,* VPN, 09/2004; scale format created for author's book, *Canine and Feline Geriatric Oncology: Honoring the Human-Animal Bond*, Blackwell Publishing, 2007. Revised for the International Veterinary Association of Pain Management (IVAPM) 2011 Palliative Care and Hospice Guidelines. Dr. Alice Villalobos & Wiley-Blackwell.

Villalobos, A., Kaplan, L. and Meyers, F. (2007). Palliative Care: End of Life "Pawspice" Care. In Canine and Feline Geriatric Oncology (eds A. Villalobos and L. Kaplan). https://doi.org/10.1002/9780470344446.ch10.

F. Discuss what an unassisted passing would look like.
G. Discuss the benefits of euthanasia when it is time.
H. Provide emotional support resources if needed, for example:
   - Lap of Love Pet Loss Support (some group activities are free; there is also individual support)
   - Losing Lulu
   - Best Friends Grieving and Loss Resources

4. Good prognosis for longer life, but *QOL is low* for the patient and family. Or the patient may pose a danger to society or be miserable to live with. These cases are especially challenging. As veterinarians, we desire to heal, and taking a life when there is still life to live carries a heavier emotional weight.

Though animals can be wonderful companions, people intrinsically have a higher value. If a domesticated animal becomes a danger to humans, it becomes a legal issue. If a child is hurt, the emotional impact is compounded. If another pet dies because of this pet, that is complex, too.

This does not mean all aggressive pets must be killed. Under proper conditions, with responsible custody, veterinary behaviorist care, medications, trainer guidance, safe zones away from other animals and people, and other support measures, some can live safely.[9] Special cases may even be rehabilitated.

Owner considerations include whether the family can provide safety for all and support the mental health of the patient. It's important to recognize that when a pet feels the need to defend itself fiercely over small things, it's not mentally healthy. If the family cannot provide this safe environment, what organizations can help take the pet? Shelters may have to kill anyway, and the environment can be even more stressful.

Keeping these considerations in mind, guidance should include offering resources to help determine a safe plan if they want to keep the pet. Provide a plan for when they are ready to kill, in a way that can be done safely, or refer them to home care services.

Emotional support must be heavily accepting and nonjudgmental, as families often feel guilty about killing a physically "healthy" pet. Place the focus on safety, the patient's emotional struggle, affirming the decision, and expressing compassion. Also, acknowledge how difficult, yet kind, this decision is.

If you find this topic challenging, it is important to only do what you are comfortable with. When you are comfortable, you can hold space for the family's healing. If moving from a nonjudgmental place isn't possible for you, please refer the family to someone who can help.

Other points to consider: our hearts go out to shelter veterinarians who must kill healthy dogs as part of their job; 366,000 shelter animals died in the first 6 months of 2025 (most of which were euthanasia).[10] For those who aren't vegan, we are grateful for the healthy animals that sustain us. These animals may not be considered family like our domestic pets, but they are equally valuable and deserve a dignified existence.

CHALLENGES

These conversations take time, easily half an hour to an hour, to cover in appropriate depth and with abundant compassion. Charge appropriately for your time. If this isn't feasible for you or your clinic, at minimum, gently guide your client with the key points A, C, and F. Discuss the patient's condition, the suspected speed of decline, and what an unassisted passing would look like. Also, offer QOL guides and resources for mobile end-of-life veterinarians to help support them through the process.

SUMMARY

Pets have their 5 freedoms, and families have financial, emotional, physical, time, and personal beliefs to consider. All these factors come into play to preserve QOL and maintain the human–animal bond. By addressing these, we fulfill our oath as veterinarians and create long-lasting connections with the families we serve.

We can help families well, from the moment they bring in their puppy or kitten for their first exam, through maintaining their healthy adult, senior, and geriatric pets, treating them when they become ill, and ultimately supporting them through that difficult time when they must make the final decision for a peaceful ending and QOD.

With your expertise and compassion, families heal faster and better. They will be more likely to return to you with their future fur babies, allowing you to restart the care journey together.

CLINICS CARE POINTS

- *Personal beliefs of staff:*
  Everyone in the clinic will feel differently about each euthanasia. Some have been with the pet and know the families for years, so they may have a harder time separating personal from professional opinions. Others have little experience, and every euthanasia hurts. Some have so much experience that they are either well adapted to handling the emotions that come with it, or they are experiencing emotional fatigue and burnout. There is a whole range of other responses as well.[11]
  Those who feel comfortable and are able to help the family will be best. Having compassion for those who are burnt out and helping build resilience for those who are more sensitive can improve team dynamics. Ultimately, all you are responsible for is guiding the family, giving resources, and being kind and compassionate when it is your turn, and making it a good death for the patient.
  When it comes to the decision, that's between you and the family. It's made in the best interest of the pet and the family. Allowing your team to know all factors can help them process and understand your decision. Still, not all employees have to be on board for you to do what is right for the family and the pet. So be kind to yourself. You are doing your very best. And if you don't have one already, please set a standard in your clinic that harassment among team members is forbidden. A team can be supportive of each other, even if they have different opinions. These cases are challenging enough on their own.
- *Personal beliefs of the family*
  Different family members may regard the patient with different levels of value. For example, if the patient is cuddly with mom, but it protects her so much that no other family member can get near her. Then, when they try to pet the patient, it bites everyone but her; she is going to value the patient more than the rest of the family will. She may also feel that her family is ready to have the end-of-life discussion before she is. In this situation, it is best to *focus on the QOL of the pet.*
  Some people with faith will have a hard time deciding when to end life and if they even should. The conversation can be heavily focused on not letting the patient suffer, and it being a kind decision and a duty of us as pet parents, natural death implications, and extending natural death by taking an animal out of the wild, medicating it, and keeping the furry family member safe is already unnatural.
  "We make the decision together in the best interest of the patient."
- *Not considering the enjoyment of the pet*
  If we can do more medically, and the family is willing and able, but the measures we are taking aren't improving the QOL for the patient, reassessing and guiding a QOL discussion is indicated for the welfare of the patient.
- *Not considering the family when making a recommendation*
  If we only focus on what we can do for the pet but neglect to consider the dynamics of the family, we place undue pressure and possibly guilt on the family.
  Instead, consider the humans who come attached to the animals we love so much. This approach will foster relationships, connection, return, referral, reduce their stress, improve healing for the family, and increase the well-being of the team.

DISCLOSURE

The author has nothing to disclose.

REFERENCES

1. Mellor D, Reid C. Original model 1994: the five domains model for animal welfare. ASPCA PRO 2025. Available at: https://www.aspcapro.org/resource/five-domains-model-animal-welfare. Accessed August 30, 2025.
2. Piotti P, Karagiannis C, Satchell L, et al. Use of the milan pet quality of life instrument (MPQL) to measure pets' quality of life during COVID-19. Animals (Basel) 2021;11(5):1336.
3. Gardner M. It's never long enough: a practical guide to caring for your geriatric dog. Rolled Toe Publishing; 2022.
4. Monteiro BP, Lascelles BDX, Murrell J, et al. 2022 WSAVA guidelines for the recognition, assessment and treatment of pain. J Small Animal Practice 2023;64(4): 175–310.
5. Lap of Love. QOL scale. 2013. Available at: https://www.lapoflove.com/how-will-i-know-it-is-time/lap-of-love-quality-of-life-scale.pdf. Accessed August 30, 2025.
6. Brooks W. Assessing quality of life and euthanasia in companion animals. Quality of life scale: the HHHHHMM scale. Veterinary Partner 2004. Available at: https://veterinarypartner.vin.com/default.aspx?pid=19239&catId=225989&id=4951966. Accessed August 30, 2025.
7. The Ohio State University Veterinary Medical Center. How will I know? Assessing quality of life and making difficult decisions for your pet. 2024. Available at: https://vmc.vet.osu.edu/sites/default/files/documents/how-will-i-know_rev_mar2024ms_0.pdf. Accessed August 30, 2025.
8. Banks F. MMVHS quality of life scale. 2012. Available at: https://mmvhs.ca/wp-content/uploads/2021/02/mmvhs-qol-chart-Form-Interactive.pdf. Accessed August 30, 2025.
9. Kleszcz A, Cholewińska P, Front G, et al. Review on selected aggression causes and the role of neurocognitive science in the diagnosis. Animals (Basel) 2022; 12(3):281.
10. Shelter Animals Count. Shelter animals count the national database. 2025 mid-year report. 2025. Available at: https://www.shelteranimalscount.org/wp-content/uploads/Shelter-Animals-Count_-2025-Mid-Year-Report_FINAL-1.pdf. Accessed August 30, 2025.
11. Cooney K, Kipperman B. Ethical and practical considerations associated with companion animal euthanasia. Animals (Basel) 2023;13(3):430.

REFERENCES

Just as Loved

Unique Species Considerations at End-of-life

Jason Doll, DVM, MPH, CVHEP

KEYWORDS

- End-of-life care • Species-specific welfare • Quality of life (QOL) assessment
- Euthanasia procedures and family-centered approach

KEY POINTS

- Unique species require tailored end-of-life assessments considering their biology, behavior, and environment.
- The Five Domains model emphasizes mental and social health alongside physical welfare for holistic care.
- Visual tools like Rainbow Mapping aid families in understanding their pet's quality of life and planning care.
- Proper preparation, sedation, and aftercare are crucial for humane euthanasia tailored to each species.
- Effective communication and understanding family dynamics are essential for compassionate end-of-life decision-making.

INTRODUCTION

Unique species (that is, noncat and dog companion animals) are like any other family member important in the assessment and treatment in respect to their end-of-life. Due to the growing popularity of these species in the home, there is a growing interest in evidence-based research on the treatment and care of these species.[1] Unfortunately, a lot of knowledge still needs to be extrapolated or inferred, many of them not just across a breed or subspecies perspective, but across that taxonomic family tree to a whole separate species or genera for comparison. This article aims to not only help with the comparisons and also the species considerations of these important furry and scaly family members.

The Five Domains, a welfare model developed in 1994 in Australia, is an important model for looking at animals not under human care in a zoologic setting, but also in the home as well.[2,3] The 4 key physical (also known as functional) domains focus on discrete aspects of how an animal interacts with not only their everyday environment,

Lap of Love Veterinary Hospice, 17804 U.S. 41, Lutz, FL 33549, USA
E-mail address: drjasond@lapoflove.com

Vet Clin Small Anim 56 (2026) 491–505
https://doi.org/10.1016/j.cvsm.2025.10.005 **vetsmall.theclinics.com**

Abbreviations	
POTZ	*preferred* optimal temperature zone
VCPR	veterinary–client–patient-relationship

but also the other animals as well as humans (**Fig. 1**). This model focuses on how these converge into a quality of life focused on mental and social health, not just physical.

As veterinarians, our goal is to promote animal welfare, especially with a species we may not work with every day. An ideal welfare state, especially with end-of-life care ultimately should focus on multiple aspects that a family can routinely focus on each day. These aspects (nutrition, environment, health/disease progression, and behavior) ultimately can help a family answer the questions, "what is their current quality of life and how can I ensure that it is best today?"

Before entering the examination room or if a home visit is possible, consider a similar schema of how to approach a canine or feline quality of life examination when faced with a unique species appointment:

- What is the patient's normal response to visitors and how are they normally handled in the most fear-free way possible?
  - Also consider how this species can show fear and how to best protect yourself (physical barriers, such as gloves or towels, or chemical barriers, such as pre-visit oral sedation).
  - Your safety is the most important. If you get hurt, it is so much more difficult to ensure that your patient and their people also do not get hurt.
- What is the family's knowledge of what is going on with their loved one and how do they approach their loved one's quality of life?
  - Who is the primary caregiver or if it is a combination of people, how do they communicate to each other what the needs are of their loved one?
  - What resources have they already used and are you familiar with those resources? This could help cultivate trust, even if the resource that they are referencing does not provide evidence-based medicine.
- What is the family's ability to administer medications or other caretaker tasks if indicated? Is this something the patient would tolerate?

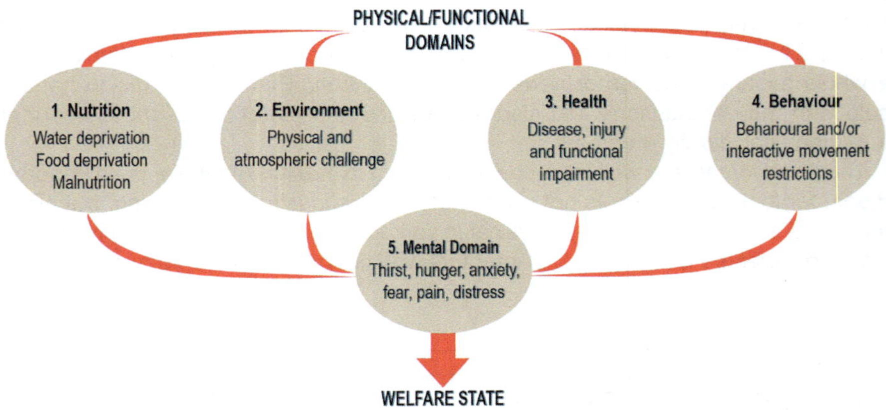

Fig. 1. The Five Domains.[2] (Mellor DJ et al., The 2020 Five Domains Model: Including Human–Animal Interactions in Assessments of Animal Welfare. Animals. 2020; 10(10):1870. https://doi.org/10.3390/ani10101870.)

- What does the end-stage disease process (or processes) look like in this species, both for conditions that have been confirmed and also if symptoms continue to manifest?
- How could this loss affect both the human and nonhuman loved ones in the home?
    - Important Consideration of the Four Budgets of Caregivers aka "taking the TEMP of the Family."[4]
        - Time
        - Emotional
        - Monetary (financial)
        - Physical

These are all aspects that we as veterinarians use to ensure that regardless of species, the overall mental state of the animal is at a net positive for the majority of their days.[3] When that starts to shift to more negative days than positive days or when overall mental state (ie, quality of life) is not where we want it to be, then medical intervention (eg, update with the veterinary professional team vs consideration for euthanasia vs other) is warranted (**Fig. 2**).

Regardless of species, having a caregiver that is not only knowledgeable about the species themselves and also of the individual is essential for knowing what a "positive welfare experience" is as well as a "negative welfare experience" is. Having knowledge of the species or taxonomic group is of course important for the veterinary profession; however, having a caregiver that is able to work with you on what their observations and care goals are is essential for not only a good quality of life and care for the patient but also for the relationship you have with their family to support with the most effective, available resources.

QUALITY OF LIFE ASSESSMENT FOR ANY SPECIES: THE RAINBOW MAPPING EXAMPLE

Quality of life assessment tools are essential to any end-of-life care conversation, especially for our unique species, however, can be very difficult to implement and disseminate. According to 111 veterinary nurses and veterinarians surveyed in the United Kingdom when asked about quality of life questionnaires, "perceived resistance from owners was the strongest barrier. Again, this reflects human medicine,

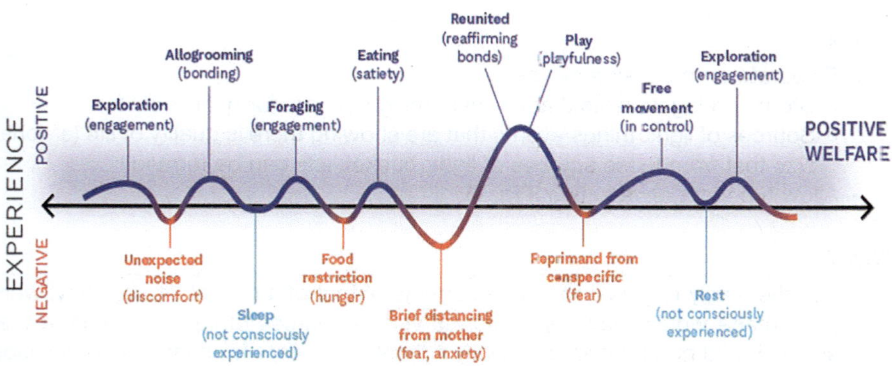

Fig. 2. Welfare experience states.[3] (Zoo and Aquarium Association Australasia (ZAA), "Conceptual Model of an Animal's Affective Experience", Zoo and Aquarium Association, 2018 https://www.zooaquarium.org.au/public/Public/Animal-Welfare/The-Five-Domains.aspx.)

where doctors expect poor patient compliance."[5] It can be truly difficult to quantify something where the answer is about quality, especially in such an emotionally charged conversation.

In the human end-of-life care world, quality of life has also posed some challenges.[6] In pediatric chronic asthma cases, having a "diary" written by the patient's parents has been reported to help understand results of interventions better.[7] In geriatrics, journey mapping is a tool that is sometimes used by physicians to provide a timeline of admissions next to functional performance scores, a unique measurement in human medicine.[8] Although it is a visual representation, this is something that is not often shared with patients and their caregivers and more for the health care team or auditing purposes.[7,8]

So many of us are visual learners, especially in veterinary medicine and those of us that love or work with animals. Participatory epidemiology is something that only can provide visual representation when discussing a complex problem, historically with understanding interventions for infectious disease.[6] These methods can also be helpful when there is not a shared spoken language and can easily be referenced later.

A participatory method can be utilized in our end-of-life care conversations as a way to not only express the difficulties of being a primary care giver, but also the wealth of resources, from medications to in-home/created products to other beings/organizations.

These are what will be known as "sources of light" that are peeking through the "storms" of navigating end-of-life care. The model for this will require a piece of paper (or this model laminated) and 2 (2) different colors of pens or dry erase markers, ideally 1 black and 1 a bright color (family favorite color, color of the feathers or scales of angel, or if the angel has a favorite color).

Step 1

- Make or have 3 circles drawn out:
  - One being the angel to emphasize that this is the center of the conversation
  - One being the "storms" (can stylize as a cloud for effect)
  - One being the "sources of light" (add rays later so family does not feel they need "a certain number" (quality over quantity of course)
  - Emphasize both are needed to create a Rainbow, our goal is to focus on the quality sources of light and mitigate the storm as much as possible
- Allow time for conversation (**Fig. 3**)

Step 2

- Elaborate on the 2 side circles:
  - Storms: things/events that are becoming concern for quality of life
  - Sources of light: things/events that are showing there is quality of life (emphasize that from these sources of light, bucket lists can be formed!)
- Allow time for conversation (**Fig. 4**)

Step 3

- Ask the family to give a rough percentage of that of a typical 24 hour day, what percentage would they say is storms versus sources of light. Emphasize that sleep should be counted, especially if there is concern for changes in cognition or sleeping patterns. Have the storms in 1 color and the sources of light in another color.
- Allow time for conversation (**Fig. 5**)

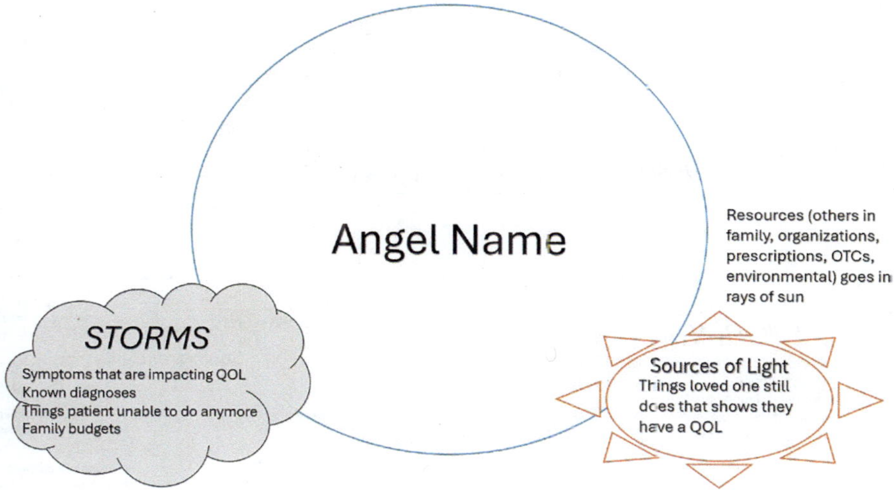

Fig. 3. Step 1 of Rainbow Mapping.

Step 4

- Take the other color and put bands/patterned bars in other wedge to show that our goal is to not only add "more sources of light as we are able" but also to emphasize to be mindful that as time/disease progresses that there can be signs of storms in the sources of light too.
- This should spark conversation about the end-of-life care plan and how caretakers, in-home veterinarians, and other veterinary professionals can help navigate these changes in both sides.
- Again, emphasize that although both storms and sources of light are needed to make a Rainbow

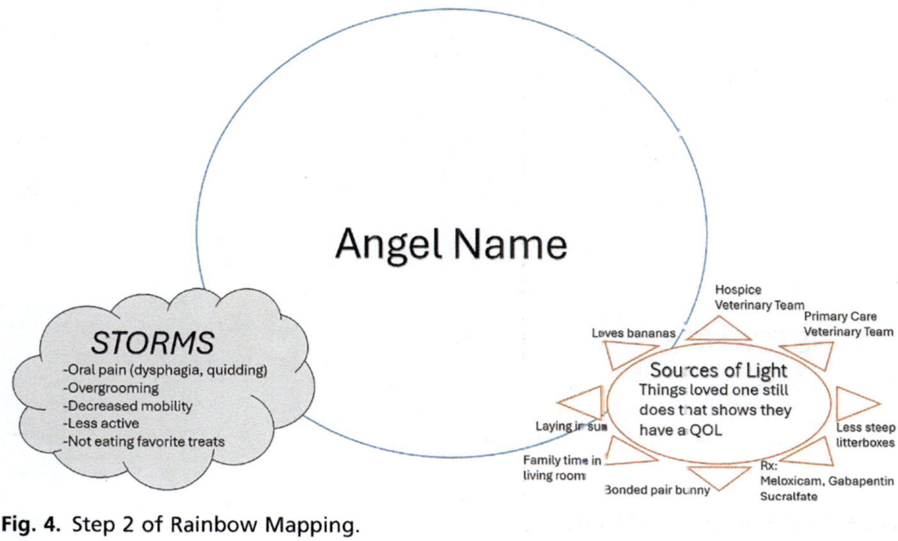

Fig. 4. Step 2 of Rainbow Mapping.

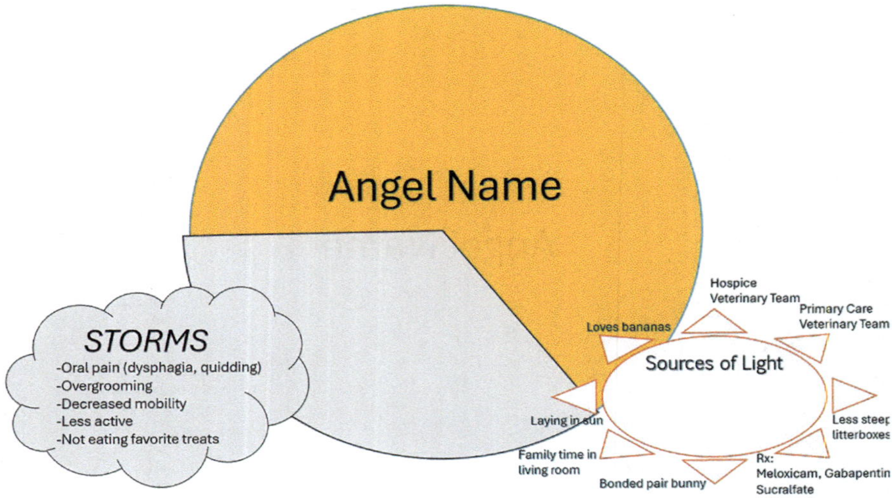

Fig. 5. Step 3 of Rainbow Mapping.

- Allow time for final thoughts and conversation (**Fig. 6**)

Overall, this novel quality of life assessment should not be in place with other, more quantifiable questionnaires but can be a good way to not only spark conversation but also provide something visual for the whole family to follow along. It could even be something that the family is given prior to an appointment as it sets the tone that end-of-life care has a unique approach that emphasizes not only the bond the family has with their loved one but also that there are ups and downs in any given day. It also serves as a reminder that they are not alone in the process and that there are things that can be done to help lessen the storms and provide more light.

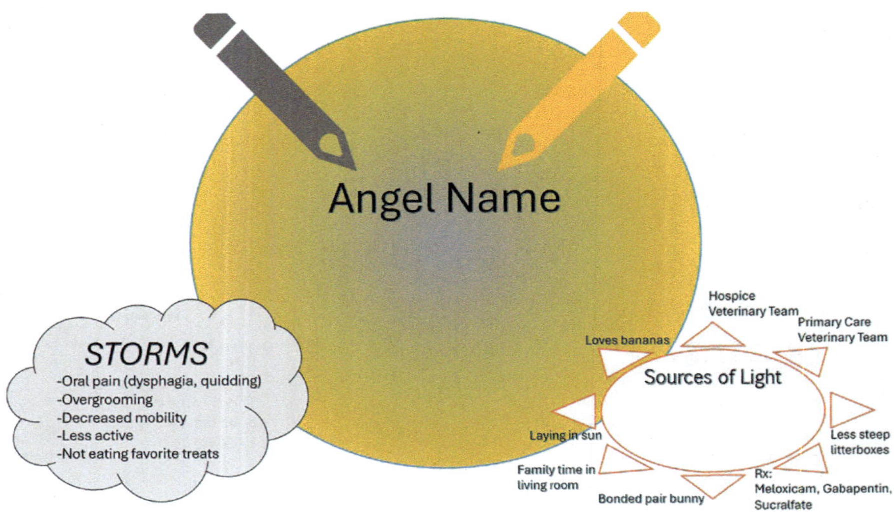

Fig. 6. Step 5 of Rainbow Mapping.

ROADMAP OF AN ANGEL APPOINTMENT

While there are many ways to approach a Euthanasia or Angel Appointment, this author has these 5 main aspects of the appointment for consideration across all species:

1. Natural history
   a. Obtain a history from the family about what their loved one has been experiencing, what symptom management and/or diagnostics have been performed.
   b. Examination of the patient: especially for an end-of-life appointment, a visual examination or abbreviated physical examination may be warranted to minimize patient stress and maximize their comfort.
   c. Quality of life assessment with the family using a scale of your choice. This is of course individual specific and should be done ideally with the primary caregivers.
2. Preparation
   a. Where in the clinic or home is the most stress-free for the patient, especially if it is a species that has not left their enclosure or safe space in their home. Consolidation of the other specifics/pets in the home where those individuals should be during the appointment. Many of these species live their entire lives in an enclosure or in a certain part of the house so moving to a new part of the home prior to sedation may cause a lot of stress.[9]
   b. What is the family's comfort in holding their loved one? Think of ways that they are able to protect themselves (teeth, claws, beaks, and so forth) to ensure not only your comfort but also the comfort of the patient and their family.
3. Sedation
   a. Oral sedation if there is a veterinary–client–patient-relationship (VCPR) prior to the appointment may be a prudent idea. If not, giving oral sedation in food or oro-transmucosal may be helpful in patients unable to initially give injectable sedation.[9]
      i. This author is based in the United States of America, so medication recommendations will be based on medications available in this geographic area.
   b. Injectable sedation with analgesics, anxiolytics, and tranquilizers not only maximize pain control but also provide the ability to give intraorgan euthanasia if a peripheral vessel is unable to be found.
4. Euthanasia
   a. Peripheral vein access can be obtained in areas anatomically similar to canine or feline venipuncture.
   b. In instances when the above is not possible, intraorgan euthanasia may be warranted.
   c. Secondary measures, such as pithing in reptiles/amphibians to ensure full cessation of neural connections.
5. Aftercare
   a. Honoring how the family would like to best remember their loved one either via cremation (flame vs aquamation) versus burial
   b. Keepsakes, such as impressions in clay or physical integumentary keepsakes, are usually best to be collected after euthanasia to ensure there is no discomfort during collection.

AVIAN

Psittacine

1. Natural history

   Psittacines are a diverse group of social, tropical, or subtropical species of over 400 species that often are very social and have a dynamic relationship with those that care for them.[10,11] Often living as long or longer than the humans that are taking care of them, these are among one of the most long-lived animals that people can keep as pets. Understanding the relationship that the family has with the individual, especially if they are pair-bonded with someone that may or may not be at the appointment, is crucial before entering the home.

Common disease processes that you may encounter with these species include cardiac disease (congestive heart failure secondary to atherosclerosis), reproductive disease (neoplasia), or organ dysfunction (liver or renal dysfunction). Since these are often long-lived birds, there are sometimes behavior issues (eg, feather picking and fearful behavior) with family members less experienced with avian care and husbandry.[10] Approach these like you would any other behavioral quality of life consultation. Remember what is the patient's not only quality of life in the environment that they are currently in and also what is the ability of possible care and comfort of their loved ones. Rehoming can be considered and is not always possible.

2. Preparation

A proper discussion of the household set-up is very important.

- Is the patient free-flight or have any feathers clipped?
- What type of enclosure do they have?
- Do they have free roam of the household? Which rooms are accessible?
- How protective are they of their space or to new people in the home?
- Are they able to be handled? If so, how?
- When are they most active?
- Can a high-value food be used as a distractor?

3. Sedation

Previsit sedation may be prudent if a VCPR is available, *gabapentin 10 mg/kg by mouth* given the night before and a couple hours prior to visit.

Once you enter the home and are able to provide a visual examination if a VCPR is not available beforehand, *intranasal midazolam (5 mg/mL) and butorphanol (10 mg/mL) via either syringe or aerosolizer attachment* (up to 0.5–1.0 mL total per nare pending there is no concern for dyspnea or respiratory disease) may be helpful in helping cause mild sedation within 10 to 15 minutes, especially for patients are unable to be fully handled.

Once able to be handled, giving *intramuscular tiletamine-zolazapam (100 mg/mL) fully reconstituted with acepromazine (10 mg/mL, telazol [tiletamine-zolazepam] [TZA]) 0.04 mg per 200 g of bird plus butorphanol 0.01 mg per 200 g of bird* in pectoral muscles to avoid accidental administration into air sacs.

An important consideration as the patient is getting sedated is that an avian can have 2 to 3 times more cervical vertebrae, so supporting the head and neck with a towel or loved one's hand as the righting reflex is lost.

4. Euthanasia

Once the patient is sedated, euthanasia solution (this author uses exclusively *pentobarbital [390 mg/mL] plus penytoin [50 mg/mL]) 1.0 mL per 500 g of bird for peripheral veins 2.0 to 3.0 mL per 2500 g of bird for intracoelomic* can be administered either peripherally or if fully anesthetized, intracoelomically.

For peripheral administration, use of the medial metatarsal vein in can be efficacious, especially in larger parrots and macaws. The cutaneous ulnar vein can also be easily accessible; however, it is best accessed in dorsal recumbency, which is not as esthetically pleasing, as well is prone to hematoma formation.

Intracoelomic option of preference is the right liver lobe, as it is larger than the left and is ventral to the keel and usually easily palpable. Access to this lobe is best if the patient is in left lateral recumbency with a 45° angle, ventral to keel. If there is a large amount of intracoelomic fat, a longer needle may be warranted. A flash is sometimes present when using this method.

5. Aftercare

A psittacine patient has large, zygodactyl (X-shaped) feet, so a larger amount of clay may be needed for footprint impressions.

Feathers can also be obtained for keepsake. Some feathers, especially the blue feathers of macaws, get their color from light rather than pigment, so the family may need to adjust the angle to get the most esthetically pleasing keepsake.

Poultry (Galliformes, Anseriformes, Ratites, and Columbiformes)

1. Natural history

These groups of birds are being combined as most of the birds in this group often can provide eggs or meat for human consumption. These can range from the smaller, flighted Columbiformes (such as pigeon and doves) to the large, flightless Ratites (such as ostriches, emus, and rheas). Even the individuals that do not have their eggs consumed can still develop reproductive diseases, such as ovarian or oviduct neoplasia. These individuals often housed either exclusively or partially outdoors, so consideration of the weather conditions is important. These individuals are often housed in groups, so knowing if there is concern for individual versus flock health disease is an important consideration.

In the United States, the Food Animal Residue Avoidance Databank is an important consideration and that the medications used should not go into the human food chain. A statement on your clinic's consent form should include a statement about this discussion and the family's understanding, especially if they are the responsible party of body aftercare (ie, burial).

2. Preparation

A proper discussion of the household set-up is very important.

- Is the patient free-flight or have any feathers clipped?
- What type of enclosure do they have? How many other birds are housed in this area? Can they be separated beforehand?
- Do they have free roam of the household or yard? Which areas are accessible?
- How protective are they of their space or to new people in the home?
- Are they able to be handled? If so, how?
- When are they most active?
- Can a high value food item be used as a distractor?

3. Sedation

Previsit sedation may be prudent if a VCPR is available, *gabapentin 10 mg/kg by mouth* given the night before and a couple hours prior to visit.[10]

Once you enter the home and are able to provide a visual examination if a VCPR is not available beforehand, *intranasal midazolam (5 mg/mL) and butorphanol (10 mg/mL) via either syringe or aerosolizer attachment* (up to 0.5–1.0 mL total per nare pending there is no concern for dyspnea or respiratory disease) may be helpful in helping cause mild sedation within 10 to 15 minutes, especially for patients that are unable to be fully handled.

Once able to be handled, giving *intramuscular tiletamine-zolazapam (100 mg/mL) fully reconstituted with acepromazine (10 mg/mL, TZA) 0.20 mL per 200 g of bird plus butorphanol 0.10 mL per 200 g of bird* in pectoral muscles to avoid accidental administration into air sacs.

An important consideration as the patient is getting sedated is that an avian can have 2 to 3 times more cervical vertebrae (especially larger waterfowl), so supporting the head and neck with a towel or loved one's hand as the righting reflex is lost.[10]

4. Euthanasia

Once the patient is sedated, euthanasia solution (this author uses exclusively *pentobarbital (390 mg/mL) plus penytoin (50 mg/mL)) 1.0 mL/2500 g of bird for peripheral veins 2.0 to 3.0 mL/2500 g of bird for intracoelomic* can be administered either peripherally or if fully anesthetized, intracoelomically.

For peripherial vein administration, use of the medial metatarsal vein in the can be efficacious, especially in larger parrots and macaws. The cutaneous ulnar vein can also be easily accessible; however, it is best accessed in dorsal recumbency, which is not as esthetically pleasing, as well is prone to hematoma formation.[10]

Intracoelomic option of preference is the right liver lobe, as it is larger than the left and is ventral to the keel and usually easily palpable. Access to this lobe is best if the patient is in left lateral recumbency with a 45° angle, ventral to keel. If there is a large amount of intracoelomic fat, a longer needle may be warranted. A flash is sometimes present when using this method.

5. Aftercare

These avian patients have large, anisodactyl (trident-shaped) feet, so a larger amount of clay may be needed for footprint impressions. Members of anseriformes often have webbing in between their toes, so making sure that part of the impression is there as well is important.

Feathers can also be obtained for keepsake and ideally to wash them with diluted peroxide or light bleach solution especially any waterfowl to reduce infectious disease risk (such as *Escherichia coli)*.

If a reportable or infectious disease is a differential, talking to the family beforehand about possible necropsy may be important and preparation of keepsakes may be the only thing that the family is able to have to remember their loved one.

SMALL MAMMALS

Hind-gut Fermenters (Lagomorpha and Rodentia)

1. Natural history

After cats and dogs, hind-gut fermenters are the most common small companion mammals that we see as pets.[1] Similar to equine patients, their lives revolve around eating vegetation and ensuring that they have proper gut health. Both lagomorphs (rabbits) and rodents are similar in that they can be very social but also very territorial of their space. Often rabbits and guinea pigs are housed in a pair bond, whereas others such as hamsters and chinchillas are often housed individually.

One of the most common end-of-life care diseases is dental disease as these species have continuously growing teeth that can impact their quality of life if growth under the gumline infiltrates their sinuses.[12] Reproductive disease is also very common, especially for rodents such as rats and mice.[13,14] Lifespans can vary based on species from a couple of years (smaller rodents such as hamsters, rats, and mice) to 4 to 8 years for midsized rodents (such as guinea pigs) or large breed rabbits to 8 to 14 years for larger rodents (chinchillas) and small breed rabbits.[12]

2. Preparation

Restraint using a towel or blanket may be helpful in the larger patients. An inverted "V" hold or use of a sock or thin fabric wrap can be helpful in the restraint of smaller rodents.[15]

3. Sedation

Previsit sedation may be prudent if a VCPR is available, *gabapentin 20 mg/kg by mouth* given the night before and a couple hours prior to visit.[16]

Similar to avians, you enter the home and are able to provide a visual examination if a VCPR is not available beforehand, *intranasal midazolam (5 mg/mL) and butorphanol (10 mg/mL) via either syringe or aerosolizer attachment* (up to 0.5–1.0 mL total per nare pending there is no concern for dyspnea or severe dental or respiratory disease) may be helpful in helping cause mild sedation within 10 to 15 minutes, especially for patients are unable to be fully handled.

Oral *pentobarbital (390 mg/mL) plus penytoin (50 mg/mL) 1.0 mL per 1000 g* in a high value food item, such as ice cream, peanut butter, or tahini, can be helpful for initial sedation.

Once able to be handled, giving *intramuscular tiletamine-zolazapam (100 mg/mL) fully reconstituted with acepromazine (10 mg/mL, TZA) 0.10 mL per 1000 g of patient plus butorphanol 0.10 mL per 1000 g of patient* in epaxial muscles. Use a larger (greater than 25 gauge) needle due to the thicker fur of lagomorphs.

4. Euthanasia

Once the patient is sedated, euthanasia solution (this author uses exclusively *pentobarbital [390 mg/mL] plus penytoin [50 mg/mL]) 1.0 mL/1000 g of patient for peripheral veins 2.0 to 3.0 mL/1000 g of patient for intraorgan* and can be administered either peripherally or if fully anesthetized, intraorgan.

For peripheral vessels, consider the cephalic or lateral saphenous for rabbits. An auricular vein is possible; however, this may be an unideal location esthetically. For rodents, a tail vein may be accessible; for larger rodents with tails, such as rats, however, intraorgan is more accessible.

For intraorgan administration, hind-gut fermenters have a relatively small thorax compared to cats and dogs, so intracardiac administration may be a little more difficult. Kidneys are often palpable for rabbits and so intrarenal administration similar to feline euthanasia is comparable. The left liver lobe of rabbits is larger than their right, so intrahepatic administration is best on right lateral recumbency. For rodents, intrahepatic or intraperitoneal is ideal due to their small size.[12]

5. Aftercare

Lagomorphs lack pawpads, so getting a paw print is often difficult, so doing a nose print can be a more effective keepsake.[12]

Rodent toes are often very small, and many families request multiple paws together with an imprint of the tail as well.

Fur is a wonderful keepsake too, just be sure that if clipping to be careful of the thinner skin that these species usually have and consider using scissors instead of clippers.

Crepuscular Small Mammals (Mustelids and Insectivores)

1. Natural history

This is a group of mammals that bring out the night life for some families. Mustelids include the ferrets, which are a type of carnivore and insectivores include hedgehogs. Both of these species are more crepuscular than nocturnal, meaning they are more active at dawn and dusk, which may be a consideration when scheduling a visit.

Some end-of-life disease processes that can affect ferrets include endocrine, such as adrenal disease or other neoplastic processes, such as insulinomas or lymphoma. A ferret's lifespan can be from 6 to 10 years.[12]

Some end-of-life disease processes that affect hedgehogs are cardiovascular and neoplasia, such as squamous cell carcinoma. A hedgehog's lifespan can be up to 8 years.[12]

2. Preparation

   For ferrets, the use of a sock or light fabric restraint may be necessary due to the very flexible body of even a sick or weak ferret to protect from bites.

   If a hedgehog rolls into a ball, putting the hedgehog in a small amount of water can help them unfold and gently scruff behind their ears to avoid quills.

3. Sedation

   Oral pentobarbital *(390 mg/mL) plus penytoin (50 mg/mL) 1.0 mL per 1000 g* in a high value food item, such as ice cream, peanut butter, or tahini, can be helpful for initial sedation.

   Once able to be handled, giving *intramuscular tiletamine-zolazapam (100 mg/mL) fully reconstituted with acepromazine (10 mg/mL, TZA) 0.10 mL per 1000 g of patient plus butorphanol 0.10 mL per 1000 g of patient* in epaxial muscles.

4. Euthanasia

   Once the patient is sedated, euthanasia solution (this author uses exclusively *pentobarbital [390 mg/mL] plus penytoin [50 mg/mL]) 2.0 to 3.0 mL per 1000 g of patient for intraorgan* and can be administered either peripherally or if fully anesthetized, intraorgan.

   Intraorgan is the most accessible for ferrets and hedgehogs. Ferrets have a much more caudal position to their heart than other carnivore species. Hedgehogs' most accessible intraorgan would be intrahepatic or intraperitoneal.

5. Aftercare

   Pawprints of these patients in clay or collection of fur or quills (removed with forceps) make for very memorable keepsakes.

HERPTILES (REPTILES AND AMPHIBIANS)

Reptiles

1. Natural history

   Among the most unique pet owners with a penchant for creating a whole ecosystem in their home is that of the reptile family. This diverse group of individuals include 2 major orders most commonly kept as companion pets: Squamata and Testudines (Chelonians).[17] The order Squamata include lizards and snakes and geriatric diseases of this order often include metabolic derangements or neoplasia (especially reproductive). Some of these members may be venomous, so ensuring that the local hospital has the antivenom of the species or similar is essential before going into a home with one. The order Testudines (Chelonians) include turtles and tortoises and are among the longest lived species, often spanning many generations of families. Their geriatric diseases also included metabolic derangements and neoplasia. Irreversible husbandry conditions (especially historic nutritional deficiencies) can also decrease quality of life, so proper historical insight is important to ensure how to best assess quality of life.

2. Preparation

   - Squamata:
     - Lizards: Gentle restraint around the neck using inverted "V" and pelvic girdle with one hand, and with the other around the pelvis and hindlimbs. A soft cloth

may be used to catch the delicate skinned geckos. Never handle a lizard by the tail as some species can drop them.[18]

- Snakes: Boas tend to be more fearful early in the evening (crepuscular), so avoid these appointment times.[19] Hold with your thumb and second finger behind the occiput and the forefinger on top of the head. Do not hold on "neck" as they have a single occiput, which can be easily dislocated. If bitten, remember the teeth angle to the back of the mouth so resist pulling back. Drops of isopropyl alcohol into the mouth encourage release. If bit, avoid ripping your finger or hand out of the mouth as could result in a deeper bite and loss of teeth into the wound.[19]

- *Chelonians*. Restrain shell slightly cranial to hind imbs or around the back of the shell between the hindlimbs (long nails can be used in fearful behavior). Some species, such as terrapins, can completely close their upper shell.[19]

Reptiles, especially those that are older or immunocompromised, are unable to regulate their own body temperature. They rely on a *preferred* optimal temperature zone (POTZ) both for intrinsic as well as extrinsic (ie, medication administration) metabolic. Most reptiles are housed with partia artificial light (Utraviolet A [UVA] 320–400 nm and Utraviolet B [UVB] 290–320 nm lights) that can help best regulate the POTZ.[19]

For maximum and effective absorption of medications, the following protocol is recommended:

1. Normal light schedule until about an hour prior to arrival.
2. Turn off light 1 hour before arrival or have appointment during part of day when light is less in use to ensure patient is as relaxed as possible.
3. Once sedation is administered, turn light back on and place patient there for 15 to 60 minutes.
4. After euthanasia and secondary measures, place under heat lamp if family is handling body aftercare (ensure that if the patient is wrapped in blankets that are not a fire hazard and not directly under lamp).
5. Leave the patient there overnight, up to 24 hours. Avoid freezing up to 24 hours if possible. Counseling the family about the decomposition process is important.

3. Sedation

Once safely handled, give *intramuscular tiletamine-zolazapam (100 mg/mL) fully reconstituted with acepromazine (10 mg/mL, TZA) 1.0 to 2.0 mL per 10 pounds of reptile* in triceps muscles for lizards and chelonians or proximal third epaxials for snakes.

4. Euthanasia

Once the patient is sedated, euthanasia solution (this author uses exclusively *pentobarbital [390 mg/mL] plus penytoin [50 mg/mL]) 1.0 mL/5000 g of reptile for peripheral veins 2.0 to 3.0 mL/5000 g of reptile for intracoelomic* can be administered either peripherally or if fully anesthetized, intracoelomically.

For peripheral administration, ventral tail vein for snakes and lizards is accessible. The carapace is the top shell is most accessible for chelonians.

For intracoelomic administration, intracardiac (cranial fourth of snake) is most accessible. If a Doppler is available, it is helpful for finding the area of heartbeat, especially for chelonians.[20]

Due to their slow metabolism, even while controlling their POTZ, a secondary measure of euthanasia is often warranted, especially if freezing for aftercare is needed. Freezing would further slow metabolism of these medications, so the secondary measure of pithing is recommended.

Pithing is an American Veterinary Medical Association approved adjunctive euthanasia technique.[9] This is best recommended to be performed away from the family as it is increased destruction of brain and spinal cord tissue. A 20 gauge needle is inserted caudally into the foramen magnum in a controlled and repetitive manner to disrupt brain stem connections within brain matter.[20] It is recommended for elevated placement of the head after pithing to ensure that any fluids do not drain out of the back of the head for esthetic purposes.

5. Aftercare

   Foot or whole body (depending on size) imprint in clay or ink can be included as a part of the keepsakes.

   Scales can also be obtained for keepsake and ideally to wash them with diluted peroxide or light bleach solution especially any waterfowl to reduce infectious disease risk (such as *Salmonella* spp).

SUMMARY

The love of an animal companion can be just as unique as the person that loves that loves them. It is important as veterinarians, especially at end-of-life, embrace this bond as it is just as strong as loving a cat or a dog. After taking your own expertise and comfort into account before helping a family of a unique species, know that you are making a difference to this family just by helping them help their favorite loved one.

CLINICS CARE POINTS

- Have confidence when conseling a family about end-of-life options and the human-animal bond with non-cat and non-dog species.
- Use Rainbow Mapping when assessing QOL for unique species.
- Use proper restraint for safety of patient, practioner, and family during euthanasia appointment.

DISCLOSURE

This author has been working as an associate veterinarian with Lap of Love Veterinary Hospice from 2021 to present (August 2025). No other disclosures.

REFERENCES

1. American Veterinary Medical Association. (2018). 2017-2018 pet ownership & demographics sourcebook. Schaumburg, IL.
2. Mellor DJ, Beausoleil NJ, Littlewood KE, et al. The 2020 five domains model: including human–animal interactions in assessments of animal welfare. Animals 2020;10:10.
3. ZAA, the five domains, zoo and aquarium association of Australia. 2023. Available at: https://www.zooaquarium.org.au/public/Public/Animal-Welfare/The-Five-Domains.aspx.
4. Gardner, Mary, and Dani McVety. "When is it time? assessing quality of life." 2016:528-531.

5. Roberts C, Blackwell EJ, Roe E, et al. Awareness and use of canine quality of life assessment tools in UK veterinary practice. Animals 2023;13(6):1105.
6. Catley A, Alders RG, Wood JLN. Participatory epidemiology: approaches, methods, experiences. Vet J 2012;191(2):151–60.
7. Stelmach I, Podlecka D, Smejda K, et al. Pediatric asthma caregiver's quality of life questionnaire is a useful tool for monitoring asthma in children. Qual Life Res 2012;21:1639–42.
8. Ly S, Runacres F, Poon P. Journey mapping as a novel approach to healthcare: a qualitative mixed methods study in palliative care. BMC Health Serv Res 2021; 21:1–9.
9. Underwood, Wendy, and Raymond Anthony. "AVMA guidelines for the euthanasia of animals: 2020 edition." Retrieved on March 2013.30 (2020): 2020-2021.
10. Miesle, Jeannine. "Overview of Avian Geriatric Disorders with Emphasis on Psittacines." 2022.
11. Pollack C. Parrot handling and restraint. LafaberVet 2010. Available at: https://lafeber.com/vet/parrot-handling/.
12. Lennox AM. End-of-life decisions: palliative care, hospice, and euthanasia for exotic animals. Veterinary Clinics: Exotic Animal Practice 2020;23(3):639–49.
13. LaFaber "Care for Senior Rabbit". 2023. Available at: https://www.lafeber.com/vet/wp-content/uploads/Senior-Rabbit-Client-Handout.pdf.
14. TeSelle E. To a long life: geriatric workups. 2023, House Rabbit Society website. Available at: http://rabbit.org/to-a-long-life-geriatric-workups/.
15. Tynes, valarie, today's veterinary practice ,Safe and humane handling of small mammals. 2023. Available at: https://todaysveterinarypractice.com/exotic-medicine/todays-technician-safe-humane-handling-of-small-mammal-patients/.
16. Conway, Rachel E., et al. "Behavioral and physiologic effects of a single dose of oral gabapentin in rabbits (Oryctolagus cuniculus)." Topics in Companion Animal Medicine 2023:100779.
17. Divers SJ. "Overview of Reptiles." merck veterinary manual. 2023. Available at: www.merckvetmanual.com/exotic-and-laboratory-animals/reptiles/overview-of-reptiles.
18. Renee CWR, Schott DVM. "Reptile Wildlife Euthanasia Techniques - LafeberVet." LafeberVet 2023. Available at: lafeber.com/vet/reptile-wildlife-euthanasia-techniques.
19. Redrobe S. "Basic approach to the reptile patient". World small animal veterinary world Congress proceedings. 2004. Available at: https://www.vin.com/apputil/content/defaultadv1.aspx?id=3852208&f5=1&f5=1.
20. Pollock C. "How to Verify Life (and Death) in Reptiles - LafeberVet." LafeberVet 2023. Available at: lafeber.com/vet/how-to-verify-life-and-death-in-reptiles.

Supporting Caregivers

Overcoming Stress, Burnout, and Burden

Mary Beth Spitznagel, PhD[a,*], Nikki E. Bennett, PhD[a],
Mark D. Carlson, DVM[b]

KEYWORDS

• Caregiver burden • Stress • Burnout • Strain

KEY POINTS

- Psychological distress is present in many owners of aging and ill companion animals due to increased caregiving responsibilities.
- Understanding and being able to identify this distress will likely facilitate communication and rapport with the client.
- The veterinary health care team is encouraged to acknowledge distress and take action within the bounds of professional competence to alleviate it.

INTRODUCTION

Caregiver Burden, Stress, and Burnout

As a natural consequence of aging, the need to tend to health issues in companion animals will often arise. Caregiver burden is a common response to the demands of providing care for a loved one with an illness.[1,2] Increased care (eg, specialized meal preparation, complicated medication regimen, coordination of health care appointments, etc.) is often required as companion animals age, become more frail, or show signs of specific disease processes. While many describe caregiving as positive or even transformative (eg, enhanced relationships, feeling useful, greater appreciation for life),[3] a wide variety of negative consequences are associated with caregiving as well.[4] The burden of caregiving includes emotional effects (eg, guilt, anger, frustration) as well as impact on daily life (eg, financial strain, physical demands of caregiving, less time for oneself).[5–7] Caregivers often "give until it hurts," sacrificing their own resources (eg, physical, emotional, financial) and self-care to provide for their loved one.[2,8]

An important component of the impact on the caregiver's life is stress.[5–7] More than 80 years ago, Hans Selye[9] characterized a "stress" response syndrome as a sequence

[a] Department of Psychological Sciences, Kent State University, PO Box 5190, Kent, OH 44242, USA; [b] Stow Kent Animal Hospital, 4559 Kent Road, Kent, OH 44240, USA
* Corresponding author.
E-mail address: mspitzna@kent.edu

Vet Clin Small Anim 56 (2026) 507–519
https://doi.org/10.1016/j.cvsm.2025.10.002 **vetsmall.theclinics.com**
0195-5616/26/

of 3 stages: alarm reaction, resistance, and exhaustion (reviewed by Rochette and colleagues;[10] **Box 1**).

The initial response to a stressor is met by immediate mobilization of our physiologic defenses to rise to the challenge of the stressor ("alarm reaction"). This short-lived reaction helps us respond to the threat and can thus be viewed favorably. The alarm reaction might occur when a caregiver first learns about a new problem or diagnosis in their loved one and must garner resources to accept and meet the challenges of caregiving.

When a stressor remains present, we begin to adapt to the chronic presence of that stressor ("resistance"). Our bodies initiate a return to a more balanced physiologic state while continuing to contend with the stressor. In terms of caregiving, coping with increased needs of the care recipient, confronting caregiving challenges as they arise, and integrating the caregiving role into a busy life are likely to characterize this stage.

With prolonged presence of the stressor (or accumulation of multiple stressors), the caregiver's resources are overwhelmed and depleted, and exhaustion sets in. Within this third stage of the stress response lies the potential for extension of stress to burnout. Burnout is a widely recognized response occurring among individuals providing care[11,12]; key to burnout is emotional exhaustion.[13] In this stage, the caregiver may experience the caregiving role as burdensome; indeed, greater burden is associated with longer duration of the caregiving role.[14]

The consequences of burden are not just stress and burnout in the caregiver, but extend to include the potential for reduced care provision for the care recipient, decreased quality of life, and deterioration of both physical and psychological health.[15] Understanding the presentation of burden in the companion animal caregiver is thus critical.

Companion Animal Caregiving

The past decade has seen significant advancement in the understanding of the psychological distress present in companion animal caregivers.

Early work demonstrating the importance of burden

Initial qualitative work examined concerns of a small group of owners of elderly or ill dogs and identified issues including the need to provide higher levels of care, emotional strain, and impact across several domains of life including work, social life, and finances.[16] Subsequent quantitative research adapted and validated a caregiver burden assessment tool from human medicine for use with companion animals.[17] This work showed that owners of a seriously ill dog or cat reported levels of caregiver burden approximately double that of individuals with a healthy dog or cat;

Box 1
Overview of Selye's 3 Stages of the Stress Response

Stage 1—Alarm
Initial mobilization of defenses to meet a challenge

Stage 2—Resistance
Adaptation to ongoing presence of stressor

Stage 3—Exhaustion
Overwhelm from prolonged stressor presence

From Selye[9] and Rochette and colleagues[10]

in fact, the average level of burden in those with a sick companion animal was within a range that is considered clinically meaningful burden for human caregiving. Associated with that greater burden was evidence of psychological distress across many spheres, including higher levels of stress, greater symptoms of depression, and anxiety and poorer quality of life. Together, these early works highlighted the importance of recognizing caregiver burden in companion animal owners.

Advances since early research

Since that initial research, the presence of burden in companion animal caregivers has been repeatedly demonstrated. From a robust initial replication of the first quantitative study showing caregiver burden in companion animal owners[8] to extension of this work in species-specific projects (eg, cat vs dog owners[18]), burden is routinely found to be present in many owners. Demonstration of this phenomenon has been repeated for owners of elderly companion animals,[19] as well as those with companion animals exhibiting dermatologic problems,[20] behavior concerns,[21] osteoarthritis,[22] cancer,[23] and cognitive dysfunction.[24]

In addition to acknowledging the presence of caregiver burden, the field is simultaneously advancing to identify potential implications of it. Beyond burden's association with psychological distress in the companion animal owner, it has the potential to influence decisions an owner makes on behalf of the companion animal, as burden is linked to factors associated with poorer treatment adherence[17] and greater consideration of euthanasia.[25] Moreover, studies have demonstrated that clients experiencing distress associated with caregiving are more likely to engage in behaviors that are, in turn, stressful for the veterinary health care team.[26,27]

Overwhelmingly, this body of research shows that caregiver burden is often present in the companion animal owners and is linked to negative outcomes that extend past the owner to the companion animal and veterinary health care team. Findings suggest that efforts to reduce caregiver burden in the veterinary context may be important. In turn, if efforts to better support owners with this experience are to succeed, identification of its presence is critical.

Identification of Burden

Not every client with an elderly or ill companion animal develops caregiver burden.[28] Alleviation of burden must thus begin with its identification. Burden can be identified in a variety of ways, including watching for specific signs of psychological distress, recognizing burden transfer behaviors in the client, and finally, formal assessment.

General signs of burnout

Significant distress might be noticeable through common physical, emotional, or behavioral signs of burnout, such as those described by Noroian and Yasko.[29] Physical signs could include fatigue, headaches, increased or decreased appetite, weight gain or loss, other gastrointestinal symptoms, sleeplessness, frequent minor illnesses, or feeling physically run-down. Emotional responses may look like irritability or impatience, rigidity, cynicism, boredom or apathy, helplessness or hopelessness, and self-dissatisfaction. Behavioral changes could appear in the form of confusion, forgetfulness, poor concentration, difficulty being productive, expressions of anger, withdrawal from others or activities, and even substance use. Although these signs can be indicative of psychological distress associated with caregiving, a veterinary health care provider might not have the opportunity to observe or be familiar enough with a given client to detect such changes. Awareness of these signs may be useful, yet other methods of burden detection are likely needed.

Burden transfer interactions

Research provides another insight into the detection of burden in the companion animal owner via burden transfer. Studies have linked distress related to companion animal caregiving to specific behaviors or interactions with veterinary staff (which in turn, are experienced as stressful by the providers[26]). The term "burden transfer" was coined to characterize a putative shift of a companion animal owner's distress to a person working in the veterinary medicine field through these interactions.[26,27] A variety of burden transfer interactions has been identified through factor analytical work and described using the acronym "DANCE" interactions: *D*aily Hassles, *A*ffect, *N*onadherent/Inconsiderate Behavior, *C*onfrontations, and *E*xcess Communication; **Table 1**.

The "Daily Hassles" domain refers to everyday behaviors from veterinary clientele, such as shopping around to compare the price of a procedure or inefficiency in decision-making. "Affect" encompasses situations in which heightened emotions are present in the client, such as when euthanasia counseling is necessary, or the client exhibits anxiety. "Nonadherent/Inconsiderate" behaviors involve rejection of necessary work-up, noncompliance with a treatment protocol, or behavior perceived as inconsiderate (eg, failing to attend a scheduled appointment). "Confrontation" includes conflicts that sometimes arise with a client, such as clients placing blame on the veterinary health care team for undesirable outcomes. Lastly, "Excess Communication" refers to times when the client asks for support that seems excessive (eg, repeatedly calling or emailing).[26] Because a higher frequency of these DANCE behaviors is strongly related to caregiver burden in the companion animal owner,[26] taking note of such behaviors may be useful in identifying caregiver burden in the owner.

Formal Assessment

Finally, burden can also be identified through formal assessment, which may range from a formal survey to a single question. Burden assessment may be conducted by the veterinarian or another member of the veterinary health care team. Several ways to measure caregiver burden have now been adapted or developed for use in general veterinary populations.

The first tool used to quantitatively examine caregiver burden in owners of seriously ill companion animals was an adaptation of the Zarit Burden Interview,[1] reduced to the

Table 1
Burden transfer DANCE behaviors

DANCE Domain	Definition	Examples
*D*aily Hassles	Everyday frustrations	Client wants impossible predictions, has difficulty making decisions, and compares costs
*A*ffect	Difficult client emotions	Client demonstrates anxiety, sadness, and grief
*N*onadherent/ Inconsiderate	Noncompliant or thoughtless behaviors	Client declines recommended treatment or work-up, no-shows for appointment
*C*onfrontations	Conflict with client	Client becomes upset, blames, and refuses to pay for services
*E*xcess communication	Greater support is needed than seems warranted	Client has a high frequency of contact (eg, calls, emails)

18 items of this tool deemed applicable to animal caregiving, and subsequently validated.[17] Considered the gold standard as the primary tool used in the research presented above, this measure (particularly if used to collect information as part of an extended intake procedure) is relatively lengthy.

Due to the length of this measure, an abbreviated version of this tool, created through statistical reduction, was validated for use with companion animal owners.[30] The resulting 7 item tool demonstrates sufficient psychometric qualities and includes reference values to help determine if a client's caregiver burden is elevated. This abbreviated instrument may be useful, yet still relies upon a measure adapted from human medicine; limitations could be present due to critical differences that exist between human and companion animal caregiving.[28]

As such, burden assessment might be best informed by the use of a measure developed explicitly to examine these issues in companion animal caregiving. Recently, psychometric development and validation of a 24-item caregiver burden questionnaire for owners of dogs, the Canine Caregiver Burden Assessment Tool (CCBAT), was created from the ground up. Items for this tool were developed through a combination of review of existing burden measures, interviews with owners, and expert input. Through statistical reduction, an abbreviated 5-item version (CCBAT-A) was created. Simultaneously, psychometric analyses were conducted for a 1-item screening item ("Overall, I have felt burdened by the care I provide for my dog") that can be followed by more in-depth conversation or assessment. These measures are available in the public domain[31]; interested readers are referred to the original source to determine the measure that best meets individual research or clinic needs.

Of note, although early assessment at the time of presentation for the companion animal's problems may be the most natural time to inquire about burden, this stage shows a lower incidence of burden.[32] Burden generally increases over time.[14] This occurs for many reasons. Care recipient needs typically increase over time, and care requirements become more complex. Additionally, the nature of the stress response—specifically that prolonged exposure to a stressor eventually elicits exhaustion (eg, Rochette and colleagues[10]) is such that longer duration of caregiving is linked to greater burden. Repeated assessment over time may thus be the best way to capture burden.

Attenuating Burden in the Companion Animal Caregiver

While methods of burden detection can identify *who* may be in need of intervention, an understanding of why burden is present is needed to inform *how* to best intervene. A prior review[8] observed that no interventions for caregiver burden in the companion animal owner had yet been researched, and cautioned against simply borrowing methods from human medicine due to differences between human and companion animal caregiving.[28] Unfortunately, several years later, the dearth of research producing effective interventions remains. Methods used in human medicine to alleviate caregiver burden, combined with knowledge about antecedents of burden in the companion animal, make for a good starting point. A solid understanding of both may thus be useful.

Successful burden interventions: lessons from human medicine

A significant body of literature examining caregiver interventions has emerged within human medicine, most prominently in dementia caregiving, though work extends also to other chronic or terminal disease states like cancer and Parkinson's disease. This work suggests many potential avenues to alleviate caregiver distress, with the caveat that different modalities of intervention may be needed, depending on the nature of that distress.

A comprehensive systematic review and meta-analysis[33] examining caregiver interventions for dementia caregivers demonstrated that for caregivers with depression, a wide variety of interventions may be effective, including psychoeducation, cognitive behavioral, acceptance and commitment therapy, behavioral activation, and mindfulness-based interventions. In contrast, that same work showed that when anxiety is the primary target, psychoeducation is the only effective intervention, while support groups appear to have the greatest impact on quality of life. Combined modalities that offer actual instrumental support, such as case management, psychoeducation, and multicomponent intervention may be necessary to move the dial on caregiver burden.

A recent review of Parkinson's disease[34] demonstrated that primary contributors to caregiver burden include longer disease duration, greater disease severity, and more negative emotion; that is, caregivers with more intense caregiving roles and negative emotions in general had the highest levels of burden. This is consistent with the dementia literature suggesting that instrumental assistance is needed to alleviate burden,[33] as well as the notion that perception of the caregiving role matters.[3] In fact, caregivers who show less positive appraisal of the caregiving role prior to intervention actually appear to benefit more from caregiver interventions over time.[35] Such findings suggest that helping caregivers change their view of this role from a burden that is difficult to a challenge to which they can rise may promote emotional satisfaction and protect against burden.

Additionally, early intervention may be key. Bayly and colleagues[36] conducted a systematic review and meta-analysis showing that early-stage caregiver intervention exerted a small positive effect on well-being in the caregiver and their ability to provide care. Interestingly, in early stage caregivers, they found no difference in effectiveness based on intervention type (individual vs group, psychotherapy vs psychoeducational vs or multicomponent), suggesting that the need for interventions to be tailored to specific outcomes could be more important with time and progression of burden.

While early caregiver interventions were typically conducted face-to-face or by telephone, recent decades have seen an evolution of interventions leveraging technological advances. Online interventions in particular offer both reach and sustainability. A systematic review and meta-analysis of online interventions for dementia caregivers supported that web-based interventions can effectively enhance caregiver self-esteem and self-mastery (ie, sense of control) as well as decrease caregiver strain.[37] Technology-based interventions are not ubiquitously beneficial—meta-analytic work examining cancer caregiver interventions suggests good potential for improvement in depressive symptoms and quality of life, but caregiver burden did not show overall improvements in this study.[38] The reason for this discrepancy is not fully clear: possibly due to dissimilarities in the interventions attempted, or to differences in the contributors to burden in these groups. Regardless, the importance of understanding the target caregiver group and specific antecedents driving burden in a given population is highlighted.

Antecedents of companion animal caregiver burden

The most successful path forward for optimizing interventions in companion animal caregivers will combine knowledge of burden interventions in human caregiving together with that of burden predictors in the companion animal context. Research has identified several potential causative and modifiable factors of caregiver burden in the companion animal owner, including the presentation of illness in the animal, reduced personal resources, negative appraisal of the caregiving role, and difficulty enacting a care plan. To date, these variables have been examined in a cross-sectional manner, so these links are cautiously interpreted.

Specifically, clinical signs and behavior changes in the animal predict correlate with burden, with particularly prominent links to weakness, perceived alteration of personality or mood, the appearance of pain or discomfort, frequent urination, and excessive sleeping/lethargy in the animal.[39] The animal's symptoms are most likely an active target of both the owner and veterinary health care team. If problems in the animal can be reduced, caregiver burden may grow lighter. However, the approach taken to this end is important. Other factors related to caregiver burden include the degree to which a treatment plan impacts day-to-day life, with greater changes to the owner's daily routine and difficulty following new routines being associated with a higher perception of burden.[40] Another work showed that a caregiver's perception that treatment is ineffective was strongly linked to burden.[32] Findings from these studies demonstrate the complex nature of caregiver burden: it arises not from a single factor, but from many, and most often in combination. In light of this, working with owners to collaboratively identify the problems of greatest concern and generate solutions that fit into the owner's life may be useful in alleviating the burden on the owner and optimizing care for the animal.

While severity of the animal's problems is related to burden, the caregiver's personal resources are important, as well. The same study that showed a link between burden and specific signs and symptoms in the animal also showed that elements like the caregiver's self-mastery and reactivity to the animal's problems are key contributors to burden.[39] An intervention that focuses on reducing the stress response in caregiving while instilling a sense of control could be helpful. Along similar lines of personal resources, active coping skills and good social support are also negatively linked to burden.[39] While these latter variables did not explicitly predict burden in larger statistical models, their correlations with burden suggest that the inclusion of elements to enhance coping and social support may be worth including in an intervention.

Relevant to personal resources, a robust negative relationship between burden and a positive caregiving appraisal has been observed in the literature,[41–43] including in companion animal caregivers.[28] As noted above, the tendency to positively appraise the caregiving experience may impact responsiveness to interventions.[35] This makes it a crucial factor when considering potential treatments for burden. However, research shows that companion animal caregivers, at baseline, exhibit a more positive appraisal of their role as caregiver compared to those caring for a human.[28] The reason for this is not known but may be due to the option of euthanasia in companion animal caregiving; whereas the companion animal owner has a choice to be a caregiver or euthanize an animal, a human caregiver may be obligated to the role due to finances or family dynamics. Regardless of the reason behind this difference, companion animal caregivers may already be at a ceiling for such effects.

Overall, the animal's specific clinical signs and behavior problems should be considered, as well as the ease with which an owner might carry out a care plan. However, individual differences in the personal resources of owners, including the level of reactivity and how well-equipped they feel to deal with these problems should not be forgotten. Appropriate targeting of specific predictors of companion animal caregiver burden will likely enhance the efficacy of any formal efforts toward prevention or intervention.

Current Recommendations

In a perfect world, veterinary clients experiencing burden could be directed to well-researched interventions and support resources in a manner similar to human caregivers, for whom myriad caregiving resources exist (eg, national caregiving organizations, local elder care agencies, websites, respite care[44]). At present, many larger veterinary networks employ veterinary social workers[45]; however, this field is certificate-based (rather than license-regulated), and standards of practice are not yet firmly established.[46,47] Gold standard approaches to working with burdened companion animal owners do not yet exist. However, several practical, evidence-informed strategies can be made for veterinary teams working with these clients:

Acknowledge burden, and avoid labeling or assuming

As previously discussed, the full spectrum of caregiving challenges extends beyond terms like "stress" or "burnout." For this reason, the term "caregiver burden" is preferred in scientific circles. However, when speaking with a client, the term "burden" can evoke defensiveness in people unfamiliar with the clinical use of the term: "My pet isn't a burden!" If you notice telltale signs of burden (eg, a client exhibiting stress and anger, expressing uncertainty or guilt[47]), let them know that it is common to feel overwhelmed by the challenges of caregiving. At the same time, avoid assuming that a burden is present. Not all owners experience caregiver burden when caring for a companion animal with chronic illness.[16,28] Choosing to care for a sick loved one can foster a sense of purpose, deepen appreciation for one's own strengths, and provide opportunities to practice patience.[3] Burden is not an inevitable outcome of providing long-term care.

Empathize with feelings and empower through knowledge

If a client confides in you about personal struggles in caregiving, use the moment to offer empathy. Acknowledge your client's trust in you and bridge the interaction into an educational moment. You could note that research shows that companion animal caregiving is often stressful for owners.[17] In addition to providing trusted resources about their pet's specific condition, your client may be interested in learning more about caregiver burden. If this is the case, consider introducing the term "burden" with caution, emphasizing that the burden of caregiving does not imply that the companion animal is a burden; rather, the term refers to personal challenges experienced when providing long-term care for a loved one. Though education alone does not typically resolve caregiver burden,[48] it is an essential step for clients to fully understand the circumstances, which is important to lowering burden.[8] For interested clients, our team has a dedicated science blog to help pet owners understand caregiver burden: www.petcaregiverburden.com.

Collaborative treatment planning

Work together with the client in a collaborative manner, keeping in mind that decision-making is, at its best, a joint effort. Collaborative care planning may help minimize caregiver burden, as research shows that when clients perceive a treatment plan as difficult to follow or disruptive to their daily routine, their burden increases.[32,40] Partnering with the client on a clear plan, giving consideration to household schedules, and developing a "back-up plan"[8] offers an opportunity to build the client's confidence as a caregiver. Other studies show that as the number of medications increases, so do burden levels.[32] This pattern holds even after controlling for disease severity, with fewer overall treatments predicting lower caregiver burden.[25] Indeed, research shows that when outcomes are equal, companion animal owners express a preference for simpler treatment.[49] Although individuals may vary (and cost may be a factor for some), the simplest effective treatment tends to be best from a burden perspective. Additionally, research shows that if owners believe an intervention is ineffective, they experience greater burden.[32] Clear communication regarding expected outcomes from treatment may be helpful. For example, if the veterinary team is focused on managing the animal's comfort, while the owner believes interventions are meant to improve specific signs or symptoms, mismatched perceptions of "success" could contribute to burden. Keep in mind that as the professional, you have a better understanding of the medicine (eg, treatment, prognosis, disease processes), while the client is the expert on this particular animal. Combining these strengths through authentic collaboration is likely in the patient's best interest.

Guide problem-solving and celebrate wins

A client's confidence in caregiving is negatively associated with caregiver burden—in other words, owners reporting low confidence in their ability to manage treatment are more likely to experience burden.[25] This lends to the importance of anticipating potential challenges that may arise. As the veterinary provider, you are well-positioned to guide problem-solving and celebrate successes. When discussing potential challenges, such as administering oral medication, proactively provide possible solutions (eg, strategies or products to facilitate ingestion of medication), and ensure the client is aware of support services (eg, educational technician appointments). Guide clients to take small, sequential steps to try different strategies as they navigate caregiver challenges[8]; if multiple new tactics are simultaneously attempted, it is difficult to discern which strategies are most useful. Lastly, simple praise or encouragement can potentially boost the client's sense of competence as a caregiver,[48] which might translate to reduced burden. Celebrating client successes in navigating caregiving challenges may be a simple way to maintain a positive veterinary–client relationship while helping to reduce caregiver burden.

Caregiving isn't just a burden—it has benefits worth understanding

Relative to human caregivers, companion animal owners often report more positive perceptions of their caregiving role.[28] Qualitative data suggest that strong attachment to a pet can help buffer against the negative aspects of caring for an aging pet.[50] Beyond the challenges of caregiving, this role can lead to positive affect from feeling needed, useful, and appreciated.[3] When working with clients providing long-term care to a pet, developing an understanding of their experiences may contribute to a stronger rapport. Asking clients about their positive experiences gives them space to reframe their burden in a way that reminds them *why* they are invested in their pet's care. Importantly, interactions should be kept within the boundaries of your professional expertise. If you do not have a degree and license in a human mental health field, efforts to help a burdened client could begin extending beyond the bounds of your competence. When in doubt, consider referring to an allied mental health provider (eg, veterinary social worker), or other provider of clinical mental health services (eg, psychologist).

While the above recommendations are informed by research, it is worth re-emphasizing that direct research of owner interventions for caregiver burden is lacking at present. Important next steps include research to develop treatments for the burden. This knowledge will be gained through carefully designed studies that facilitate our understanding of what works for whom.

Emerging Treatments

While there is a paucity of companion animal caregiver burden intervention research, the past 2 decades of human caregiving research might be informative. As described above, in recent years, low-cost, technology-based interventions have taken center-stage. Interventions using such modalities are demonstrably effective, similar to face-to-face interventions for human caregiving relationships, and far easier to scale up for broad use.[51] Due to common caregiver challenges, such as financial strain, difficulty leaving the home, and lack of time, it is crucial that readily available and cost-effective interventions be developed.

Using human caregiving research to inform companion animal caregiver interventions may be useful. For example, drawing upon work described by Ploeg and colleagues,[37] web-based interventions for caregiver strain could be successful, though this is suggested with caution as Li and colleagues found no change in burden following web-based caregiver interventions.[38] When treatments are less successful, it is due to a lack of specific intervention components (eg, social support, case management)? Future research should focus on additive study designs, starting with a basic intervention and adding components to determine if effectiveness is increased. Companion animal caregiver interventions will likely be most successful if developed by drawing upon lessons learned in human caregiving research while being mindful of caregiver differences in these populations[28] and focusing on known predictors of burden in pet owners.[39]

In summary, technology-based interventions present a potentially cost-effective, scalable method to alleviate caregiver burden in companion animal owners. Multicomponent interventions that include educational materials about the specific disease and pet caregiving, connection with other pet caregivers, and existing evidence pointing to modifiable risk factors for pet caregiver burden will be important.

SUMMARY

In conclusion, psychological distress is present in many (though not all) owners of elderly or ill companion animals. Challenges of caregiving can elicit caregiver burden, stress, and burnout. The veterinary healthcare team can play an important role in supporting clients by recognizing and understanding burden, and taking action within the appropriate bounds of competence to facilitate the reduction of burden.

CLINICS CARE POINTS

- Caregiver stress, burnout, and burden can occur in owners providing care for an elderly or ill companion animal.
- Identify presence of distress through watching for specific signs, recognizing burden transfer behaviors, and/or formal assessment of caregiver burden.
- When burden is present, acknowledge it, empathize with the client's feelings while empowering them through knowledge, and focus on collaborative treatment planning with a problem-solving focus.
- Understanding and supporting clients experiencing burden is an important piece of the veterinarian-client relationship, but a mental health provider is best equipped to help someone with mental health problems; when in doubt, refer out.

DISCLOSURES

Dr M.B. Spitznagel and Dr M.D. Carlson have received honoraria for presenting scientific work related to caregiver burden and/or workshops for veterinary professionals to reduce burden transfer. Dr M.B. Spitznagel holds current grant funding from Zoetis LLC. Dr M.B. Spitznagel and Dr N.E. Bennett both receive salary support through the National Institute for Occupational Safety and Health, United States and the Centers for Disease Control, United States (R01OH012580).

REFERENCES

1. Zarit SH, Reever KE, Bach-Peterson J. Relatives of the impaired elderly: correlates of feelings of burden. Gerontol 1980;20:649–55.
2. Tremont G. Family caregiving in dementia. Med Health R I 2011;94(2):36–8.
3. Tarlow BJ, Wisniewski SR, Belle SH, et al. Positive aspects of caregiving: contributions of the REACH project to the development of new measures for Alzheimer's caregiving. Res Aging 2004;26:429–53.
4. Paradise M, McCade D, Hickie IB, et al. Caregiver burden in mild cognitive impairment. Aging Ment Health 2014;19:72–8.
5. Martin JT, Chapman KR, Was C, et al. Factors of dementia caregiver burden differentially contribute to desire to institutionalize. J Geriatr Psychiatr Neurol 2022;35(4): 594–600.
6. Patrick KS, Gunstad J, Martin JT, et al. Specific agitation behaviour in dementia differentially contribute to aspects of caregiver burden. Psychogeriatrics 2020; 22(5):688–98.
7. Springate BA, Tremont G. Dimensions of caregiver burden in dementia: impact of demographic, mood, and care recipient variables. Am J Geriatr Psychiatr 2014; 22(3):294–300.
8. Spitznagel MB, Carlson MD. Caregiver burden and veterinary client well-being. Vet Clin North Am Small Anim Pract 2019;49(3):431–44.
9. Selye H. Stress and the general adaptation syndrome. Br Med J 1950;1(4667): 1383–92.
10. Rochette L, Dogon G, Vergely C. Stress: eight decades after its definition by Hans Selye "Stress is the spice of life.". Brain Sci 2023;13(2):310.
11. Maslach C. Burnout: the cost of caring. Englewood Cliffs (NJ): Prentice-Hall; 1982.
12. Edu-Valsania S, Laguia A, Moriano JA. Burnout: a review of theory and measurement. Int J Environ Res Publ Health 2022;19(3):1780.
13. Maslach C, Jackson SE. MBI: maslach burnout inventory. Manual. Palo Alto (CA): University of California, Consulting Psychologists Press; 1981.
14. Kim H, Chang M, Rose K, et al. Predictors of caregiver burden in caregivers of individuals with dementia. J Adv Nurs 2011;68:846–55.
15. Liu Z, Heffernan C, Tan J. Caregiver burden: a concept analysis. Int J Nurs Sci 2020;7(4):438–45.
16. Christiansen SB, Kristensen AT, Sandoe P, et al. Looking after chronically ill dogs: impact on the caregiver's life. Anthrozoös 2013;26:519–33.
17. Spitznagel MB, Jacobson DM, Cox MD, et al. Caregiver burden in owners of a sick companion animal: a cross-sectional observational study. Vet Rec 2017;181-(12):321.
18. Spitznagel MB, Gober M, Patrick K. Caregiver burden in cat owners: a cross-sectional observational study. J Feline Med Surg 2023;25(1). https://doi.org/10.1177/1098612X221145835.
19. Spitznagel MB, Anderson JR, Marchitelli B, et al. Owner quality of life, caregiver burden and anticipatory grief: how they differ, why it matters. Vet Rec 2021; 188(2):e74.
20. Spitznagel MB, Solc M, Chapman KR, et al. Caregiver burden in the veterinary dermatology client: comparison to healthy controls and relationship to quality of life. Vet Dermatol 2018;30(1):3-e2.

21. Kuntz K, Ballantyne KC, Cousins E, et al. Assessment of caregiver burden in owners of dogs with behavioral problems and factors related to its presence. J Vet Behav 2023;64-65:41–6.
22. Spitznagel MB, Patrick K, Gober MW, et al. Relationships among owner consideration of euthanasia, caregiver burden, and treatment satisfaction in canine osteoarthritis. Vet J 2022;286:105868.
23. Silva PTRF, Coura FM, Costa-Val AP. Caregiver burden in small animal clinics: a comparative analysis of dermatological and oncological cases. Animals 2024; 14(2):276.
24. Taylor TL, Smith BP, Hazel SJ. Guardians' perceptions of caring for a dog with canine cognitive dysfunction. Vet Rec 2024;194(2):e3266.
25. Spitznagel MB, Marchitelli B, Gardner M, et al. Euthanasia from the veterinary client's perspective: psychosocial contributors to euthanasia decision making vet Clin North am small. Anim Pract 2020;50(3):591–605.
26. Spitznagel MB, Ben-Porath YS, Rishniw M, et al. Development and validation of a Burden transfer inventory for predicting veterinarian stress related to client behavior. J Am Vet Med Assoc 2019;254(1):133–44.
27. Spitznagel MB, Updegraff A, Twohig MP, et al. Reducing occupational distress in veterinary medicine personnel with acceptance and commitment training: a pilot study. N Z Vet J 2022;70(6):319–25.
28. Britton K, Galioto R, Tremont G, et al. Caregiving for a companion animal compared to a family member: burden and positive experiences in caregivers. Front Vet Sci 2018;5:325.
29. Noroian EL, Yasko J. Care for the critical care-giver: strategies for the prevention of burnout. Dimens Crit Care Nurs 1982;1(2):97–102.
30. Spitznagel MB, Mueller MK, Fraychak T, et al. Validation of an abbreviated instrument to assess veterinary client caregiver burden. J Vet Intern Med 2019;33(3): 1251–9.
31. Spitznagel MB, Martin J, Knudsen E, et al. Development and psychometric validation of a canine caregiver burden assessment tool. Under review.
32. Shaevitz MH, Tullius JA, Callahan RT, et al. Early caregiver burden in owners of pets with suspected cancer: owner psychosocial outcomes, communication behavior, and treatment factors. J Vet Intern Med 2020;34(6):2636–44.
33. Sun Y, Ji M, Leng M, et al. Comparative efficacy of 11 non-pharmacological interventions on depression, anxiety, quality of life, and caregiver burden for informal caregivers of people with dementia: a systematic review and network meta-analysis. Int J Nurs Stud 2022;129:104204.
34. Zhao Y, Wu W, Wu J, et al. Risk factors and intervention of caregiver burden in Parkinson's disease: a systematic review and meta-analysis. Qual Life Res 2024;33(7): 1753–66.
35. Hilgeman MM, Allen RS, DeCoster J, et al. Positive aspects of caregiving as a moderator of treatment outcome over 12 months. Psychol Aging 2007;22(2): 361–71.
36. Bayly M, Morgan D, Elliot V, et al. Does early-stage intervention improve caregiver well-being or their ability to provide care to persons with mild dementia or mild cognitive impairment? A systematic review and meta-analysis. Psychol Aging 2021;36(7):834–54.
37. Ploeg J, Ali MU, Markle-Reid M, et al. Caregiver-focused, web-based interventions: systematic review and meta-Analysis (part 2). J Med Internet Res 2018;20-(10):e11247.

38. Li Y, Li J, Zhang Y, et al. The effectiveness of e-Health interventions on caregiver burden, depression, and quality of life in informal caregivers of patients with cancer: a systematic review and meta-analysis of randomized controlled trials. Int J Nurs Stud 2022;127:104179.
39. Spitznagel MB, Jacobson DM, Cox MD, et al. Predicting caregiver burden in general veterinary clients: contribution of companion animal clinical signs and problem behaviors. Vet J 2018;236:23–30.
40. Spitznagel MB, Cox MD, Jacobson DM, et al. Assessment of caregiver burden and associations with psychosocial function, veterinary service use, and factors related to treatment plan adherence among owners of dogs and cats. J Am Vet Med Assoc 2019;254(1):124–32.
41. Abdollahpour I, Nedjat S, Salimi Y. Positive aspects of caregiving and caregiver burden: a study of caregivers of patients with dementia. J Geriatr Psychiatr Neurol 2018;31(1):34–8.
42. Cousins E, Patrick K, Chapman K, et al. The indirect effect of positive aspects of caregiving on the relationship between cognitive decline and dementia caregiver burden. Psychogeriatrics 2023;23(4):603–8.
43. Fauziana R, Sambasivam R, Vaingankar JA, et al. Positive caregiving characteristics as a mediator of caregiving burden and satisfaction with life in caregivers of older adults. J Geriatr Psychiatr Neurol 2018;31(6):329–35.
44. Swartz K, Collins LG. Caregiver care. Am Fam Physician 2019;99(11):699–706.
45. Vincent A, Rauktis M, Maxwell L, et al. Caring for those who care for our pets: veterinary social workers' perceived role in veterinary medicine. Soc Work Ment Health 2024;22(6):788–806.
46. Hoy-Gerlach J, Ojha M, Arkow P. Social workers in animal shelters: a strategy toward reducing occupational stress among animal shelter workers. Front Vet Sci 2021;8:734396.
47. Vincent A, Rauktis ME, Maxwell L, et al. The role and scope of practice of veterinary social workers in animal shelters. Pets 2025;2(1):6.
48. Tremont G, Davis JD, Spitznagel MB. Understanding and managing caregiver burden in cerebrovascular disease. In: Vascular dementia: cerebrovascular mechanisms and clinical management. Totowa (NJ): Humana; 2005. p. 305–21.
49. Spitznagel MB, Martin J, Updegraff J, et al. Assessment of owner perceptions of caregiver burden, veterinarian-client relationship and satisfaction with the provider in canine pruritus: an experimental vignette study. Vet Dermatol 2024;35(1):81–91.
50. Taylor TL, Smith BP, Hazel SJ. Guardians' perceptions of caring for a dog with canine cognitive dysfunction. Vet Rec 2024;194(2):e3266.
51. Shin JY, Choi SW. Interventions to promote caregiver resilience. Curr Opin Support Palliat Care 2020;14(1):60–6.

Euthanasia

The Ending Matters Most

Sara Lynch, DVM, MPH[a,b]

KEYWORDS

• Humane euthanasia • Good death • Dying well • Pet loss

KEY POINTS

- Humane euthanasia is a complex aspect of pet ownership and veterinary care; when used appropriately and with sensitivity to the needs of the pet and owner, euthanasia can provide a peaceful end to physical and mental suffering for the veterinary patient.
- Much like the themes important to the human experience of "dying well," the priorities at the end phases of an animal's life should include veterinary support and effective communication, validation of the decision by the pet's family, a painless death in a comfortable environment, and appropriate options for aftercare of the body.
- Negative feelings experienced during a euthanasia appointment can have long-lasting effects on the pet owner, including feelings of guilt and prolonged grief.
- The preservation of the human–animal bond should be of utmost importance at the end of a pet's life—this can be achieved by a veterinarian providing medical knowledge, empathy, and sensitivity to the needs of both the pet and the owner throughout the euthanasia appointment.

INTRODUCTION

While most veterinary education builds on skills to maintain patients' quality of life through preventative care, surgeries, and treatment plans, we should never dismiss the fact that an equally vital part of our training is meant to prevent unnecessary suffering and ensure a good quality of death. Veterinarians are the only health professionals who are granted the unique responsibility of providing end-of-life measures for our patients through humane euthanasia, and the sacredness of this responsibility is not to be underestimated. Moreover, veterinarians find themselves in a unique medical professional role—they are the clinician for the patient and therefore the animal's advocate first and foremost, but undeniably, there is also have a responsibility to provide compassionate support and communication for the pet family. For many clinicians, this can be a massive learning curve as many veterinarians graduate with no significant training on how to provide support to owners during end-of-life stages of the pet's life.

[a] Lap of Love Veterinary Hospice, Memphis, TN, USA; [b] Lap of Love Veterinary Hospice, 17804 US-41, Lutz, FL 33549, USA
E-mail address: drsally@lapoflove.com

Vet Clin Small Anim 56 (2026) 521–533
https://doi.org/10.1016/j.cvsm.2025.09.031 vetsmall.theclinics.com

Appointments that are dedicated to the performance of humane euthanasia should be conducted with medicine in mind, but the central focus should be the preservation of the human–animal bond. Whether euthanasia is being considered for reasons of age-related changes, a life-limiting diagnosis, severe behavior concerns, or sudden trauma, there is always space and time to acknowledge the sacredness of the bond between the pet and their human on the hardest day.

DISCUSSION

It is common knowledge in the veterinary community that the word *euthanasia* comes from the Greek *euthanatos*, which means "easy death." Various definitions have been added which emphasize "dying well," or "a good death." But what does an "easy" or "good" death look like, and how do we translate that into actions to make those final moments calm, peaceful, and loving for both the pet and the human family members?

When "dying well" or "good death" is researched in human medicine and human hospice, there are several repeated themes that are considered of great importance to patients, caregivers of the dying, and medical professionals managing the health of the patient.[1,2] These include[1,2]

- Effective communication and relationships with medical providers
- Support of family, particularly family acceptance and preparation for death
- Feelings of life completion and having had lived well, including the ability to say goodbye and find closure at the end
- Relief of pain, a painless dying process, and dying in a familiar/comforting place

Obviously, due to the inability to verbally communicate with our animal companions, it is impossible to say with certainty whether our patients would concur with these end-of-life priorities and to examine that concept would likely lead to a variety of different conversations. However, the decision to euthanize a beloved pet is not made strictly based on the severity of the animal's physical health, nor is euthanasia solely the veterinarian's choice. Ultimately, the decision to euthanize comes down to the pet's prognosis, the primary caregiver's goals, and the support of the veterinarian; this can create a challenge for veterinarians who must consider the needs of the family unit as a whole when determining what "dying well" for pets may look like.

In a survey by Clooney and colleagues, pet owners reported positive experience associations when the following criteria were met before, during, and after a pet's euthanasia[3]:

- Being at home in a familiar environment to decrease the pet's anxiety
- The ability to prepare for the euthanasia appointment and having a preeuthanasia appointment in which the need for and procedure of euthanasia was explained
- Owners were able to present throughout the euthanasia allowing for constant physical closeness
- The pet was well sedated prior to euthanasia
- Allowance of time for privacy before and after euthanasia
- Respectful and thoughtful care for the pet's body following euthanasia

Between the human and veterinary medicine aspects of "dying well," we can clearly see common themes, including the need for clear communication from medical providers, support for both the patient and the caregivers, relief of pain and anxiety, and emotional and psychological closure for the family.

Today, pets are more so considered family members than ever before, and many owners report the loss of a pet to be equal to or harder than the loss of human family member.[4–6] People want the same level of attention, care, and prioritization for their pets as they do for their human family members, especially when both the people and the pets are at their most vulnerable.

Effective Communication in the Practice of Humane Euthanasia

Compassionate communication to ensure a good quality of death starts long before the day of the goodbye.[3] In cases of pets who have been diagnosed with severe, chronic, or congenital health concerns, communication and continuity of care are extremely important to caretakers.[3,6] Becoming educated on disease progression, how a pet's present and future quality of life may be affected by both treatment and disease progression, and what challenges home care can mean may be important to families considering euthanasia.[3,6] Veterinary professionals should not only provide information on disease, treatment, and prognosis, but they should also be prepared to acknowledge and respond to owners' concerns, questions, and needs for options.

Most pet owners do not have a medical background, and many may never have experienced caring for a pet with significant health concerns, so reducing medical jargon and providing written information and summaries can reduce client overwhelm.[6] This is especially applicable in situations where the pet's diagnosis is life-limiting, making hospice or euthanasia the only appropriate options.

Starting the Conversation

While it can be a delicate conversation to have, it is the responsibility of the veterinarian to initiate the conversation surrounding humane euthanasia when appropriate and applicable.[7,8] This serves 3 important purposes:

1. The veterinarian is taking the pressure off the client by providing professional, supportive guidance to consider euthanasia in the event of a poor diagnosis, congenital disease, advancing clinical signs, or chronic decline that is no longer controlled by medications or recommended therapies.[7]
2. The veterinarian can prevent unnecessary physical and mental suffering for the pet, avoid emergencies due to acute decline, and protect the human–animal bond from strain and stress related to worsening clinical signs.[7]
3. The family has the potential benefit of sharing intentional time with their pet. This means that they can complete a bucket list, gather family members who may live out of town if desired, and plan for a day of love and a pain-free passing for their pet.

The initial conversation can be pivotal in not only the next steps for the pet but also how the family handles their emotions, including guilt, anticipatory grief, and prolonged grief following euthanasia. Decision-making regarding the whys, hows, and whens of end of life should be made in an inclusive manner between the veterinarian and the pet owner, and always with the pet's welfare as the center focus. Owners who feel excluded from the veterinarian's euthanasia decision-making process are more likely to experience intense and prolonged grief due to feelings of distrust and loss of control.[9] These negative associations with veterinary care and humane euthanasia may in turn affect the health outcomes of other or future pets within the grieving family.

Communication During the Euthanasia Appointment

In the veterinary industry, the best thing that a clinician can do is acknowledge each pet as they would their own. There is no time that this gesture is more significant to an owner than the day of a pet's euthanasia. Using the pet's name, gender, and showing physical affection for that animal is paramount from the start. For a grieving family, hearing acknowledgment of how special, beautiful, and precious their best friend provides joy and helps them to share memories when it is sometimes needed most.

Necessary communications including consent forms, decisions regarding body care, and requests for keepsakes should all be addressed prior to drug administration. Care should be taken with each of these topics, and it should be acknowledged with the owner that taking care of these concerns first will allow complete focus to remain on their pet without interruptions through the rest of the appointment time.

Even if a family has been through a beloved pet's euthanasia before, it is important to walk through an explanation of the procedure with them. This can be particularly important if children are present; communicating with all family members may require slight variations in terminology or wording, so considering who is in the room can be helpful. In a quiet, calm tone, explain the process of euthanasia and reiterate support for this difficult decision.

Example of Euthanasia Explanation:

"I know this is a very hard day, but I can see that your sweet friend is tired in their body. This is a very fair, loving, and time-appropriate decision, as hard as it may be.

I am going to give (insert pet's name) two injections—the first is a combination of good pain control and anesthetics. This will just go under his/her skin. He/she is allowed to tell me if I am being rude, but most pets don't mind this injection too much. If you would like, we can offer him/her some really yummy treats as a happy distraction. I am giving this injection first to allow your sweet friend to become very comfortable—no pain, no nausea, no anxiety, just nice, comfortable sleep. I want him/her to feel like he/she is on a cloud. You can snuggle with him/her and talk to him/her as they fall asleep if you would like to, but it is also okay to take whatever space you need. When I can tickle his/her toes and put a potty pad under his/her bum without bothering them, I will place a small IV at the back leg. This will give me access to the bloodstream so that I can administer the last injection, which is an overdose of an anesthetic that works on the central nervous system. He/she will go so deeply to sleep that their body will forget to do its normal reflexes, and the heart and lungs will follow. This is a sleeping death—there is no pain or worry.

There are two very common things that we may see as our friend passes—these things can happen in natural death or when we are helping them on their way—the first one is that he/she may let go of their bladder. This is why I am going to put the potty pad under his/her bum—I want to protect his/her dignity just as you have been doing all their lives. The second thing that we commonly see is that our pets' eyes often remain open when they pass—this is because of the natural relaxation of the facial muscles, and it does not mean that they are awake or aware. If (insert pet's name here) shows any other changes as he/she finds her way over the Rainbow bridge, I am right here and will address them. I will do for him/her whatever I do for my own pets. It's okay to ask questions if you have any. Do you understand why I am supporting you on this decision?"

Before administering sedation, it may be helpful to reiterate your support for this important decision. It can also be important to communicate with the family regarding the speed at which the pet may become sedated—this will vary depending on medications and route of administration. Some families will want a moment or two to share with their pet while they are still conscious. In trying not to rush a family, it may be appropriate to acknowledge how hard it is to be "ready" for the first step of euthanasia with phrases like,

"I know that there is no such thing as 'ready,' but when you feel as prepared as possible, I will give (insert pet's name) his/her sedation so he/she can start feeling comfortable."

Or, "I understand it's hard to feel ready, but (insert pet's name) is ready. He/she has done such a good job taking care of you, and he/she is ready to rest."

Once sedation has taken effect, it may be appropriate to remark on how comfortable the pet looks sleeping. Beyond that, keep communication brief and only on an as-needed basis. Gently inform the family when you are administering the euthanasia solution, but keep this brief and in a calm, quiet tone. While it can be important to allow the family to have some say or expectation in how soon before the euthanasia solution is administered following sedation, ultimately, the decision of "when" is the veterinarian's responsibility. Medical knowledge gives the clinician the understanding that the pet's body may not remain stable under anesthesia, resulting in possible physical changes such as increased respiratory effort, involuntary vocalization, muscle spasm, stretching, etc. While painless, such changes can be perceived as suffering in the eyes of owners and should be avoided when possible. It is also unnecessary to make the responsibility of the "when" of the final injection the client's; this is the most pivotal time for their focus to be completely on their pet without interruption. In a 2024 survey of owners whose pets required CPR, an overwhelming 84% stated that they thought that the veterinarian should make the decision to stop resuscitation efforts.[10] This reflects trust that clients place in the medical professional to make decisions that are in the best interest of their pet, as well as the emotional toll that making such decisions can have on pet owners.[10]

When the euthanasia solution injection is completed, the veterinarian should auscultate the chest for heart sounds. Once death is confirmed, the family can be assured with phrases like:

"He has his angel wings on now."

"She is free now – her body is no holding her back anymore."

"He is at peace. He found his way easily."

Especially if children are present, it may be appropriate to preemptively ask the parents about the use of verbiage that includes religious undertones or suggestions, such as heaven or angels. Not all families want this kind of verbiage or imagery to be a part of their pet's passing—it is important to be sensitive to cultural and spiritual variations in how death may be perceived. If needed, be frank but kind with words like,

"She's passed now. Her heart and lungs have stopped working. It was a seamless transition."

From diagnosis to the final day, effective, compassionate communication can make a significant difference in how a family navigates the last mile of their pet's life.

Communication during the euthanasia appointment

1. Reaffirm the decision for a peaceful passing.
2. Explain the procedure and allow for questions.
3. Give verbal permission to family to leave or step away if needed.
4. Warn of possible muscle relaxation:
   a. Bladder relaxation
   b. Eyes may remain open.
5. Let the family know when you are administering the euthanasia solution.
6. Reassure family if respiratory or muscular changes are observed during the dying process.
7. Confirm pet's passing via auscultation and gently inform the family.

Support of the Family and Preparation for Death

Veterinarians are advocates for their patients first and foremost. Our medical knowledge guides our concerns for prognosis and possible ongoing or worsening struggling or suffering, but we are also advocating for our clients in how end-of-life occurs to help avoid emergencies, dissolution of the human–animal bond, and prolonged or complicated grief. Essentially, we are working from a big picture perspective. Clients and their families, however, are not.

Often, if a pet is still eating, drinking, going to the bathroom, etc., there can be significant doubt and disconnect between the physical nature of disease progression and the appropriate time to euthanize; this timeline may vary not only between the family members and the veterinarian, but between individual family members. This is why communication and education beyond disease diagnosis are so important.

Many families may need time to process the news of the pet's condition and digest the information in a safe setting, and this often means taking their pet home with palliative, hospice, or comfort care measures in place. By supporting the pet physically, the veterinarian can mentally and emotionally support the family members who are likely in a state of anticipatory grief.

Obviously, sending a terminally ill patient home is not always medically appropriate. Concerns including oxygen-dependency, uncontrolled pain, and severe dehydration create physical boundaries for in-home care for most animals. However, when it is possible to manage clinical signs with options like oral medications, long-acting injectables, environmental safety recommendations, and fluid boluses, the ability to send a patient home, even for a short time, can be highly beneficial to all involved. Giving a family and a pet time together at the end of a pet's life is sometimes the most important gift that our medical knowledge can provide.

When considering euthanasia, families need to

- Understand prognosis of disease and what clinical signs may develop in an estimated timeline.
- Be clear on treatment options and what side effects may occur.
- Have tools available for management of lifestyle changes at home.
- Be able to monitor quality of life so that the decision to euthanize feels not simply necessary, but as "right" as possible for all involved.
- Understand that they are supported in the decision to euthanize at any time.

Feelings of Life Completion and Having Had Lived Well

The human desire to reflect back on a life well lived is one of the conditions that many people find important, whether they are the patient or the caregiver.[1,2] While we are still understanding the ability of animals to share in this experience of feeling "accomplished in life," the overall benefit of reflection on the years shared for the pet's family members is undeniable.

Celebrations of a beloved pet's life can be crucial to the family's acceptance and preparation for their pet's euthanasia and may decrease long-term grief. If possible, time spent at home under hospice or comfort care offers families the opportunity for completing a bucket list, taking photographs, allowing for special treats and meals, and sharing stories of the pet's life. In many cases, this time can also provide feelings of acceptance and reconfirmation of the decision to provide a peaceful passing by allowing families time to acknowledge the victories of their pet's life.

On the other hand, a pet that rallies with the stimulation of family presence, favorite meals, and favorite toys may create doubt about how soon to euthanize—it can be important for veterinarians to preemptively communicate the importance of a good day at the end of a good life, and to explain that a rally is not the same as recovery from age-related decline or disease. This proactive approach to supportive communication can prevent back peddling on the timing of euthanasia.

Relief of Pain in a Comforting Environment

The need for a calm, comfortable, and stress-free transition is the very foundation of end-of-life care for humans and animals alike.[1–3,6–8] This concept should be applied to the entirety of the pet's euthanasia, which means that during the appointment, anxiety and pain should not only be abated but should be prevented wherever possible.

Creating a safe environment

It is important to consider the option to provide euthanasia services in the home when able. The theme of the desire to die at home or in a comforting environment is a core concern among human patients and their caregivers,[1,2] and many pet owners express the desire to meet that same criteria for their pets in the interest of keeping anxiety as low as possible.[3,7,8] While in-home euthanasia may be preferable, it is not always possible for a variety of reasons including the hospitalization of the pet due to instability, availability of mobile services, and cost concerns. Therefore, making efforts to establish a comfortable, safe environment for pets and families seeking euthanasia can make a significant difference in how the family experiences the final moments with their pet.[11]

Having a designated comfort room can add value to a clinic even if euthanasia rates are relatively low.[11] Ideally, comfort rooms are larger than average examination rooms, allowing for multiple family members (and possibly other pets) to be present.[11] Comfortable furniture such as small couches, oversized chairs, and floor cushions can allow family members to sit together in a more home-like setting.[11] Biophilic elements that promote comfort for all senses should be included in these rooms when available: soft, adjustable lighting, calming music or nature sounds, gentle aromas like diluted lavender, and clean, soft blankets and pet beds are all excellent options to consider.[11] In addition, comfort rooms should be fully equipped for management of comfort and hygiene needs for both humans and animals. Items like potty pads, wet wipes, Kleenex, small trash receptacles, bottled water, and hand sanitizer should be easily available to avoid multiple requests or interruptions.[11]

To ensure privacy and avoid distractions, comfort rooms should be away from high-traffic areas like bathrooms, staff break rooms, and reception.[11] Using window shades and door signs help to maintain privacy and alert staff to be respectful when the room is in use.[11] In addition, materials including clay, cookie-cutters, paper, ink, paint, and paintbrushes should all be readily available for keepsakes like clay or ink paw prints or nose prints. Containers for collection of the pet's hair are also items to consider.

Veterinarians should be prepared to bring in all necessary medications and medical supplies when they enter the room in a designated, low-profile medical kit, bag, or basket. While it may be appropriate to leave some medical supplies in the room, at no point should controlled substances, needles, or used syringes be left in a room that is unattended by a veterinary staff member, especially if there are children or other pets in the room.

Content of Medical Kits

Stethoscope

Injection supplies

Predrawn sedatives and euthanasia solution

Flush

Vet wrap

Bandage Scissors

Rubbing alcohol

Clipper blades

Spinal needles for use at alternative injection sites if necessary

All medical supplies should be kept out of sight of the pet and the family until necessary to avoid increasing anxiety.

Having high-value food options like Vienna sausages, chocolate, tuna, and baby food can be very much appreciated, as seeing a pet enjoy a well-deserved last treat can mean the world to many families, and the higher the value, the better the result often is.

It is important to note that while a designated comfort room is preferable, a traditional exam room can easily be utilized with some of the additions mentioned above added. Any measures taken to remove the sterile nature of the clinic setting can make a significant difference in the family's experience.

Avoid separation whenever possible

Understandably, when a family seeks euthanasia, whether due to an emergency or a chronic decline, both the pet and family may be in a sensitive state, and any separation of pet and owner will likely increase feelings of insecurity and fear. Remember, this is the last day that this family has to spend with the pet that they have shared a lifetime of love with; whenever possible, keeping the family together is vital to the human–animal bond and prevents escalating anxiety for both the humans and the pet. As much as possible, avoid separating the pet from their family. Some options to avoid separating the pet from their family include having all necessary paperwork prepared and completed in the comfort room, including taking payment, administering sedation subcutaneously, and using a butterfly needle instead of an indwelling IV.

The sedation process and euthanasia solution administration

Even in healthy animals, the stimuli of a veterinary clinic (other animals, various smells, new people, etc) can be overwhelming and trigger the instinctual, adaptive behaviors of fight, flight, or freeze.[12,13] In animals who are not feeling well, pain and anxiety may increase these responses and increase the risk of aggression or misdirection toward owners and clinic staff. Therefore, a noninvasive method of effective sedation is a hugely important part of the euthanasia appointment protocol. Depending on the pet's disease process, behavioral changes (anxiety level), and pain level, recommending a premedication protocol that the owner can administer before driving to the clinic may be helpful for the entire family. To achieve the best effects of any anxiolytic or anesthetics, medications should be administered when the pet is in a calm state, and not aroused or overly stimulated.[12,13]

Sedation prior to the final injection of euthanasia is meant to provide the initial relief from pain, nausea, anxiety, and exhaustion to the pet. Still, it can also be a source of relief for the owner.[3,8] Opioids, dissociates, and benzodiazepines should be considered for use in combination to provide effective sedation and analgesia while decreasing the risk of excitatory stages of anesthesia. Depending on what options are available, various combinations of anesthetics and analgesics like ketamine, telazol, dexmedetomidine, butorphanol, midazolam, xylazine, and acepromazine should be considered, keeping in mind the pet's age, species, breed, and health concern. Tailoring sedation choices to each patient can make all the difference in the effects. According to the AVMA 2020 Guidelines on Euthanasia, providing sedation prior to euthanasia in companion animals allows for the benefits of comfort for the pet and owner, increased safety for staff by reducing the need for restraint, and an overall decrease in stress during the appointment.[14] It is also important to note that the AVMA euthanasia guidelines require that unconscious sedation be achieved prior to injection of euthanasia solution in mammals and birds when using alternative routes (intrahepatic, intrarenal, intracardiac, etc.) to prevent unnecessary pain and discomfort to the animal.[14]

Just as important to sedation success as the chosen anesthetics and analgesics is the route of administration. While gaining intravascular access early in the euthanasia appointment may be clinic protocol, the necessity of an indwelling IV should be considered on a case-by-case basis. The removal of the pet from the family, patient pain during IV placement, and technical challenges due to possible low blood pressure or dehydration are anxiety-inducing aspects of euthanasia appointments which can in turn effect the client's perception of the "dying well" experience. Generally, any aspect of the euthanasia that is interpreted as negative or anxiety-inducing for the owners can not only affect the experience of that appointment but may also induce feelings of guilt, resulting in prolonged grief.[8]

In a survey conducted by Kogan and colleagues in 2023, clients responded to how specific aspects of the euthanasia appointment may contribute to a negative effect on the overall experience with the following reported to have had "large" to "extreme" negative impacts[8]:

"Client hearing their pet, in what sounds like distress, if out of sight"[8]

"The pet appearing to be in distress when it is returned to the room"[8]

"Client not allowed to be with their pet during the entire procedure"[8]

As an alternative to early IV placement for drug administration, sedatives mentioned above can be given intramuscular or subcutaneously for efficient and effective results. Typically, combining sedatives into one syringe, using the smallest needle possible, and providing a positive distraction of high-value food or owner attention can allow for injection with minimal restraint and reaction. With this sedation process, the pet will typically become relaxed and pain-free over approximately 3 to 10 minutes; these calming effects often provide a significant relief to pet owners who may have been monitoring their pet's clinical signs for days or weeks. Achieving a peaceful and deep sedation allows for a painless experience for the pet, a peaceful "last look" for the owners, and an opportunity for IV placement without resistance or restraint. With the family focused on their comfortable pet, the veterinarian can gain IV access with an IV or butterfly needle at various venous sites. While the cephalic vein is typically most used for drug administration, attempting to obtain IV access at the lateral saphenous vein may allow for an equally advantageous option for the veterinarian and allow more space for the family to gather at the pet's head. It is worth reacknowledging that a family's ability to be with their pet throughout the euthanasia appointment, to maintain physical contact with their pet, and to know that their pet's death is painless are among the aspects of euthanasia that matter most to owners.

Tips for Smooth Intramuscular (IM) or Subcutaneous (SQ) Sedation

1. Combine selected sedatives into one syringe.
2. Use a new needle that is the smallest gauge possible for injection.
3. Gently pinch or massage the skin of the scruff.
4. Consider application of lidocaine gel at the injection site.
5. Provide high-value food treat or a distracting physical touch.
6. Push syringe contents slowly to avoid a sudden/severe response to drug administration.

In the moments after

Once a peaceful passing has been confirmed for the pet, certain steps need to be taken to continue to ensure the owner's comfort in their time of active grieving. Most families wish to have some time with their pet's body in private. This can be important for the grieving process and should be respected as part of the "dying well" experience.[8] Before exiting the room, veterinary staff members should.

1. Ensure that the pet's body is in a natural position (close eyes if possible, place the tongue into the mouth if needed)
2. Make sure that the pet is clean and remove any soiled potty pads or blankets. Use wet wipes to clean the body as needed, and place clean pads under the pet.
3. Gently warn of possible muscle twitching, which may occur even several minutes following death.
4. Provide a method of communicating any needs that arise with the clinic staff—remote doorbells are an easy way for clients to alert staff to their needs.
5. Communicate next steps so that the family knows what to expect when they feel ready to move forward:

"Take any time you need or want to be present with (insert pet's name) and your family. When you are ready, myself or (provide the name of a specific staff member) will come back into the room, and we will make some keepsakes if you would like."

It can be reassuring for the family if the veterinarian gently touches the pet on their way out of the room, as it communicates love for that animal, just as was expressed when the pet was living.

After a family has had the time that they need with the pet's body, it may be preferable to make keepsakes (clay or ink paws or nose prints, hair clippings, etc) to send home the same day. Creating keepsakes in the moment can often be bittersweet and bring some joy where it is much needed. Additionally, be sure to remove and collect any collars, leashes, or halters that the family may wish to keep. Providing a velvet pouch in which items like ink prints, hair clippings, and collars can be placed is an added touch to help provide some sense of privacy and respect as the family exits the clinic.

Meeting expectations for body care

Respectful care of the pet's body is significant to pet owners, though it often may be considered an after-thought.[3,8,15] Gentle handling of the body, ensuring that personal items like toys or blankets remain with the body, and the length of time between death and final resting state (burial, cremation) have all been identified as common owner concerns and sources of anxiety following their pet's passing.[15] Information provided to families regarding their pet's aftercare, whether cremation, aquamation, or burial at a pet cemetery should be up-to-date and accurate, especially about contact information and expectations for returns of cremains to ensure confidence and reduce worry.

A family's last view of their pet is one that will stay with them in memory and will likely play a substantial role in the processing of grief. Under no circumstances should a pet's body be placed into a body bag with the owner present. Additionally, the pet's body should never be alone in the exam or comfort room; seeing a caring team member remain present with their pet's body as a family departs can allow them to feel more secure and at ease about the standard of aftercare.

End with support and reassurance

Just as the appointment began, the euthanasia appointment should end with the veterinarian's reinforcement of support and assurance of the exceedingly difficult decision that was made together. Acknowledgments of the family's care for their pet through its life, especially on the day that mattered most, can help mitigate negative emotions, abate grief without dismissing it, and help ensure a better long-term memory of the euthanasia experience.

In a 2025 study by Silva and colleagues, surveys found that owners of euthanized pets experienced lower levels of guilt, but more grief when compared to owners whose pets died without the assistance of euthanasia.[8] In contrast, owners of non-euthanized pets reported feeling more intense levels of guilt but with less grief.[8] These findings suggest that owners who felt actively engaged in decision-making and had perceived support from their veterinarian team were able to move forward with euthanasia before advanced suffering of the pet occurred.[8] Feelings of less guilt may be related to the decision to euthanize being made in the interest of the pet; however, the increased or prolonged grief may have been the result of the experience of anticipatory grief leading up to euthanasia.

Conversely, owners whose pets died naturally are suspected to have carried a higher emotional burden due to a lack of adequate veterinary support regarding the decision surrounding euthanasia; without support, prolonged suffering for the pet may have been observed leaving the owner with difficult memories of their pet's final days.[8] These findings highlight the need for veterinarians to provide compassionate and informed support through each step of the end-of-life process.

Having resources for pet loss grief counseling and recommended reading materials readily available for clients regardless of how their pet passed can leave an impression of care and concern.

SUMMARY

The multifaceted nature of how both humans and animals "die well" relies heavily on the guidance and communication skills of the medical professionals involved in the patient's care. While providing support to patients and their caregivers during such a vulnerable time is a vital aspect of both human and veterinary medicine, the added responsibility of providing humane euthanasia falls uniquely to veterinarians.

Animal euthanasia has been a necessary and important aspect of veterinary medicine for centuries, and the human influence on its evolution to today's standards is undeniable.[16] Now more than ever, the pet-owning population has a need for the standard of their pet's death to be like that of a human family member's death, particularly when it comes to support from their veterinary providers, prevention of their pet's pain and anxiety, the gentleness of that animal's passing, and respectful body care. Making efforts to meet and even to exceed these standards can prevent unnecessary animal suffering, ensure client satisfaction, and, most importantly, preserve the human–animal bond when it may be at its most fragile.

CLINICS CARE POINTS

- When appropriate, discussions regarding euthanasia should be initiated by the veterinarian to prevent unnecessary or prolonged suffering for the pet.
- Providing client education on the diagnosis and disease progression is important to helping families understand how their pet's present and future quality of life will be affected by health concerns.
- Establishing an environment of comfort, safety, and privacy is vital to the euthanasia experience in the clinic setting—while a comfort room is ideal, converting an examination room with warm lighting, soft blankets, and a sound machine can help reduce anxiety in both the pets and their owners.
- During the euthanasia appointment, pets should remain with their owners. Separation has been linked to increased negative feelings in owners, especially if they suspect the pet has been in distress during the separation.
- Use of IM or SQ sedation to allow the pet to become pain-free and comfortable without the need for an indwelling IV catheter can be a significant source of relief for owners; sedation also allows for ease of IV administration without restraint or discomfort for the pet.
- Veterinarians and veterinary care providers should be prepared to explain the euthanasia procedure, answer questions from owners, ensure gentle body care, and provide resources for pet loss support as needed.

DISCLOSURES

The author has nothing to disclose.

REFERENCES

1. Zaman M, Espinal-Arango S, Mohapatra A, et al. What would it take to die well? A systematic review of systematic reviews on the conditions for a good death. Lancet Healthy Longev 2021;2(9):e593–600.
2. Meier EA, Gallegos JV, Thomas LP, et al. Defining a good death (successful dying): literature review and a call for research and public dialogue. Am J Geriatr Psychiatr 2016;24(4):261–71.
3. Cooney K, Kogan L. How pet owners define a "good death". wwwdvm360com 2022;53:12. Available at: https://www.dvm360.com/view/how-pet-owners-define-a-good-death-.
4. The graduate review the graduate review a deep dive into pet bereavement: implications for mental health professionals. Available at: https://vc.bridgew.edu/cgi/viewcontent.cgi?article=1316&context=grad_rev.
5. Crossley M, Rolland C. Overcoming the social stigma of losing a pet: considerations for counseling professionals. Human-Animal Interactions 2022;2022:1–9. Available at: https://www.cabidigitallibrary.org/doi/epdf/10.1079/hai.2022.0022.
6. Hoummady S, Chaise L, Guillot M, et al. All pet owners are not the same: end-of-Life caregiver expectations and profiles. Top Companion Anim Med 2025;65: 100960. https://doi.org/10.1016/j.tcam.2025.100960.

7. Cooney K, Kipperman B. Ethical and practical considerations associated with companion animal euthanasia. Animals (Basel) 2023;13(3):430.
8. Kogan LR, Cooney KA. Defining a "Good Death": exploring Veterinarians' Pprceptions of Ccmpanion Aaimal Eethanasia. Animals (Basel) 2023;13(13):2117.
9. Silva MV, Santos RR, Barbosa M. Euthanasia and prolonged grief: a cross-sectional study with bereaved pet owners. J Vet Behav 2025;79:60–7.
10. Bertram L, Kuo K, Hofmeister E, et al. Small animal veterinary clients prefer veterinarians to decide when to terminate resuscitation and to be informed after cardiopulmonary resuscitation efforts. J Am Vet Med Assoc 2024;262(4):535–42.
11. Euthanasia comfort rooms. CAETA. 2021. Available at: https://caetainternational.com/euthanasia-comfort-rooms/.
12. Herron ME, Shreyer T. The pet-friendly veterinary practice: a guide for practitioners. Vet Clin North Am Small Anim Pract 2014;44(3):451–81.
13. Riemer S, Heritier C, Windschnurer I, et al. A review on mitigating fear and aggression in dogs and cats in a veterinary setting. Animals (Basel) 2021;11(1):158.
14. Leary S, Johnson C, AVMA Guidelines for the Euthanasia of Animals: 2020 Edition. 2020. Available at: https://www.avma.org/sites/default/files/2020-02/Guidelines-on-Euthanasia-2020.pdf (Accessed 2 August 2025).
15. Cooney KA, Kogan LR, Brooks SL, et al. Pet owners' expectations for pet end-of-life support and after-death body care: exploration and practical applications. Top Companion Anim Med 2021;43:100503. https://doi.org/10.1016/j.tcam.2020.10050317.
16. Cooney K. Historical perspective of euthanasia in veterinary medicine. Vet Clin North Am Small Anim Pract 2020;50(3):489–502.

Post-euthanasia

How to Provide Continued Support

Rebecca K. Frank, DVM, CVHEP, CT (Certified in Thanatology: Death, Dying, Loss, and Bereavement)

KEYWORDS

• Bereavement • Grief • Post-euthanasia • Attachement theory
• Continuing bonds theory

KEY POINTS

- Understanding different types of grief, including anticipatory and disenfranchised grief, helps veterinarians support pet owners effectively.
- Various grief theories, such as attachment, continuing bonds, and the dual process model, provide frameworks to comprehend individual grief responses.
- Veterinarians can assist grief journeys by ensuring seamless euthanasia procedures, offering reassurance, and facilitating memorialization options.
- Follow-up through cards, calls, and resources strengthens trust and helps clients process their loss.
- Providing clients with additional support resources and training staff in compassionate communication enhances grief support without acting as counselors.

GRIEF, BEREAVEMENT, AND PET LOSS

Often people know the feeling of a word but are unable to define it. Most veterinarians can imagine what it feels like to be grieved. Many of us see it weekly, if not daily, in our clients in whom we may have to give a grave diagnosis, or help a beloved family member say goodbye. But what exactly are grief and bereavement? Grief is an emotional response to the loss of something that includes physiologic, behavioral, cognitive, and spiritual dimensions. Grief is not necessarily limited to feelings at the loss of another living creature. It can also be employed at the loss of a job, the loss of beloved item or heirloom, and even the loss of an opportunity. Bereavement refers to the state of that loss. Thus, when you lose something, you are bereaved, and your response to that loss is your grief. Additionally, the active adjustment to that loss is grieving, or grief work.[1]

Pet owners fit these definitions, along with a few variations of grief as well. For example, prior to bereavement, a pet owner may go through a period of anticipatory grief. In other words, they begin to react to a loss that has not occurred yet, due to a

Lap of Love, PO Box 4063, Reading, PA 19606, USA
E-mail address: drbecky@lapoflove.com

Vet Clin Small Anim 56 (2026) 535–543
https://doi.org/10.1016/j.cvsm.2025.10.003 vetsmall.theclinics.com

poor prognosis, or even the existential realization that they will outlive their pet. Or perhaps they are already experiencing some pre-losses, like their pet no longer enjoying being held, or no longer able to play like they used to. The bond with their pet is already changing, which forces change and adjustment.

Another type of grief pet owners often deal with is disenfranchised grief. Disenfranchised grief occurs when their grief is not supported, or cannot be acknowledged.[2] Pet owners may have friends, family, or social contacts that do not recognize the bond with their pet, thereby not acknowledging the loss. Their social supports may also see their grief as non-normative in these ways.[3] As veterinarians, we often see this in the unhelpful friend or partner who does not want the pet owner to grieve so hard or so openly, as it makes them uncomfortable to see the loss of a bond they frankly do not understand. We could have a bingo card filled with unhelpful phrases like "Don't cry-we can get another cat," or "Well at least he had a good long life," or even "Why are you like this? It was just a dog."

Sometimes even veterinarians do not know what to do in the face of grief. A client may be crying loudly, screaming, or even completely unemotional and uncommunicative. We sometimes wonder what must be going through a client's mind and are unsure how to help. Reassurance? A hug? As veterinarians, we want to fix, but sometimes we cannot. In the next section, we will, however, explore current grief theories to help understand what a client may be experiencing.

PAST AND CURRENT GRIEF STYLES AND THEORIES

Entire textbooks are written on grief theories, and we will not be rewriting them here. However, giving veterinarians tools and a brief overlay may help us in the times where we may not understand someone else's grief. First, we must dispel some myths. For example, in western culture, Kubler-Ross's paper on the stages of grief is pervasive in pop culture. While it has its place as a foundational grief theory, the paper itself was actually looking at 400 terminally ill human patients and how they responded to the fact that they were dying. In pop culture, it has been inappropriately applied to generalized bereavement. Not everyone goes through "Denial, Anger, Bargaining, Depression, and Acceptance."[1] In fact, it was never Kubler-Ross's intent that her publication be applied to people grieving. While dying people may have things to impart on the still living, it was not meant to be a model for how to grieve.[4]

Other foundational grief theories that are a bit closer to the mark are Attachment Theory and Tasks of Mourning. Started in the 1960s and still an important and developing research position, attachment theory originally looked at how infants reacted to the absence of their caregiver, and how these reactions may reflect grief later on in life.[5] An infant who is consistently and reliably taken care of is much more flexible and responsive when they are uncomfortable. A person with a secure attachment to their pet may have less complicated grief than a person who is anxiously attached. When care is less reliable, anxious attachment shows up as clinging or an inability to let go of a relationship. On the other hand, an avoidantly attached individual will not show outward signs of distress at discomfort. Finally, a disorganized attachment style develops as erratic behavior and is thought to be a reflection of a difficult or even abusive environment.[6]

Attachment theory has even gone so far as to be researched in conjunction with pet loss. In a 2016 study, Eckert and colleagues described various attachment styles in accordance with Attachment theory as they explored the intensity of grief following the death of a pet. In the discussion, they found that grief was not tied to a species, and that the loss of a pet was quite comparable to the loss of a human. Furthermore, the closeness of an individual with whom they lost seemed the best predictor of the intensity of their grief.[7] While attachment still may play a role in grief, it has also been incorporated into the contemporary Dual Process Model.[1]

Tasks of Mourning, a foundational theory put forth in 1982 by J. William Worden presents 4 tasks that may be different for each mourner, but each mourner works through in their bereavement. Task 1 is to accept the loss. Task 2 is processing the pain of that loss. Task 3 is to adjust to a world without what they lost. Task 4 is to remember the loss while still engaging in the world.[8] Unlike one of the first theories of grief, proposed by Freud, which insisted that those who continued to remember a lost loved one were morbid or unhealthy, Tasks of Mourning proposes that remembering can be healthy. As this theory has continued to be reworked, there have been influences to how people handle these tasks of mourning, which include the attachment style, type of relationship, the circumstances of the death, cultural and personal factors, as well as an individual's personality. This theory has also been instrumental in forming contemporary grief theories.

Continuing Bonds: This contemporary grief theory proposes that a grief journey is not about forgetting and moving on, like Freud and much of the western world thinks is supposed to happen, but that the bond with a deceased loved one is still intentionally ongoing, even dynamic, and can change over time.[9] In some cultures, this is more supported. For example, the Qingming Festival in China, or Dia de los Muertos in Mexico are good examples of this continuing bond being supported in a social context. While some western cultures may see this as unhealthy, we need to keep in mind that the continued bond may have both positive and negative effects on the bereaved. Where we may see this most often is online, where one's social community helps maintain that bond through memorials and supporting one another.[1] Application of this in the veterinary world would perhaps look like having a memorial page for clients to share and support one another.

Dual Process Model: This contemporary grief theory focuses on fluctuations over time as an individual is in a bereaved state, and works toward re-entering the world. The 2 states in this theory are "loss-orientation" and "restoration-orientation." In the former, the bereaved individual's focus is on the loss, doing grief work, and processing the emotions and consequences of the loss. In restoration-orientation, the individual is focused on dealing with the changes in their life that comes with the loss, like changed responsibilities, having to take time off work, and feelings of isolation due to their bereaved state. In this model, the individual will oscillate between these states, and both states are necessary for them to find a new normal.[10] Unlike the later Two Track Model, which has two paths walking in tandem, this model dictates you may jump between loss and restoration. It is best to think of this as feeling the loss, and doing grief work in the loss-orientation, and then in restoration orientation, dealing with the consequences of being in that loss-orientation for a period of time. Individuals may be more prone to one state or the other, and in a family one's state may affect other family members. We can see this in the room where one partner may be preoccupied with the loss itself, and the emotions it elicits, while the other partner may be stressed about how they are going to drive home in this state. Another example would be taking a few days off for bereavement to deal with a loss, and then coming back to work and having to interact and deal with people and tasks you missed while you were dealing with your loss.

Meaning Reconstruction: Developed in conjunction with several researchers, this contemporary grief theory is developed around the idea that humans do not just experience loss, but they attach meaning to the loss to help them understand it. This theory is most helpful in the face of traumatic loss: the hit by car dog, the cat that got into lilies, and so forth.[1] With time, a bereaved individual engages in sense-making (creating a narrative about life), benefit finding (seeking positive gains in the loss), and identity change (individual now sees themselves in a different way). While the meaning reconstruction may be limited to what society sees as legitimate, it has opened the way for new therapies, such as narrative therapy.[1] A good example of this would be a person who tragically lost their pet, and uses the empathy and care they learn from the experience to start a Pet Loss Support Group at a local church. In starting the group, they may reframe their loss, which was once a net negative, into something more of a net positive as they grow and see how they help others.

Two-track Model of Bereavement: Like the Dual Process Model, this contemporary grief theory sees death as being a "double process event."[1] What that means is that grief moves along these 2 tracks in tandem, and an individual can work on both tracks together, unlike the Dual Process Model, which oscillates. Track 1 deals with the biopsychosocial functioning after loss. That is, it focuses on the individual's adaptation of their emotional, cognitive, interpersonal, and biological states to a loss. Track 2 is similar to the Continuing Bonds theory, in that it focuses on how the relationship with the deceased is changed over time, as well as how the individual views themselves after the loss. One track is not more important than the other, and they move together.[1,11] To help visualize this, think of the client who is very upset by the loss of their cat, processing how they hospiced him with cancer. To help her explore her feelings about this, she puts together a shadow box of his pictures and pawprint so it can help her feel like he is close, and bring back some of the good memories she has of him, instead of just him dying of cancer. This helps her maintain that bond with her cat, while simultaneously helping to process her strong feelings over his loss.

Adaptive Grief Styles: This contemporary grief theory came about in looking at gender differences in grief, social acceptance of them, and how there is no set style of grief in relation to gender. As the theory developed, there was movement away from categorizing styles as masculine or feminine, and replacing them with the terms "instrumental" and "intuitive." Instrumental grievers are less likely to display outward emotion, and the painful emotions they experience are more of an intellectual experience. They may tend toward discussing problems rather than feelings. These are the individuals who want to know what they can expect in a euthanasia, and if they can wrap their pet in their favorite blanket for burial. Intuitive grievers experience grief as very profound and painful feelings. They are more likely to display and discuss their feelings. These individuals may express how difficult the decision to euthanize was, or discuss how they are feeling in that moment, and how they feel about those feelings (eg, the woman who says she feels bad about being relieved after the euthanasia). In addition, you may see blended grievers, which incorporate both functional styles. Because of societal pressures, you may see individuals fighting their natural style.[12] For example, think of the man who is trying hard not to cry, or the woman asking if she is strange or judged for not openly weeping. This is considered to be "dissonant." These individuals feel pressured to grieve a certain way due to current cultural norms surrounding grief where they live.

HOW TO ASSIST THE GRIEF JOURNEY AS A VET

By now, you probably recognize how the different grief theories fit into what you have seen in practice. But how do we as veterinarians set a family up to have an uncomplicated grief journey, when we are not counselors?

Set Yourself Up for Success

Most veterinarians can remember someone telling us that the most important appointments we have with a family are the first and the last. As touched on in the euthanasia article, getting the details right for a seamless transition is key. Here are a few details you will want to have on hand.

a. Choose and inspect an aftercare specialist you trust. In a 2021 survey, pet owners were found to rely heavily on the guidance of veterinary teams when it came to deciding and having questions about how they would like their pet's body cared for postmortem.[13] Go to the actual crematory, meet the owners/staff, and be prepared to share that information if the family leaves their pet with you for cremation. Be ready to give them a timeline, and how a crematory will keep track of their pet and not mix it up with any others. Vetting a crematory is imperative to maintaining the trust between veterinarians and families. If you are unsure where to start, visit the Web site for the International Association of Pet Cemeteries and Crematories. Accreditation through this association helps maintain high standards in caring for the pets we entrust to our aftercare specialists.[14] In researching, you will quickly find not all crematories and aftercare are the same. A few things to look for to set yourself up for success include:
   1. Tracking for private cremation. This can look like a metal tag, or some other chip system that will prevent any pet from being mixed up with another.
   2. Multiple labels for each pet. That is, there may be software, as well as physical paper or tags that can and should be cross-checked in order to make sure a pet is cared for in accordance with the wishes of the owner.
   3. Excellent documentation. A good crematory should have the ability to produce and keep track of financial records and licenses in accordance with its operation. To not be able to produce these is a red flag.
   4. Several options for families to choose from: While you may opt for a standard urn for a standard price, a good aftercare specialist knows that the bond between pets and their families is individual, and having different aftercare options is a reflection of that. Communal cremations with a memorial site, different urns or urn options (like jewelry), or even viewed cremation are excellent options for an aftercare specialist to offer.
   5. Superior communication. While we may not expect an aftercare specialist to be available 24/7, we do expect them to be responsive and prompt in a reasonable period. We also want them to be kind and understanding with pet owners who may call in to check on the progress of their pet. Being lost in the unknown can make grief worse for families, thus steadfast and prompt communication with families and vets is key.
   6. Upright core values. An aftercare specialist should exemplify the care and quality of their work in every step, from courteous communication when a pet is transferred to their care, to the final return to a vet or the family. The last thing someone grieving wants to feel or suspect is that the aftercare specialist does not care about them or their pet.

b. Having a list of local alternative options for families for body care is also helpful if the family perhaps wishes to have a burial or even taxidermy for their pet. Having just a little bit of knowledge on these alternatives and being able to explain them to families who have questions can deepen the trust they have with you. For example, for a family that wishes to taxidermy, encourage them to make sure their taxidermist is aware of the euthanasia solution, or even how to handle the pet after. In some processes, too much petting can cause a pet's hair to fall out over time.

c. For burials, having information on local ordinances, or even a sheet on burial tips with the Web site for them to check is helpful. Some states have a timeline in which a pet must be buried, and some towns ban any pet being buried.
d. Have a price list for reception to go over, so it is not a surprise when the family arrives with their beloved pet. Make sure reception is ready with that paperwork so the family does not have to deal with it when they are sobbing. Double check, and draw attention to the most important parts of the paperwork: Aftercare option is properly selected, pet's name is spelled correctly, financial information is correct.
e. Have a room ready for the family to go into. This may not always be practical in the case of an emergency, but privacy in these tender moments is valued by most families.
f. Have resources available to your front staff for when you may not be available, including emergencies and in-home euthanasia as alternative options.
g. A good trend now in many US practices is having a candle or light to let people in the waiting area know to keep their voices down, as a family is saying goodbye.
h. Train yourself and front staff on how to compassionately handle grieving families. There are many resources out there for this sort of training!

Be Ready with Reassurance

a. As veterinarians, this is where we can really shine. Our medical knowledge gives us insight into a pet's condition, and bridges the family's understanding with what the pet is experiencing. By translating this prognosis into understandable terms, the family can feel more affirmed with their decisions.
b. If open to it, a hand on the shoulder or the upper arm can provide grounding when a family member is falling apart. If you are unsure, it is always ok to ask if a grieving person would like a hug. Asking permission does not lessen the sentiment and compassion.
c. Reassurance is especially impactful in complicated euthanasias like behavioral euthanasia or juvenile euthanasia. Disenfranchisement is much more common in these situations, so understanding and affirmation of the decision from a veterinary professional vastly helps with the narrative in a grieving family member's mind. This gives them a foundation to build their grief journey on. Remember that you may be the only person in their life who holds space for them to grieve a commonly disenfranchised loss.
d. Use your best verbiage that is authentic and supportive. This might take some trial and error to what feels comfortable to you. Here are some common supporting phrases that help a grieving owner feel understood:
   i. "14 years is amazing, but it's never long enough, is it?"
   ii. "It's ok to cry; tears just mean that you care."
   iii. "You're allowed to cry and feel sad; I can tell you loved him so very much, and this is going to hurt for a while."
   iv. "You've done an amazing job getting him this far. It's ok to be free of his pain now."
   v. "Together we are helping her not to hurt anymore. You're not alone."
   vi. "There is nothing wrong with grieving. Grief is simply all the love we want to give them, with nowhere to put it anymore."
e. Above all, keep in mind that no matter what you say, you will not cure their grief. Be kind to yourself, this is not a problem to "fix." You can only support them as much as they let you.

Memorialization

a. As mentioned in several of the theories, maintaining a bond with the deceased is part of the grief journey for many people. Offering a pawprint, ink nose-print, lock of fur, or even a picture frame can be useful for your clinic. Build the cost into the base price so families do not feel nickel and dimed. Many crematories do this as well as an alternative, but when a family leaves you with their pet, having something for them to carry out that belongs to their pet cannot be understated. They are already leaving without their pet, and they will be all too aware of empty hands on the way to their car. This need not be limited to private cremations either; a communal cremation or burial deserve keepsakes as well. Do not be afraid to try different products until you find one that works for you and your staff. Practice making pawprints, nose-prints, and so forth, because these are the last pieces of a pet a family may have, and may play an integral part of the continuing bond with their loved one.

b. If a family is looking for something unique or different, having a list to give them of some unique Web sites or local alternatives is great to have on hand. Many things can be done with ashes, from jewelry to suncatchers. Places selling memorial plaques and stones are useful for those doing home burials. Stuffed animal replicas are great for children or anyone who misses seeing their loved one. Having a paper to hand families if they ask can be useful.
c. Reserve judgment; some things like taxidermy, keeping teeth, or even cryogenically freezing tissue for cloning may seem strange for us, but for a grieving family it may be how they wish to lovingly remember their pet. As mentioned prior, knowing a little bit about these processes can even help guide a family in deciding what is the best way to remember their pet. Keep in mind that what may seem strange to us may be perfect for that individual, or even normal in that individual's culture. For example, at various times in history, death masks were made of the deceased. This practice would seem quite strange in many places now, but certain cultures and individuals may still access the continuing bond with their loved one by having a death mask made.[15] Unless it is something which may harm an individual, it is best to be curious and understanding of the many ways in which continuing bonds may occur with memorialization.
d. Children can often be left out of the process, so a small stuffed animal or memorial coloring book is often very appreciated by families who are saying goodbye, and help them feel included. Sometimes families will look to the veterinary team for guidance as to whether or not children should be present, or if they should even bring up memorialization with a child. It is often best to refer to the temperament of the child, if they want to be there, and for the very young, will they distract from a grieving guardian. There are many books and resources as to how to discuss death with children, but a general rule of thumb is that ages 6 and up may wish to attend, and exposing them to death or death practices in a supportive and understanding environment does no lasting harm.
e. Online memorials are quite popular from social media to funeral homes. Giving the family the information to set up a memorial online, even if it is just a link to the crematory memorial page may be quite appreciated. It is best to ask permission, but online obituaries and tributes on a clinic's page can help a family feel supported and remembered.

Follow-up

a. Veterinarians care about patients, and one of the best ways to follow-up is a handwritten card. Some of the best have little messages from the staff that are heartfelt. In fact, from many clients, a card is the minimum of what is expected.
b. An email may also be appreciated, especially if it has a link to a memorial option either on your Web site or your aftercare specialist's. A good rule of thumb is to

send the email the following day, when a grieving individual is starting their life without their pet.

c. Some families may request a phone call, and while this is probably not doable for every client, those special ones may be worth the effort. It does not have to be long-just a few minutes to check in, express condolences and see if you can answer any questions they may have.
d. Do not be surprised if the family does not come to pick up ashes right away. It may be very painful for them to come back to the place they said goodbye, and handling this in an empathetic manner is always in the best interest of both the family and your staff.

Additional resources for clients

While the majority of euthanasia experiences result in uncomplicated grief, there may be exceptions, and some pet owners may need additional help in their grief journeys. Most veterinarians are not trained in social work. We are not trained in counseling services, and to extend without proper training may do more damage than good. However, we are human, and we can at least give a pet owner the resources they may need to help them in their grief. If a client reaches out because they are struggling you can provide a list of people and places that may help them.

When compiling your list you will want to pay attention to a few key things to make sure that it is helpful.

1. While it may be impractical to call and vet every counseling agency in your area, you can often check if counselors have a specialty on their Web sites. Stick with those who specialize in grief, or have extensive grief training. Being mismatched with a counselor who has very little grief training can do more harm than good.
2. Check with local vet collages. Some have pet loss support groups.
3. Check with local In Home Euthanasia practitioners. Some may be running groups, or know of additional resources.
4. Sometimes churches or a local pet shelter may also offer in person pet loss support groups.
5. Your aftercare specialist may also host or know of local pet loss support groups.
6. National end of life veterinary companies may also have their own groups and pet loss support you can utilize. Lap of Love, for example, offers pet loss support groups, as well as individual sessions to help those who have lost pets.
7. Have a plan for the clients who may not be safe to drive home after an appointment. For those that threaten self-harm, question, persuade and refer (QPR) training among the staff can be very beneficial when facing these crises that veterinary school did not teach us to manage.

As veterinarians, we cannot expect to make every client feel better after euthanasia. That is not how grief works. We can, however, do a lot to set a pet owner up to begin that grief journey on the right foot, and cement the trust they have in us. We can be supportive through our roles as facilitators and animal advocates. These small touches and interactions uplift us, as well as the entire veterinary community as a whole, letting pet owners know that we care.

CLINICS CARE POINTS

- Be aware that everyone grieves differently. It is important to stay non-judgemental of grief responses.

- There is nothing you will say to make grief all better, but you can still support a client in a bereaved state to make their grief journey smoother.
- Be aware of community support so that you can refer a client for qualified help should they seek it.
- Finding your own style and words takes time, but as long as you are sincere, most clients will respond favorably.

DISCLOSURE

The author of the article has nothing to disclose.

REFERENCES

1. Servaty-Seib HL, Chapple HS. Handbook of Thanatology: the essential body of knowledge for the study of death, dying, and bereavement. 3rd Edition. New York (NY): Association for Death Education and Counseling; 2021.
2. Corr CA, Corr DM, Doka KJ. Death and dying, life and living. 8th Edition. Boston (MA): Cengage; 2018.
3. Doka KJ. Disenfranchised grief: new directions, challenges, and strategies for practice. Champaigne (IL): Research Press; 2002.
4. Stroebe M, Schut H, Boerner K. Cautioning health-care professionals: bereaved persons are misguided through stages of grief. Omega J Death Dying 2017;74(4): 455–73.
5. Ainsworth MDS, Blehar MC, Waters E, et al. Patterns of attachment: a psychological study of a strange situation. Mahwah (NJ): Erlbaum Associates; 1978.
6. Main M, Solomon J. Discovery of a new, insecure disorganized/disoriented attachment pattern. In: Brazelton TB, Yogman MW, editors. Affective development in infancy. Ablex Publishing; 1986. p. 95–124.
7. Eckerd LM, Barnett JE, Jett-Davis L. Grief following pet and human loss: closeness is key. Death Stud 2016;40(5):275–82.
8. Worden JW. Grief counseling and grief therapy: a handbook for the mental health practitioner. 5th edition. New York: Springer; 2018.
9. Silverman PR, Klass D. Introduction: what is the problem?. In: Klass D, Silverman PR, Nickman S, editors. Continuing bonds: new understanding of grief. New York: Taylor & Francis; 1996. p. 73–86.
10. Stroebe MS, Schut H. The dual process model of coping with bereavement: overview and update. Grief Matters: The Australian Journal of Grief and Bereavement 2008;11:1–4.
11. Rubin SS, Malkinson R, Witztum E. The two-track model of bereavement and continuing bonds. In: Klass D, Steffen EM, editors. Continuing bonds in bereavement. Oxford: Routledge; 2018. p. 17–30.
12. Doka KJ, Martin TL. Grieving beyond gender: understanding the ways men and women mourn. 2nd edition. Oxford: Routledge; 2010.
13. Cooney KA, Kogan LR, Brooks SL, et al. Pet owners' expectations for pet end-of-life support and after-death body care: exploration and practical applications. Top Companion Anim Med 2021;43:100503.
14. International Association of PET cemeteries and Crematories. 2023. Available at: https://www.iaopc.com/. Accessed August 13, 2025.
15. Kathleen K, mask Death. Encyclopædia britannica. Available at: https://www.britannica.com/topic/death-mask. Accessed August 13, 2025.

Appendix: Resources

- *Senior vs. Geriatric: Unpacking the Fragility of Aging by Dr. Adelman and Dr. Tarantino*

  Recommended Reading:

  - Morris Animal Foundation Golden Retriever Lifetime Study: morrisanimalfoundation.org/golden-retriever-lifetime-study
  - The Dog Aging Project: dogagingproject.org/
  - "It's Never Long Enough" and "Nine Lives are Not Enough" Dr Mary Gardner - available on online bookstores and Amazon.

- *Movement Is Medicine: How Rehabilitation Revitalizes Aging Pets by Dr. Alvarez*

  Recommended Products:

  Harnesses:

  Help'em Up

  https://www.helpemup.com

  Best for dogs who are weak in both rear and front legs. Helps owners assist dogs getting in/out of vehicles. Best harness for lifting a dog.

  Limitations: cost, many owners struggle getting it on correctly (many buckles), needs to be adjusted daily, can cause sores if hind harness is left on, fit is more challenging for small/toy breeds

  Walk About

  https://www.walkaboutharnesses.com/

  For dogs with rear limb weakness only. Washable and easy to put on

  Limitations: can get easily soiled when the dog is urinating/defecating

  Ginger Lead

  https://www.gingerlead.com/

  Easy to use and well tolerated. Doesn't cause sores

  Limitations: does not support the pelvis, may cause dogs to urinate due to increased abdominal pressure

  Ruff Wear

  https://ruffwear.com/

  Great overall harness with good quality.

  Limitations: not supportive for dogs with limb weakness. Cost

  Beds:

  Big Barker

  https://bigbarker.com/

  Very supportive orthopedic bed. Demonstrated research showing improved sleep patterns. Waterproof liner. Removable washable cover

  Limitation: can be difficult to navigate due to size (dog has to step up); may be too firm for some dogs, cost.

  Bully Beds

  https://bullybeds.com/

  Versatile and supportive. Removable washable cover. Chew proof version

  Limitation: not for smaller dogs, cost

  K9 Ballistics

Vet Clin Small Anim 56 (2026) 545–548
https://doi.org/10.1016/j.cvsm.2025.10.006 vetsmall.theclinics.com
0195-5616/26/

https://k9ballistics.com/
Variety of sizes available, while still durable and supportive. Available for small breeds. Ideal for dogs that may trip with taller/deeper mattresses
Limitation: cost
Affordable alternative: buy egg crate and/or memory foam, cut to size large enough for the dog to stand and turn around comfortably. Buy water-proof liner (or use disposable pads) and cover with a comfy blanket or sheet

Booties:
Pawz rubber boots
https://pawzdogboots.com/
Increases grip while still allowing sensory feedback
Limitations: can increase risk of pododermatitis and limb edema due to constriction; does not last more than a few uses
Ruff wear boots and shoes
https://ruffwear.com/
Very durable, good traction, long lasting
Limitations: decreases sensory sensation, may increase tripping if not fitted correctly, cost

Nail grips:
Dr. Buzby's Toe Grips
https://toegrips.com/
Improves traction for dogs with mild weakness
Limitations: difficult to apply, may cause nail bed irritation/infection, can fall off, not appropriate for dogs with significant neurologic deficits
Dr. McHenry's Toe Treads
https://dogtoetreads.com/
Longer lasting, improves traction for dogs with mild weakness, faster application- only 2 treads on each paw
Limitations: requires training to apply appropriately, cost, special tools needed (dremmel); not appropriate for dogs with significant neurologic deficits

- *Sensory Decline: Real-World Tactics for Managing Vision & Hearing Loss by Dr. Tarantino and Dr. Adelman*

  Recommended Reading:
  - Living With Blind Dogs: A Resource Book and Training Guide for the
  - Owners of Blind and Low-Vision Dogs – by Cariline Levin
  - Blind Devotion: Enhancing the Lives of Blind and Visually Impaired Dogs – by Cathy Symons

  Product Recommendations:
  - Drinkwell Original Pet Fountain (PetSafe) store.petsafe.net/drinkwell-original-fountain
  - SightScent Sight and Scent Mapping Program sightscent.com/index.html
  - Babble Ball (Pet Qwerks) - found through many online retailers
  - Or make your own snuffle mat: pawsocute.com/dogs/5-diy-snuffle-mats-dogs-fido-will-love-4/
  - Ocu-Glo - ocuglo.com/
  - Wobble Wag Giggle Ball (As Seen On TV) asseenontvwebstore.com/Wobble-Wag-Giggle-p/wobble-wag.htm
  - Muffin's Halo Guide for Blind Dogs muffinshalo.com
- *Addressing Cognitive Dysfunction: Education, Diagnosis, and Practical Care by Dr Lynch*

Recommended Reading:
- DISHAA Tool for differential diagnosis of Canine Cognitive Dysfunction Syndrome: https://www.purinainstitute.com/science-of-nutrition/advancing-brain-health/cognitive-dysfunction-syndrome#dishaa
- CADES Assessment tools PDF for canine and feline cognitive dysfunction syndrome: https://www.hillsvet.com/content/dam/cp-sites/hills/hills-vet/en_us/pdf/303489_US_Co_Condition_Cognitive_Assessment_Tool_r2v2.pdf
- CCDR Rating Scale PDF: https://acglo.com/wp-content/uploads/sites/232/2022/04/ACGLO-CCDR-scale-1.pdf

- *Client Education: Empowering Pet Owners Through the Geriatric Journey by Dr. Garcia*

  Recommended Reading:
  - Blog on Marketing for Tips & Tricks specific to veterinary practices: https://ericgarciafl.com/blog/
  - Blog on Marketing for Tips & Tricks specific to veterinary practices: https://tapir.vet/blog/
  - Book: "Free Marketing: 101 Low and No Cost Ways to Grow Your Business Online and Off" written by by Jim Cockrum
  - Book: Blackwell's Five-Minute Veterinary Practice Management Consult, 4th Edition
- *Goals of Care: Prioritizing What Truly Matters at Life's End by Dr. Frank and Dr. Welch*

  Recommended Reading:
  - 2016 AAHA/IAAHPC End-of-Life Care Guidelines: https://www.aaha.org/wp-content/uploads/globalassets/02-guidelines/end-of-life-care/2016_aaha_iaahpc_eolc_guidelines.pdf
  - 2023 AAFP/IAAHPC Feline Hospice and Palliative Care Guidelines: https://journals.sagepub.com/doi/epdf/10.1177/1098612X231201683
  - Serious Veterinary Illness Conversation Guide: https://cdn.sanity.io/files/0vv8moc6/dvm360/37d47f8bf314c2a16fc1926479305496d900509f.pdf
- *Veterinary Hospice: Enhancing Quality Without Prolonging Suffering by Dr. Carmack*

  Recommended Reading:
  - IAAHPC: https://iaahpc.org/
    - Hospice Guidelines: https://iaahpc.org/veterinary-guidelines/
  - QoL Scales:
    - Dr. Alice Villalobos' HHHHHMM Scale
    - The Ohio State University: "How will I know?" (scale on p. 7)
    - Lap of Love
    - Midtown Mobile Veterinary Hospice Services
  - University of Tennessee End of Life Goals & Values Worksheet
  - Client-Specific Outcome Measures
  - QoL Calendars:
    - Lap of Love
    - Caring Pathways
- *Guiding End-of-Life Decisions and Quality of Life Assessments by Dr. Moen*

  Recommended Reading:
  - Dr. Alice Villalobos' HHHHHMM
    - https://360petmedical.com/wp-content/uploads/2020/03/Quality-of-Life-Scale.pdf

  - Gardner M., McVety D. Treatment and Care of the Geriatric Veterinary Patient. Wiley Blackwell; 2017
  - Gardner M. Geriatric Dog Health and Care Journal. A complete Toolkit for the Geriatric Dog Caregiver. Rolled Toe Publishing; 2021
  - Gardner M. Nine Lives Are Not Enough: A Practical Guide to Caring for Your Geriatric Cat. Rolled Toe Publishing; 2022
  - Shanan A., Pierce J., Shearer T. Hospice and Palliative Care for Companion Animals Principles and Practice. Wiley Blackwell; 2017, 2023 (second edition)
- *Just as Loved: Unique Species Considerations by Dr. Doll*
  Recommended Reading:
  - Grimace Scales of Hind Gut Fermenters
    - https://nc3rs.org.uk/3rs-resources/grimace-scales
    - Mouse, Rat, and Rabbit pain scales, which were initially developed for animals in research facilities and can be very helpful when assessing pain and discomfort
  - Association of Avian Veterinarians
    - https://www.aav.org
    - Care Guides for families
      - Senior Bird article (https://cdn.ymaws.com/www.aav.org/resource/collection/AE20E93E-0F61-4C20-AB88-E237BD795B43/AAV-care-for-senior-parrots.pdf)
  - Association of Exotic Mammal Veterinarians
    - https://aemv.org/
    - Husbandry guides for families
  - Association of Reptile and Amphibian Veterinarians
    - https://arav.org/
- *Supporting Caregivers: Overcoming Stress, Burden, and Burnout by Dr. Spitznagel, Dr. Bennett and Dr. Carlson*
  Recommended Reading:
  - Science blog dedicated to helping pet owners understand caregiver burden: www.petcaregiverburden.com
  - Abbreviated caregiver burden assessment tool: Validation of an abbreviated instrument to assess veterinary client caregiver burden - PMC
- *Euthanasia: The Ending matters most by Dr. Lynch*
  Recommended Reading:
  - In Home Euthanasia Directory vetangel.com
- *Post Euthanasia: How to Provide Continued Support by Dr. Frank*
  Recommended Reading:
  - Lap of Love Pet Loss Support Groups https://www.lapoflove.com/our-services/pet-loss-support

Mary Gardner, DVM
CEO & Co-Founder, Lap of Love Veterinary Hospice, North Palm Beach, FL, USA

E-mail address:
drmary@lapoflove.com

9780443432163